PLACEMENT LEARNING IN
Medical **Nursing**

Senior Commissioning Editor: Ninette Premdas/Mairi McCubbin
Development Editor: Sally Davies/Carole McMurray
Project Manager: Andrew Riley
Designer/Design Direction: Charles Gray/Miles Hitchen
Illustration Manager: Merlyn Harvey

Placement Learning in

Medical **Nursing**

A guide for students in practice

Maggie Maxfield BSc(Hons) MA RGN
Practice Experience Facilitator, Newham University Hospital NHS Trust,
London, UK

Michelle Parker BN(Hons) MSc RN
Consultant Nurse for Older People, Newham University Hospital NHS Trust,
London, UK

Series Editor:
Karen Holland BSc(Hons) MSc CertEd SRN
Research Fellow, School of
Nursing, Midwifery and Social Work,
University of Salford, Salford, UK

Student Adviser:
Philippa Sharp
Student Nurse, Division of
Nursing, University of
Nottingham, Nottingham, UK

BAILLIÈRE TINDALL

ELSEVIER

Edinburgh London New York Oxford Philadelphia St Louis Sydney Toronto 2012

BAILLIÈRE
TINDALL
ELSEVIER

© 2012 Elsevier Ltd. All rights reserved.

ISBN 978-0-7020-4302-4

British Library Cataloguing in Publication Data
A catalogue record for this book is available from the British Library

Library of Congress Cataloging in Publication Data
A catalog record for this book is available from the Library of Congress

Notices
Knowledge and best practice in this field are constantly changing. As new research and experience broaden our understanding, changes in research methods, professional practices, or medical treatment may become necessary.

Practitioners and researchers must always rely on their own experience and knowledge in evaluating and using any information, methods, compounds, or experiments described herein. In using such information or methods they should be mindful of their own safety and the safety of others, including parties for whom they have a professional responsibility.

With respect to any drug or pharmaceutical products identified, readers are advised to check the most current information provided (i) on procedures featured or (ii) by the manufacturer of each product to be administered, to verify the recommended dose or formula, the method and duration of administration, and contraindications. It is the responsibility of practitioners, relying on their own experience and knowledge of their patients, to make diagnoses, to determine dosages and the best treatment for each individual patient, and to take all appropriate safety precautions.

To the fullest extent of the law, neither the Publisher nor the authors, contributors, or editors, assume any liability for any injury and/or damage to persons or property as a matter of products liability, negligence or otherwise, or from any use or operation of any methods, products, instructions, or ideas contained in the material herein.

Printed in China

Contents

Section 1
Preparation for practice placement experience 1

Section 2
Placement learning opportunities 51

Contents

Series Preface

Learning to become a nurse is a journey which sees the student engaging in challenging and life-changing experiences as well as developing their skills and knowledge base in order to be able to practice as a competent and accountable practitioner. To be able to do this requires engagement with others in two different yet complimentary environments, namely the clinical and the University, with the ultimate aim of learning the required knowledge and skills to be able to care for patients, clients and their families in whatever field of practice the student chooses to pursue. The clinical placement becomes the centre of this integrated learning experience.

Tracey Levett-Jones and Sharon Bourgeois (2007) point out however that 'there is plenty of evidence, anecdotal and empirical, to suggest that clinical placements can be both tremendous and terrible' but that it is at the same time 'one of the most exciting journeys of your life'. Whilst their book focuses on helping you though this journey in relation to the more 'general' aspects of learning and coping when undertaking your clinical experiences, this book, and others in this series, sets out to help you gain maximum learning from specific placement learning opportunities and placements.

The focus to each book is the actual nature of the placements, the client/patient groups you may encounter and the fundamentals of care they might require, together with evidence-based knowledge and skills that underpin that care. Whilst the general structure of each book might be different, the underpinning principles will be the same in each.

In order to ensure that the learning undertaken in University is linked to that in practice there will be reference to academic regulations, specific learning responsibilities such as meeting with personal tutors, mentor-student relationships, placement expectations and the importance of professional accountability.

Each book will also outline how your experiences in practice will help you to achieve the specific learning outcomes and competencies as specified by the United Kingdom (UK) Nursing and Midwifery Council (NMC). Although the books are primarily aimed at the UK student, the general principles underpinning the care practice described and the underpinning evidence base throughout are valid for all student nurses who are required by their respective international professional organisations to gain experience in a number of clinical environments in order to become competent to practice as a registered qualified nurse.

Nursing is a challenging and rewarding profession. The books offer a foundation of knowledge and learning to support you on your professional journey and their content is based on the editors and authors experiences of engaging with students and colleagues in this learning experience. In addition their content draws on personal experience of working with service users and carers as to what is best practice in caring for people at various stages of life and with various health problems. The ultimate aim is to enable you to use them as 'pocket guides' to learning in a range of clinical placements and specific planned placement learning opportunities, and share their content with those who manage this learning experience in practice .We hope that you find them a valued resource and companion during your journey to becoming a qualified nurse.

Karen Holland
Series Editor

Student Foreword

Like most students, I have experienced a range of feelings on starting a new placement: the fears and excitement of what experiences you will have, who you are going to meet and work with, what you will learn, and the responsibilities that come with being that bit further along in your training. These are all feelings that are part of our education and training and contribute to the student's growth as a nurse and as an individual. What is expected of you during a placement is another persistent anxiety, in particular, how you can get the best from that specific placement and how you achieve the gold standard of truly incorporating theory into your practice in an effective and useful way.

Most placement experiences vary in length from introductory 2-week placements to full 18 week hub-and-spoke model placements. It can take a significant amount of the placement time to settle in, understand the way that particular clinical area works and develop an effective professional relationship with your mentor and other members of staff that enables you to learn and achieve.

This series of books makes the gap between what is taught in the University and practiced in clinical placements much smaller and less frightening. It provides guidance on achieving the Nursing and Midwifery Council (NMC) outcomes and competencies, which are essential for becoming a registered nurse, using case studies and real examples to help you. Knowledge of what opportunities to seek in particular clinical areas and how best to achieve them helps considerably, especially when there is so much else to think about. The series also provides a number of opportunities to recap essential knowledge needed for that area (very useful as lectures can seem a long time ago!). For student nurses setting out on that journey to those nearly ending, these books are a valuable resource and support and will help you overcome these sudden panic attacks when you suddenly think 'what do I do now?'. Enjoy them as I have enjoyed being able to have an opportunity to contribute to their development.

Philippa Sharp
3rd Year Student Nurse
University of Nottingham

Student Foreword

Contributors

Anne Claydon MSc RN
Nurse Consultant, Newham University Hospital NHS Trust, London, UK

Maggie Maxfield BSc(Hons) MA RGN
Practice Experience Facilitator, Newham University Hospital NHS Trust, London, UK

Maria Mercer RGN
Lead TB Clinical Nurse Specialist Newham University Hospital NHS Trust, London, UK

Michelle Parker BN(Hons) MSc RN
Consultant Nurse for Older People, Newham University Hospital NHS Trust, London, UK

Brian Thornton RN
Greenway Centre, Newham University Hospital NHS Trust, London, UK

Introduction

If you are reading this book then you will be about to embark on a medical placement experience. You may be feeling a mixture of emotions from deep terror to excitement. Let us reassure you that this is completely normal and your feelings will alter depending on a variety of factors, including your level of experience, the number of learning outcomes you need to achieve and whereabouts you are in your course.

The aim of this book is to introduce you to medical nursing and the various environments that you may find yourself in during a medical placement and to help you get the most out of your placement experience. We hope that this book will help you throughout the course of your medical placement and also provide you with helpful strategies for future placements.

We want you to find your medical placement enjoyable and hopefully you will be able to use the information in this book to enhance your practice experience. We appreciate that medical wards can throw up difficult situations and the aspects we have written about should help you to appreciate the complexities of medical nursing. We hope this book provides a step-by-step guide.

How to use this book

The book is divided into four sections. In each section, you will find activities and reflections aimed at developing your knowledge of medical nursing practices and understanding the experience of the patient with medical health problems. You will be directed to articles, policy documents, national guidelines and other texts that will help you to continue to expand your knowledge in specific areas.

There are also many suggestions as to how your medical nursing experiences can contribute to completing your placement learning outcomes. Many of your learning outcomes will have been developed to meet the requirements of the Nursing and Midwifery Council, which can be found in the NMC (2010) *Essential Skills Clusters* and the NMC (2010) *Proficiencies for Pre-Registration Nursing Education*. Each chapter will guide you to the relevant domain of the proficiencies and section of the skills clusters. Inevitably, there will be other competencies within these documents that can be met throughout your placement and it is recommended that you access these documents along with your university learning outcomes before you commence your placement to make yourself familiar with what is expected. The documents can be found at http://www.nmc-uk.org/.

Section 1: Preparation for practice placement experience

In this section, we will focus on what you need to do and to learn about prior to commencing what has been identified as a 'medical' placement. It will enable you to gain new knowledge if you have not previously experienced such a placement, and update your knowledge if you have.

As well as focusing on general preparation for placement issues which apply to any placement, you will find relevant sections that require active engagement in searching evidence, reading about procedures and, most importantly, anatomy and physiology which we believe are essential in understanding what happens at all stages of a patient's experience of their care.

We will also introduce you to the principles of medical nursing and what a medical placement might look like.

> *When you are on the ward, you are seen as an authoritative figure when you are in uniform and you may think 'I'm just a student nurse', but to them you are a nurse. Your actions speak louder than words and your words and actions could change a patient forever.*
>
> (Emma Hankin, first-year student)

Section 2: Placement learning opportunities

This section will focus on helping you take advantage of the learning opportunities within your medical placements. The journey of the medical patient is complex, and this section will focus upon the different journeys patients might experience across a broad range of medical placements, and for you to understand how national policy drivers affect the delivery and provision of health care. It will also explore common aspects of care delivery across medical placement learning pathways, from admission to discharge.

Each chapter will aim to help you identify learning opportunities that you can develop and link to the learning outcomes for your nurse training programme while you are on your medical placement learning pathway. We hope that you get the most out of your placement learning pathway and that you find this section informative and useful while you are in your practice learning environment.

Section 3: Case studies

In this section, we will be helping you to integrate what we have discussed in earlier chapters through a series of case studies, each focusing on a different kind of patient care experience. Clinical nurse specialists in cardiology, HIV, tuberculosis and diabetes, who are experts in their specialties, have either written or contributed to provide evidence-based case studies for you to read. We asked the clinical nurse specialists to provide the rationale for care to enable you to understand why a patient might require a particular nursing action. All of the case studies are fictitious and in no way reflect a real patient story.

During your programme, you will be asked to provide case studies and we hope that the examples in this section will help you to link theory to the practice.

Section 4: Consolidating your learning

This section aims to help you consolidate your learning at the end of your medical placement. We hope that it has furnished you with different experiences, skills and knowledge. It is really important to take time to think about where you were, where you are now and where you would like to be. It is very easy to just rush headlong into the next unit/module/placement/exam without taking time to look back and reflect.

We have provided some aspects that are worth considering once you have completed any placement, and also referred back to areas that we have covered in the earlier sections to help you bridge theory and practice. We have provided you with some revision questions and some exam scenarios to help you.

> *The 8 months have been tough, demanding and hard work, as I am sure*

so will many more months be, but I can truly say that I love my job, am proud to be a nurse, and am 100% happy that I have chosen to work on a medical ward at the start of my career.

(Nicola Cooper, newly registered nurse)

We hope that this book has helped you to get the most out of your medical placement and that you enjoy the rest of your nurse programme, which is only the beginning of a rewarding and varied career where you continue to learn something new every day.

Acknowledgements

When we were approached by Karen many months ago to write this book we had no idea what lay ahead. It has been a steep learning curve for us both and we could not have completed this book without the support, advice and encouragement of many colleagues, family and friends.

In particular we would like to thank Karen Holland, Series Editor, and Sally Davies at Elsevier for their advice and support, keeping us on track and for making our journey easier.

We would like to thank all those who contributed in any way, especially Angela Marney Claire McMullen and Rafael Ripoll for their contributions to Chapters 12, 7 and 13 respectively, students Nicola Cooper, Emma Hankin and Patricia Moyo for their reflections and feedback and all our colleagues who have provided us with moral support over the last 12 months. Finally, we would like to thank our families for their love and support and continuing to be there for us.

Acknowledgments

Section 1. Preparation for practice placement experience

1

Medical nursing in context

Reflections of a newly qualified nurse
> *Working on a medical ward, no one day is the same. There is not one set 'type' of patient that we look after, and although the medical ward on which I work is meant to be a respiratory medical ward, there is a huge and varied range of conditions and illnesses that we treat. When coming on duty, there is always the anticipation of not knowing what patients I will be looking after, what skills I will need to look after them and overall what my day will be bringing.*
>
> *Caring for patients with a variety of illnesses, some of which can be acutely ill having come straight from A&E or ITU, is challenging, interesting and rewarding, and continuously develops my nursing skills and knowledge.*

CHAPTER AIMS

- To introduce the student to terminology they may come ascross in medical nursing
- To introduce the student to various healthcare personnel they may meet during a medical placement
- To consider key principles of medical nursing
- To determine what knowledge and skills the student will need to understand in order to care for a patient with a medical condition

Introduction

This chapter aims to give you a basis on which to begin to build your learning outcomes for a medical placement. It will help you to start to understand the role of the nurse in medicine and the other key professionals involved. It is also an opportunity to ensure that your knowledge of medical conditions is up to date in preparation for the many varied and exciting opportunities that await you in your medical placement.

Medicine and medical nursing

Medicine and medical nursing can be characterised by the non-invasive nature of its diagnostic investigations and treatments. Advancing technology in imaging techniques has meant that many conditions can be diagnosed by X-ray or scanning leading to prompt treatment and care. The ever increasing development of drug therapies has also meant that many previously untreatable acute and long-term conditions can now be cured or managed much more successfully. This has resulted in a better quality of life for many of those living with long-term conditions.

 Activity

The following online resource follows the development of significant advances in medicine such as medical imaging, the discovery of penicillin, insulin and other drug therapies. Spend some time looking through the resources and developing your knowledge of what medicine is all about.

http://resources.schoolscience.co.uk/ abpi/history/history10.html (accessed July 2011).

Who's who on a medical placement

Nursing patients with medical conditions requires a team approach, therefore it is important that you begin to understand the roles of all the different professionals who may be involved in the care of the medical patient in your placement area. Table 1.1 explains some of the main healthcare professionals you will be working alongside. In order to complete your learning outcomes and competencies for your medical placement, you will need to work with a range of professionals and with different members of the nursing team in your placement area. This will not only ensure that you succeed in achieving your outcomes

Table 1.1 Who's who on a medical placement

Matron	The matron will be a registered nurse with experience in the specialty for which they cover. They will usually have worked as a ward manager or senior sister previously. They have overall responsibility for a number of ward areas Department of Health – Modern matrons in the NHS – a progress report on the role of the modern matron: http://www.dh.gov.uk/en/Publicationsandstatistics/ Publications/PublicationsPolicyAndGuidance/DH_4008127
Ward manager, senior sister, charge nurse	The ward manager/sister or charge nurse is a registered nurse with experience in the specialty of the ward. This person is in charge of the ward and you will be accountable to them during your placement. The ward manager is responsible for ensuring that the care delivered is of high quality and that the staffing and supplies are appropriate for the area. They will also be in charge of the shift when they are on duty The Nursing and Midwifery Council: http://www.nmc-uk.org/
Senior registered nurse, junior sister, senior staff nurse	A senior registered nurse or junior sister will deputise in the absence of the ward manager and will usually be in charge of the shift when they are on duty The Nursing and Midwifery Council: http://www.nmc-uk.org/

Table 1.1 Who's who on a medical placement — cont'd

Registered nurse (RN), staff nurse	The RNs or staff nurses will make up most of the staffing establishment on the ward and will have varying levels of experience The Nursing and Midwifery Council: http://www.nmc-uk.org/
Healthcare assistant (HCA), healthcare support worker (HCSW)	HCAs/HCSWs are non-registered staff who support the RNs and provide basic care to patients. They may or may not have had any formal training NHS Careers Website detailing the role of the healthcare assistant: http://www.nhscareers.nhs.uk/details/Default.aspx?Id=485
Assistant practitioner	This is a relatively new role which requires the person to have completed a foundation degree or similar qualification. They are usually trained in a variety of clinical skills, e.g. cannulation and catheterisation, so that they can provide increased support to the RNs on the ward NHS Careers Website detailing the role of the assistant practitioner: http://www.nhscareers.nhs.uk/details/Default.aspx?Id=2030
Phlebotomist	The phlebotomist will usually attend the ward daily to take blood samples requested by doctors or nursing staff NHS Careers Website detailing the role of the phlebotomist: http://www.nhscareers.nhs.uk/details/Default.aspx?Id=252
Physiotherapist (physio/PT)	The physio may be attached to one ward or cover a number of areas. Nursing or medical staff will refer any patients to them for assessment and assistance with mobility, rehabilitation and respiratory problems The Chartered Society of Physiotherapy: http://www.csp.org.uk/
Occupational therapist (OT)	The OT will also usually cover a number of different ward areas. Their role is to maximise people's independence through a variety of methods including adaptive equipment and home modification. Nursing and medical staff will refer patients to them for assessment of their needs while planning for discharge The British Association of Occupational Therapists: http://www.cot.co.uk/Homepage/
Speech and language therapist (SLT/SALT)	The SLT will cover a number of ward areas and will receive referrals from nursing or medical staff to assess patients who may be having problems with swallowing or communication difficulties The Royal College of Speech and Language Therapists: http://www.rcslt.org/

Continued

Table 1.1 Who's who on a medical placement—cont'd	
Ward clerk/ward receptionist	The ward clerk will be based on the ward and will usually be at a reception desk, nurses' station or an office on the ward. They will be an invaluable source of information about anything, from knowing how to contact a member of the team to where things are kept on the ward. Their role varies but may include greeting visitors to the ward, answering telephone queries, requesting and maintaining patient notes while they are on the ward and general administrative duties NHS Careers Website explaining the role of the ward clerk: http://www.nhscareers.nhs.uk/details/Default.aspx?Id=782
Housekeeper	The ward housekeeper will be responsible for ensuring that the ward environment is kept clean and tidy (although a domestic team will also provide the cleaning). They may be responsible for ensuring that stock levels are maintained and that equipment is in good working order
Social worker (SW)	Social workers are usually allocated to individual patients but may be attached to a particular ward or area. Patients who may require support to look after themselves when they are discharged should be referred to the social worker for assessment The General Social Care Council: http://www.gscc.org.uk/
Clinical nurse specialists, e.g. tissue viability nurse, diabetes nurse specialist	A clinical nurse specialist is a registered nurse in a senior position who has developed their knowledge and skills within a particular clinical specialty to an advanced level The Nursing and Midwifery Council: http://www.nmc-uk.org/
Radiographer	A radiographer is a registered practitioner who produces images of different internal body parts using a range of techniques such as X-ray, computed tomography (CT) scanning and magnetic resonance imaging (MRI) scans The Society of Radiographers: http://www.sor.org/
Consultant physician	A consultant physician is a doctor with many years of experience and specialist knowledge and skills in a particular area of medicine, e.g. endocrinology or gastroenterology. They will have passed special exams (MRCP) to become a member of the Royal College of Physicians The Royal College of Physicians: http://www.rcplondon.ac.uk/

(All Websites last accessed July 2011)

but will also ensure that you have
a rounded and varied experience within
your medical placement. The following
quote from a third-year final placement
student shows the benefit of working as
part of a team:

> *When my mentor was away I would then
> work with any senior member of staff.
> This made me realise that there is a pool
> of knowledge in these qualified nurses.
> For one to get this knowledge, one needed
> to take initiative, be proactive and
> challenging. This also enabled me to be
> able to work in a multidisciplinary team
> which I found very interesting as we
> exchanged ideas.*

 Activity

Look at the resources alongside each
profession in Table 1.1 to learn more
about their roles, training and
professional values.

Common medical health problems

Before you begin your medical placement it
will be helpful to understand some of the
common health problems patients on a
medical ward may have. This will help you
to know what to expect, understand
some of the terminology used and have an
insight into what your patient and their
family/carers are experiencing. This
section covers many of the common
conditions you will come across and
some of the basic information you will
need to know.

Respiratory health problems

 Activity

Begin by revising the normal anatomy
and physiology of the respiratory
system (see further reading list for a
selection of physiology books to use).

Table 1.2 gives examples of some common
respiratory health problems you may come
across on your medical placement along
with resources to help you learn more about
each of them.

 Activity

Using the resources alongside each
health problem and other resources of
your own, find out the following for each
health problem:
1. Common signs and symptoms.
2. Treatment and prognosis.
3. An example of how it feels for a
   person to have the problem (see the
   Website list at the end of the chapter
   for useful examples of patients
   sharing experiences).

Neurological health problems

 Activity

Begin by revising the normal anatomy
and physiology of the brain and central
nervous system.

Table 1.3 lists some of the common
neurological health problems you will come
across in your medical placement along
with resources to help you learn more about
each of them.

Table 1.2 Common respiratory health problems

Chronic obstructive pulmonary disease (COPD)	COPD is characterised by obstruction of airflow into the lungs. It is usually progressive and irreversible. It includes chronic bronchitis and emphysema. The main cause of COPD is smoking Chronic bronchitis is 'inflammation of the bronchi', resulting in increased mucus production obstructing the airways, producing phlegm and a cough Emphysema results from the alveoli in the lungs losing their elasticity causing them to narrow and obstruct the airways. Symptoms include shortness of breath National Institute for Health and Clinical Excellence (NICE) guideline – Chronic obstructive pulmonary disease: management of chronic obstructive pulmonary disease in adults in primary and secondary care: http://guidance.nice.org.uk/CG101/Guidance/pdf/English British Lung Foundation: http://www.lunguk.org British Thoracic Society: http://www.brit-thoracic.org.uk
Asthma	Asthma is a reversible obstructive disease of the lower airway, characterised by inflammation of the airways and increased mucus production. This can be caused by an internal trigger, e.g. stress, or an external trigger, e.g. pollen. Symptoms include wheezing, coughing, difficulty in breathing and chest tightness Asthma UK: http://www.asthma.org.uk
Tuberculosis (TB)	TB is a bacterial infection caused by *Mycobacterium tuberculosis*. Respiratory TB is the most common infection but it can affect other parts of the body. Symptoms of respiratory TB include fever, cough, night sweats, weight loss and blood-stained sputum NICE guideline – Clinical diagnosis and management of tuberculosis, and measures for its prevention and control: http://guidance.nice.org.uk/CG33/
Pneumonia	Pneumonia is inflammation of a part or all of one or both lungs, usually caused by infection NHS Choices information and video on pneumococcal disease and its effects: http://www.nhs.uk/conditions/pneumonia/Pages/Introduction.aspx NHS Choices information and patient story video on the experience of having pneumonia: http://www.nhs.uk/Conditions/Pneumonia/Pages/Symptoms.aspx

(All Websites last accessed July 2011)

Table 1.3 Common neurological health problems

Cerebral vascular accident (CVA) or stroke, transient ischaemic attack (TIA)	A stroke happens when the blood supply to a part of the brain is interrupted by either a clot (ischaemic stroke) or a bleed (haemorrhagic stroke) resulting in the brain cells in that part of the brain dying. Symptoms include weakness of one or more limbs, problems with speech and facial drooping. Stroke is a medical emergency A TIA is when the blood supply to a part of the brain is interrupted temporarily and the symptoms of the stroke resolve usually within minutes or hours. A TIA is an important warning sign that a person could be at risk of a stroke The Stroke Association: http://www.stroke.org.uk NICE guideline – Stroke, diagnosis and initial management of acute stroke & transient ischaemic attack: http://guidance.nice.org.uk/CG68/NICEGuidance/pdf/English NICE quality standards for stroke: http://www.nice.org.uk/guidance/qualitystandards/stroke/strokequalitystandard.jsp The National Stroke Strategy from the Department of Health: http://www.dh.gov.uk/en/Publicationsandstatistics/Publications/PublicationsPolicyAndGuidance/DH_081062 NHS Choices Website: look at the videos to help you spot the signs of a stroke and hear the story of a stroke survivor: http://www.nhs.uk/NHSEngland/NSF/Pages/Nationalstrokestrategy.aspx
Multiple sclerosis (MS)	Multiple sclerosis is a chronic progressive disease characterised by the destruction of the myelin sheath which surrounds the peripheral nerves, affecting the ability of the nerve cells and brain to communicate with each other. Symptoms include dizziness, fatigue, visual problems, problems with balance, numbness, pins and needles, stiffness of muscles or muscle spasms, speech and swallowing problems The Multiple Sclerosis Society: http://www.mssociety.org.uk Department of Health – The national service framework for long-term conditions: http://www.dh.gov.uk/en/Publicationsandstatistics/Publications/PublicationsPolicyAndGuidance/DH_4105361 NICE guideline – Multiple sclerosis: management and treatment of multiple sclerosis in primary and secondary care: http://guidance.nice.org.uk/CG8/NICEGuidance/pdf/English NHS Choices Website information and a video about living with MS: http://www.nhs.uk/Conditions/Multiple-sclerosis/Pages/Living-with.aspx
Epilepsy	Epilepsy is a tendency to have recurrent seizures (fits) caused by a sudden burst of electrical activity within the brain disrupting the normal communication between brain cells

Continued

Table 1.3 Common neurological health problems—cont'd

	Epilepsy Action: http://www.epilepsy.org.uk NICE guideline – The epilepsies: the diagnosis and management of the epilepsies in adults and children in primary and secondary care: http://guidance.nice.org.uk/CG20/NICEGuidance/pdf/English NHS Choices Website for information about epilepsy and a video of a person living with epilepsy: http://www.nhs.uk/conditions/Epilepsy/Pages/Introduction.aspx
Dementia	Dementia is a progressive syndrome characterised by memory loss, problems with thinking, judgement, understanding and language. There are many different types of dementia. The most common type of dementia in the UK is Alzheimer's disease. The second most common type in the UK is vascular dementia The Alzheimer's Disease Society: http://www.alzheimers.org.uk NICE guideline – Dementia: supporting people with dementia and their carers in health and social care: http://guidance.nice.org.uk/CG42/NICEGuidance/pdf/English NICE dementia quality standards: http://www.nice.org.uk/guidance/qualitystandards/dementia/dementiaqualitystandard.jsp Social Care Institute for Excellence Dementia Gateway: http://www.scie.org.uk/publications/dementia/index.asp The National Mental Health Development Unit: Let's Respect resources: http://www.nmhdu.org.uk/our-work/mhep/later-life/lets-respect/

(All Websites last accessed July 2011)

Cardiac health problems

 Activity

Begin by revising the normal anatomy and physiology of the cardiovascular system. The following Website, which includes a video of how the heart works, may help:

http://www.bhf.org.uk/heart-health/how-your-heart-works.aspx (accessed July 2011).

Table 1.4 lists some of the common cardiac health problems you will come across in your medical placement along with some resources to help you learn more about them.

 Activity

Using the resources in Table 1.3 and any of your own resources, for each of the conditions:

1. Find out how it feels to be living with these neurological health problems (you may also want to look at some of the videos on http://www.patientvoices.org (accessed July 2011) or the ones in the Website list at the end of the chapter).

2. Think about how these health problems would affect your ability to work, study and maintain relationships.

Activity

Using the resources in Table 1.4 and any of your own resources, for each of the above conditions:
1. Find out how each health problem could be prevented.
2. What health and lifestyle advice might you give to a patient at risk of developing these health problems?

Table 1.4 Common cardiac health problems

Heart failure	Heart failure is a result of the heart no longer pumping effectively, usually as a result of damage to the heart muscle, e.g. a heart attack. This results in an accumulation of blood and fluid within organs and tissues. Some patients may have either left-sided heart failure (left ventricular failure) or right-sided heart failure depending on where the damage to the heart muscle is The British Heart Foundation information about living with heart failure: http://www.bhf.org.uk/heart-health/conditions/heart-failure.aspx
Atrial fibrillation (AF)	Atrial fibrillation is characterised by a rapid and abnormal heart rhythm as a result of the right atrium of the heart quivering rather than contracting. It can be caused by hypertension, heart valve disease, overactive thyroid and excessive alcohol. Atrial fibrillation is a major cause of stroke The British Heart Foundation. Read about atrial fibrillation and listen to the examples of a normal and abnormal heart rhythm: http://www.bhf.org.uk/heart-health/conditions/atrial-fibrillation.aspx
Hypertension	Hypertension or high blood pressure is when blood pressure is constantly elevated, usually above 140 mmHg/85 mmHg. Listen to this podcast to learn more about what high blood pressure is: http://soundcloud.com/bhf/blood-pressure-the-facts
Pulmonary embolism (PE)	A pulmonary embolism is the result of a blood clot blocking the blood supply to the lungs. It is an emergency and can result in sudden death in some cases NHS Choices Website with information on pulmonary embolism: http://www.nhs.uk/conditions/pulmonary-embolism/pages/introduction.aspx
Deep vein thrombosis (DVT)	A DVT is the result of a blood clot forming in a vein in the leg. It increases the risk of developing a pulmonary embolus NHS Choices Website with information about DVT, its treatment and prevention: http://www.nhs.uk/conditions/Deep-vein-thrombosis/Pages/Introduction.aspx NICE guideline – Venous thromboembolism – reducing the risk: http://guidance.nice.org.uk/CG92/Guidance/pdf/English

(All Websites last accessed July 2011)

Problems affecting kidney function

 Activity

Begin by revising the normal anatomy and physiology of the renal system.

Table 1.5 lists some of the common kidney (renal) health problems you will come across in your medical placement along with some resources to help you learn more about them.

 Activity

Using the resources in Table 1.5 and any of your own resources, find out:
1. How these health problems may affect the regular medications a person takes.
2. How they might affect a person's nutritional and fluid intake.

Endocrine and gastrointestinal health problems

 Activity

Begin by revising the normal anatomy and physiology of the endocrine and gastrointestinal systems.

Table 1.6 lists some of the common endocrine and gastrointestinal health problems you will come across in your medical placement along with some resources to help you learn more about them.

 Activity

Using the resources in Table 1.6 and any of your own resources, find out how common the conditions are and what resources and support are available to patients living with these health problems in your own area.

Table 1.5 Common kidney (renal) health problems

Acute kidney injury (AKI)	Acute kidney injury is a sudden and rapid decrease in kidney function resulting in an inability to maintain fluid, electrolyte and acid–base balance. It is staged 1–3 reflecting the extent of the kidney damage. AKI is often reversible The Renal Association Website with clinical practice guidelines for the diagnosis, treatment and management of AKI: http://www.renal.org/Clinical/GuidelinesSection/AcuteKidneyInjury.aspx
Chronic kidney disease (CKD)	Progressive and irreversible decrease in kidney function resulting in an inability of the kidneys to maintain fluid, electrolyte and acid–base balance. It is staged 1–5 with stage 5 being complete kidney failure requiring transplantation or dialysis The Renal Association Website with clinical practice guidelines on the detection, monitoring and care of patients with CKD: http://www.renal.org/Clinical/GuidelinesSection/Detection-

Table 1.5 Common kidney (renal) health problems—cont'd

	Monitoring-and-Care-of-Patients-with-CKD.aspx Kidney Dialysis Information Centre Website aimed at helping those living with dialysis: http://www.kidneydialysis.org.uk/ A video on You Tube uploaded by NHS Choices about living with dialysis: http://www.youtube.com/watch?v=WZosHub0MOQ NICE quality standards for chronic kidney disease: http://www.nice.org.uk/aboutnice/qualitystandards/qualitystandards.jsp
Pyelonephritis	An acute or chronic bacterial infection of the kidney which has ascended from the urinary tract. A severe kidney infection is often referred to as urosepsis

(All Websites last accessed July 2011)

Haematological health problems

 Activity

Begin by revising the normal anatomy and physiology of the haematological system.

Table 1.7 lists some of the common haematological health problems you will come across in your medical placement along with some resources to help you learn more about them.

The role of the nurse in a medical setting

Many of the core skills required for caring for a patient with medical problems will be the same whichever area of nursing you choose to work in. As you progress through your training you will find that your transferable skills are invaluable in helping you to settle in and adapt to a new placement area. However, all areas will work in a slightly different way depending on the local policy and procedures, and the needs of your patients will change depending on why they are in hospital and the medical conditions they have.

In medical nursing you are likely to be presented with a group of patients with widely differing medical problems and your ability to manage this diverse group of patients is a skill you will soon start to acquire.

Dignity

Dignity should be a key consideration in the planning and delivery of care to your patients. You are probably aware of the

Table 1.6 Common endocrine and gastrointestinal health problems

Diabetes mellitus	Diabetes is a long-term condition caused by having too much glucose (sugar) in the blood. It is classified as type 1 or type 2. Type 1 diabetes occurs when the body fails to produce insulin, which must be replaced by daily injections. Type 2 diabetes occurs when the body does not produce enough insulin or the body cells are unable to react to the

Continued

Table 1.6 Common endocrine and gastrointestinal health problems—cont'd

	insulin produced (insulin resistance). Type 2 is more common, its onset tends to be later in life and it is associated with obesity NICE quality standards for diabetes: http://www.nice.org.uk/guidance/qualitystandards/diabetesinadults/diabetesinadultsqualitystandard.jsp Diabetes UK Website with information about living with diabetes: http://www.diabetes.org.uk
Alcoholic liver disease	Alcoholic liver disease is the term used to describe a range of conditions and symptoms that develop when the liver has been extensively damaged by alcohol. There are three stages of alcoholic liver disease – alcoholic fatty liver disease, alcoholic hepatitis and cirrhosis NHS Choices Website that describes the stages of alcoholic liver disease, its symptoms and management: http://www.nhs.uk/conditions/liver_disease_(alcoholic)/pages/introduction.aspx The British Liver Trust Website which includes information about how the liver works and how to look after your liver: http://www.britishlivertrust.org.uk/home/the-liver.aspx
Peptic ulcer disease	Peptic ulcer disease is the term used to refer to an open sore in either the stomach (a gastric ulcer) or the duodenum (a duodenal ulcer) NHS Choices Website with information about peptic ulcer disease: http://www.nhs.uk/conditions/peptic-ulcer/pages/introduction.aspx NICE guideline – Managing dyspepsia in adults in primary care. Dyspepsia refers to the symptoms of epigastric pain, heartburn and other upper gastrointestinal symptoms that are associated with peptic ulcer disease: http://guidance.nice.org.uk/CG17
Crohn's disease, ulcerative colitis	Crohn's disease is a chronic inflammatory condition that can affect all or any portion of the gastrointestinal tract. It commonly affects the lower part of the small intestine and large intestine. The inflammation extends through all layers of the intestine wall. It has a wide range of symptoms which can remit and relapse Ulcerative colitis is a chronic inflammatory condition affecting the lining of the large intestine causing diarrhoea and rectal bleeding A Website designed to provide resources to patients and health professionals on inflammatory bowel disorders such as Crohn's disease and colitis: http://www.crohns.org.uk/ Crohn's and Colitis UK Website for people living with inflammatory bowel conditions: http://www.nacc.org.uk/content/home.asp

(All Websites last accessed July 2011)

Table 1.7 Common haematological health problems	
Anaemia	Anaemia is a decrease in the number of red blood cells or amount of haemoglobin carried by red blood cells. There are many different types of anaemia including iron-deficiency anaemia and pernicious anaemia (vitamin B_{12} deficiency) The Pernicious Anaemia Society Website provides advice and support for those with pernicious anaemia: http://www.pernicious-anaemia-society.org/ NHS Choices Website where a search for anaemia will bring up the many different types of anaemia, their causes, symptoms and treatment: http://www.nhs.uk
Sickle cell anaemia	Sickle cell anaemia is a genetic disorder where red blood cells can become hard, sticky and sickle (crescent) shaped causing premature death of the blood cells and anaemia. A sickle cell crisis occurs when blood cells clog up a blood vessel, reducing oxygen supply and causing damage to nearby tissues and organs The Sickle Cell Society Website providing information and support to people with Sickle cell anaemia: http://www.sicklecellsociety.org/ NHS Choices Website containing information about sickle cell anaemia and a video of a person with sickle cell talking about how they cope with the disease: http://www.nhs.uk/conditions/sickle-cell-anaemia/pages/introduction.aspx
Human immuno-deficiency virus (HIV), acquired immunodeficiency syndrome (AIDS)	HIV is a retrovirus which attacks the body's own immune system, leaving the body susceptible to infection and other serious illness such as cancer. HIV infects CD4 cells which are responsible for fighting infection and, although the body will continue to produce CD4 cells, as they are destroyed by the virus they will decline in number leading to failure of the immune system AIDS is the term used to describe this late stage of HIV when the immune system has failed and the person has contracted a serious life-threatening illness such as pneumonia NHS Choices Website with information about how HIV is contracted and how it attacks the immune system: http://www.nhs.uk/conditions/hiv/pages/introduction.aspx Health Talk Online Website which includes real life stories of people living with HIV: http://www.healthtalkonline.org/Intensive_care/HIV/People/Stories

(All Websites last accessed July 2011)

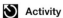 **Activity**

Using the resources in Table 1.7 and any of your own resources, find out what the risk factors are for the health problems and who may be more likely to suffer from them.

many media stories in recent years in the UK describing episodes of care where patients' dignity was not maintained.

 Activity

Look at the following link to read about some of the dignity issues that have been highlighted in the media recently: http://www.bbc.co.uk/search/news/?q=dignity%20in%20NHS (accessed July 2011).

Most nurses will say that they always treat their patients as individuals and respect their dignity, however it is important to take time to really think about this.

There are a number of different definitions of dignity. Here are two examples.

 Reflection point

What does dignity mean to you?

Think of your own personal experiences of hospital or primary care. This could be when you were a patient or when a close friend or relative was in hospital. What was important to you or your loved one in this situation?

How did staff ensure that your dignity was maintained or, if they didn't, what could they have done differently?

The Royal College of Nursing (RCN; 2008a) definition of dignity:

Dignity is concerned with how people feel, think and behave in relation to the worth or value of themselves and others. To treat someone with dignity is to treat them as being of worth, in a way that is respectful of them as valued individuals. In care situations dignity may be promoted or diminished by: the physical environment; organisational culture; the attitudes and behaviour of the nursing team and others; and the way in which care activities are carried out. When dignity is present people feel in control, valued, confident, comfortable and able to make decisions for themselves. When dignity is absent people feel devalued and lacking in control and comfort. They may lack confidence and be unable to make decisions for themselves. They may feel humiliated, embarrassed or ashamed. Dignity applies equally to those who have capacity and to those who lack it. Everyone has equal worth as human beings and must be treated as if they are able to feel, think and behave in relation to their own worth or value. The nursing team should, therefore, treat all people in all settings, and of any health status, with dignity, and dignified care should continue after death.*

The Social Care Institute for Excellence (2009) definition is based on the standard dictionary definition of dignity:

A state, quality or manner worthy of esteem or respect; and (by extension) self-respect. Dignity in care, therefore, means the kind of care, in any setting, which supports and promotes, and does not undermine, a person's self-respect regardless of any difference.

The following link will take you to the Social Care Institute for Excellence Dignity in Care Website which has, among other resources, an overview of selected research on what dignity means: http://www.dignityincare.org.uk (accessed July 2011).

 Reflection point

Have a look at these different definitions. How closely do they match your own definition of dignity?

The RCN (2008b), in their 'Dignity at the heart of everything we do' campaign, suggests using the three Ps when considering dignity – places, people, processes (Box 1.1).

Maintaining a patient's dignity can be very difficult within the medical ward and sometimes you may have to act as a patient's advocate while caring for them.

It is important that nurses feel able to challenge each other and colleagues if they feel that a patient's dignity is being compromised. For example, it is easy to become complacent and forget that all patients are individuals with feelings and needs.

Meeting the cultural and spiritual needs of patients

An important part of maintaining dignity is meeting the cultural and spiritual needs of your patients. You are likely to meet many patients with differing values and beliefs

 Activity

Dignity scenarios:

1. A patient has been incontinent and is receiving a wash when the doctor arrives wanting to examine the patient:
   a. Using the three Ps in Box 1.1, identify how your patient's dignity may be compromised.
   b. If you were involved or a witness to this scenario, what might you do?
2. During handover, a colleague's voice can be overheard by all the patients discussing the elimination needs of your patient:
   a. Using the three Ps, identify how your patient's dignity may be compromised.
   b. If you were involved or a witness to this scenario, what might you do?

Box 1.1 The three Ps

Places

This involves thinking about the physical environment in which you are providing care (e.g. privacy, cleanliness) and the organisation in which you work (e.g. positive staff attitudes, good leadership, teamwork and resources).

People

This involves looking at yourself and others and the way in which you communicate with each other and with patients and visitors (e.g. listening, being polite, introducing yourself, providing information and explanations, challenging undignified practice, role modelling and reflecting on your behaviour).

Processes

This involves reflecting on the way we provide care to patients (e.g. respecting privacy, not entering rooms or bed spaces without knocking, maintaining confidentiality, including patients in their care, not discriminating against patients).

based upon their religious, cultural, spiritual and personal backgrounds.

How will you know the cultural and spiritual needs of your patients? Having a basic knowledge of the main religious and cultural groups in the geographical area of your placement will help you begin to understand your patients' needs but it is important to remember that no two patients are alike. Patients who are members of the same religious group or from the same cultural background may have widely differing beliefs on the same issues, and how they wish their needs to be met while they are in hospital may also be very different. The best way to find out what your patients' needs are is to ask them. If your patients are not able to tell you themselves then you could ask someone who knows them well. The following Websites may be a good starting place as they have information about the beliefs of the main religious groups and some good practice guidelines for cultural awareness in health care: http://www.ethnicityonline.net and http://www.culturediversity.org/ (accessed July 2011).

Your placement area will link with a chaplaincy service which is designed to provide patients and staff with support whatever their religious beliefs. They will be able to access religious leaders within the community from different religions for patients and their families if requested.

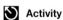 **Activity**

Find out about the predominant cultural groups in the geographical area of your placement.

Now do some research about these groups – do they have any specific cultural or religious needs that would need to be taken into account if they were in hospital? Do they have any specific beliefs or values about health and illness?

Nursing models and the nursing process

The final section of this chapter will introduce you to the concept of nursing models and the nursing process. You will find that these underpin the way nursing care is planned, delivered and evaluated wherever your medical nursing placement may be. A good understanding of these before you begin your placement will help you to identify where your learning needs are in relation to assessing and planning patient care as these are a key part of the organisational aspects of care, essential

Activity

When you begin your placement, find out how to contact the chaplaincy service and, if possible, arrange to meet with someone from the chaplaincy service to talk about the patients in your placement area and the types of requests or needs they frequently have.

skills cluster (Nursing and Midwifery Council 2010) that many of your competencies and learning outcomes will be based on.

Nursing models are theoretical frameworks designed to assist you in systematically assessing your patients' needs and planning their care appropriately. There are many different nursing models, and different placement areas will use different ones to base their patient care on. Before you commence your placement it is useful to be aware of the more popular models used.

One of the most widely used models in the UK is the Roper, Logan and Tierney activities of daily living model of nursing. This model is based on the model of living and acknowledging the indisputable fact that patients/clients still have to continue 'living' while they are receiving nursing care (Roper et al 2000). It sees the individual as being on a continuum between dependence and independence in each of the 12 activities of daily living. Where the individual is on the continuum can be influenced by five factors: biological, psychological, sociocultural, environmental and politicoeconomic (Holland et al 2008). Each of these factors needs to be taken into consideration when assessing your patient.

 Activity

Read up on the following three nursing models. Look at the differences between the three and take note of the assumptions they are based on and how they are used in practice:

1. Roper, Logan and Tierney's activities of daily living model (Roper et al 2000).
2. Orem's self-care model (Cavanagh 1991).
3. Roy's adaptation model (Roy 2008).

The 12 activities of daily living are:
- Maintaining a safe environment
- Communication
- Breathing
- Eating and drinking
- Eliminating
- Personal cleansing and dressing
- Controlling body temperature
- Mobilising
- Working and playing
- Expressing sexuality
- Sleeping
- Dying.

The nursing process was first introduced in the 1960s as a way of describing the systematic process used by nurses to provide care (Yura & Walsh 1967, Habermann & Uys

2005). The nursing process has four phases: assessment, planning, implementation and evaluation.

Assessment Assessing your patient allows you an opportunity to determine what their actual and potential problems may be. Some of these problems may be related to their medical problem, for example shortness of breath due to a chest infection, but others may relate to your patient's psychological, social, spiritual or cultural needs. This is where nursing assessment differs from the medical model which is

Reflection point

Look back at some of the conditions referred to earlier in the chapter. Consider how each of the following conditions may affect a patient's ability to maintain their independence in the 12 activities of daily living:

1. Chronic obstructive pulmonary disease.
2. Heart failure.
3. Crohn's disease.

based purely on the medical needs of the patient. Consequently, your assessment needs to be based on a discussion you have with your patient about their current needs and their perceived needs relating to what is happening to them.

Planning Following your assessment, you can then plan the goals you expect your patient to achieve. Ideally these would be set in conjunction with the patient but this may not always be possible, especially early in their admission when they are acutely unwell. By setting goals with your patient, they know what to expect and can feel part of the care process which in turn enables them to have control over what is happening to them. If they are not able to be involved in the setting of goals, try as often as possible to ensure they are aware of the goals you have set. The goals you set may be short term, but can also be longer term goals depending on the needs of the patient and the length of time they are expected to stay in hospital.

Implementation Once you have set a goal to achieve, you need to carry out appropriate interventions to help your patient reach their goal. Some of these goals will be task orientated, for example giving an appropriate medication; others may involve educating your patient about lifestyle factors that affect their health or ways to manage their condition in the long term. It is essential that all your interventions are evidence-based.

Evaluation The final part of the process is evaluating the plan you have made to determine whether or not progress has been made or a goal has been reached. Again, your patient is an integral part of the evaluation as they will be able to tell you how they are feeling in relation to the problems identified initially and whether they feel these are still problems for them.

The nursing process does not end after the problems have been evaluated. It is a continuous cycle of evaluating, identifying what are still actual or potential problems and planning and intervening to achieve your goals. As your patient's condition can change very quickly, you will find yourself completing this cycle on a daily basis, sometimes even more often.

The nursing process can be applied to many nursing actions, not just planning care. For example, a patient tells you they need to go to the toilet – you immediately assess how they are going to get to the toilet and plan what you need to do to meet their immediate need. You then put that into action, for example supporting the patient to walk to the toilet or providing a commode, and evaluating whether that was the best course of action.

By applying the process to all of the patient's actual and potential needs, we are ensuring that the care they receive is planned with the patient, evidence-based and based on what the patient actually feels is a problem, and regularly reviewed and updated. Documenting this care on care plans ensures that all members of the team are aware of the patient needs and how to meet them and provides us with a structure to evidence what we have done for the patient as accountable practitioners. You will find more information on assessing patients and care planning in Chapter 5.

Summary

This introductory chapter to medical nursing should have given you the opportunity to ensure that your knowledge of medical conditions is up to date, allowing you to begin applying this knowledge in practice once you commence your medical placement. You should also now be able to begin to plan the kinds of learning opportunities that are available to you within the team caring for a medical patient. As you now commence your placement, you can build on your knowledge of nursing models and the nursing process and develop your skills in assessing, planning, implementing and evaluating the care of a medical patient.

References

Cavanagh, S.J., 1991. Orem's model in action. Nursing models in action. Macmillan, Basingstoke.

Habermann, M., Uys, L.R., 2005. The nursing process: a global concept. Churchill Livingstone, Edinburgh.

Holland, K., Jenkins, J., Solomon, J., et al., 2008. Applying the Roper–Logan–Tierney model in practice, 2nd ed. Churchill Livingstone, Edinburgh.

Nursing and Midwifery Council, 2010. Standards for pre-registration nursing education. NMC, London.

Roper, N., Logan, W., Tierney, A., 2000. The Roper–Logan–Tierney model of nursing. Churchill Livingstone, Edinburgh.

Roy, C., 2008. The Roy adaptation model, third ed. Pearson Education, London.

Royal College of Nursing, 2008a. Defending dignity: opportunities and challenges for nursing. RCN, London. http://www.ren. org.uk/dignity (accessed July 2011).

Royal College of Nursing, 2008b. Dignity: a pocket guide. RCN, London. http://www. rcn.org.uk/dignity (accessed July 2011).

Yura, H., Walsh, M.B., 1967. The nursing process. Appleton–Century–Crofts, Norwalk.

Holland, K., Hogg, C., 2010. Cultural awareness in nursing and health care: an introductory text, 2nd ed. Hodder Arnold, London.

Montegue, S., Watson, R., Herbert, R., 2005. Physiology for nursing practice, 3rd ed. Elsevier, Edinburgh.

Pearson, A., Vaughan, B., Fitzgerald, M., 2005. Nursing models for practice, third ed. Butterworth Heinemann, Oxford.

Social Care Institute for Excellence, 2009. Background research: overview of selected research – what 'dignity' means. SCIE, London. Online. Available at: http://www. scie.org.uk/publications/guides/guide15/ backgroundresearch/selectedresearch/ whatdignitymeans.asp (accessed July 2011).

Further reading

Cutcliffe, J.R., Hyrkäs, K., McKenna, H.P., 2009. Nursing models: application to practice. Quay Books, London.

Websites

Department of Health Website with both patient experiences and professional information: http://www.nhs.uk/Video/ Pages/coping-with-stress.aspx (accessed July 2011).

Department of Health You Tube site; http://www.youtube.com/user/ departmentofhealth (accessed July 2011).

2 Medical placements

CHAPTER AIMS

- To consider what a medical placement is and what it might look like
- To consider learning opportunities which might be gained
- To explore the various types of placements and the specific learning experiences to be gained in these

Introduction

The previous chapter has explored what medical nursing is and its principles, however this chapter aims to develop your understanding of what a medical placement is and what it might look like. During your pre-registration education and training you will spend 50% of your programme in placement learning, providing nursing care in a range of environments for patients with varying levels of dependency (Nursing and Midwifery Council (NMC) 2010). Many of you will experience medical placements as part of your programme of study to meet your learning outcomes specific to your field of practice. A placement should be a minimum of 4 continuous weeks of placement to meet the NMC Standards for assessment of learning but you may find that you have a placement base which facilitates a more 'hub and spoke' approach to learning. This approach can help you to ensure that you have a greater understanding of the patient journey within your area.

An example of a hub and spoke model of practice learning opportunities could be that you are placed on a medical ward which specialises in the care of patients with respiratory health problems (conditions). Your main placement would be on the medical ward but you might spend time with some of the clinical nurse specialists and teams that might be involved within your patient journey, for example a community tuberculosis team, the pharmacist and physiotherapist.

Historically student nurses would be placed on a medical ward and that would be their medical placement. However, this does not reflect the whole patient journey with regards to their health problems and it is important that you are able to understand what that patient journey might incorporate and mean for the patient. It is also necessary to understand the nursing input within the different medical environments and to ensure that you have placement learning pathways that reflect that journey. All of the medical placements outlined below could be NHS or non-NHS, and universities will have agreements with non-NHS placements such as independent hospitals and voluntary agencies for students to undertake placements there.

It is important for you to understand that not all health care is delivered within the context of the NHS and that patients have choices regarding where they would like to be cared for. You may find that you have some preconceived ideas about independent non-NHS care, however, until you experience a placement, you will not be able to have a real idea about what occurs there and the learning opportunities that these placements can provide. An independent hospital will have many of the placements that an NHS hospital has and will provide medical care within wards, specialist wards, clinics and high-dependency units and will liaise with many other healthcare disciplines. Nursing, wherever it takes place, comes under the guidance and policies of the NMC and Department of Health.

So, what is a medical placement? It could be any of the following:

- Medical ward, general.
- Medical ward, specialist.
- Acute medical admissions ward.
- Medical high-dependency ward.
- Virtual ward.
- Intermediate care.
- Medical day care.
- Out-patient department.
- Genitourinary medical unit.

Medical general, medical specialist and acute medical admissions wards

A medical ward can be defined as an area where in-patients are admitted under the care of a physician for investigation or treatment of medical conditions not requiring surgical intervention. Medical wards can vary dramatically: a district

general hospital may have a number of medical wards that care for patients with a range of medical conditions; alternatively, a large teaching hospital may have specialist wards which may have far more specific admission criteria.

⬣ Activity

Consider these different medical specialties and find out what 'body systems' they are usually associated with. Use a nursing dictionary to help you identify the medical conditions that you might find here:

- Haematology.
- Endocrinology.
- Gastroenterology.
- Respiratory.
- Coronary care.
- Neurology.
- Renal.

The age of the patients cared for on a medical ward will vary. Some organisations will operate an integrated medicine and older people service; this means that patients of any age will be admitted to the ward depending on their medical problem so you may have patients aged 18 and 88 on the same ward. If this is the case, it is important that your knowledge and skills of caring for older people are up-to-date. Other organisations will have dedicated older people's wards, but even where this is the case, some older people may be nursed on medical wards while waiting for a bed on an older people's ward or because of their specific medical needs.

Ward environments will differ greatly from one hospital to another with some wards looking glossy, modern and high tech in comparison to other wards looking more run down. Do not let this put you off – remember, it is the patients and the standards of care on the ward that matter, not how up-to-date it looks.

Most acute hospital trusts will have mixed sex wards rather than female or male wards, but within the wards patients will be nursed in single sex environments. So the ward will be divided into bays with designated female and male bays and separate bathroom and toilet facilities for men and women. Most wards also have a number of single rooms to enable patients to be isolated if they have an infection, for example MRSA, or require privacy, for example at the end of life.

Wards tend to be arranged around either a central nurses' station or around a number of smaller nurses' stations. It is at these nurses' stations that patient notes and forms, care plans, assessment documents, etc. are usually to be found. Wards will also have a treatment or clinical room where medicines and clinical supplies are kept, a stock room where dressings and other supplies are stored and a sluice room where commodes, bed pans, etc. are kept and waste products are disposed. Individual wards will have their own storing systems so it is important that you are orientated to where everything is kept and that you have appropriate access to any storage areas.

See the Guardian newspaper for a brief history of hospital wards:
http://www.guardian.co.uk/science/gallery/2009/apr/27/nhs-design?intcmp=239 (accessed July 2011).

Medical wards are notoriously busy areas as often there can be a number of different medical teams attending the ward to see patients at the same time. There may be allied health professionals and medical students using the same placement areas. Patients are usually admitted via the accident and emergency (A&E) department or the out-patient department and some patients will be transferred to your ward from neighbouring wards or hospitals. There also tends to be less of a routine than

on a surgical ward, as patients are coming and going to investigations and tests at any time. Patients will attend a number of different departments within the hospital as their conditions are investigated. These are likely to include X-ray, computed tomography/magnetic resonance imaging scan, ultrasound scan, endoscopy, bronchoscopy, out-patient appointments and possibly other hospitals if the investigations required are not provided at the hospital.

You may also find yourself placed on a medical admissions unit. Acute medical admissions or acute assessment units are short-stay departments and sometimes are part of the A&E department. It helps A&E departments to meet their targets and provides an area where patients can be stabilised and a place where further assessment by the team can take place. These are fast paced areas caring for patients with a whole range of medical problems. Sometimes patients are discharged home from the acute medical admissions unit and at other times the patients are transferred to an acute medical ward or alternative setting. A range of patients will be admitted to this ward and the learning opportunities are vast. You will be caring for patients with acute and long-term conditions, for example a patient who has just taken an overdose of their medication or someone who has long-term respiratory problems and has a care package within the community.

Activity

'Long-term conditions' is a phrase that is commonly used. Try to find out what conditions are 'long term' and think about some of the medical placements that you might meet them on. Use your university clinical placement learning Website to help you if possible.

Medical high-dependency ward

Medical high-dependency units are often found within acute hospitals and you will immediately notice that the ratio of registered nurses to patients is increased and that there is more technical equipment within the ward environment, for example cardiac monitors, intravenous pumps and non-invasive ventilation. Initially the environment can seem frightening, however the mentors within the area will be used to having students and will usually have a welcome pack and learning opportunities pack that will guide you. First-year students don't tend to undertake placements within this environment and, therefore, students can bring their existing communication and clinical skills and develop them further during their placement time.

Virtual ward

Virtual wards provide support in the community for people with complex medical and social needs and are now being introduced across many areas of the UK. People are cared for by a team of staff as they would be in hospital, however there is no physical building. The virtual ward aims to provide multidisciplinary case management and prevent admission to secondary care (acute hospital wards) and to enhance communication for all those involved in the care. The patient is at the centre of the care. There are different models for virtual wards with some being nurse led and others GP led. Doctors and the virtual ward team will agree who should be admitted to the virtual ward and risk assessments will be undertaken (Lewis 2010).

A community matron or senior nurse will often lead the day-to-day clinical work and office-based ward rounds will occur. Frequency of patient reviews depends on their circumstances and their stability. The ward team will have an administrator, doctors, allied health professionals, health visitors, pharmacists, social workers and community nurses. Patients are discharged from the ward when a patient has been assessed by the whole team. Patients with long-term medical conditions, for example chronic obstructive pulmonary disease, could be admitted to the virtual ward with the aim that they can stay at home but still require acute care.

Intermediate care

Intermediate care is a term to represent a range of services, including integrated health and/or social care, which is agreed by the team to help patients recover more speedily from their illness. The aim of intermediate care is also to prevent readmission to hospital, prevent admission to residential care and to help patients to live as independently as possible (Department of Health 2010). The intermediate care service is normally time limited to 6 weeks and care is provided by a multidisciplinary team. The service aims to help patients to regain their confidence and has an active focus on therapy, recovery and rehabilitation. The service targets patients that may face long hospital stays. There are several examples of intermediate care: community hospitals, hospital at home schemes, rapid response teams, outreach teams, nurse-led units and day hospitals. An example of one of these teams is the respiratory early discharge service which is made up of nurse-led teams who liaise with the community matron. They provide holistic care for the patient with long-term respiratory conditions and will often come into a medical ward to assess a patient to determine whether they could care for them holistically at home and shorten their length of stay within the acute hospital ward.

The team also provides health education to the patient at home and liaises with other support agencies.

The aim of the virtual ward and intermediate care is to help patients who have often required a high-intensity use of healthcare services to remain at home longer and to have more choice about their health care. *The NHS Improvement Plan* (Department of Health 2004) described a new clinical role of community matron and is central to the government's policy for the management of people with long-term conditions.

 Activity

Using the Internet or your university student Website, find out where intermediate care and virtual wards exist within your placement areas. What do the Websites tell you about the care and service that they provide?

Useful Websites that tell you more about intermediate care include the following:

NHS Choices Website for patients: http://www.nhs.uk/Livewell/ Staywellover50/Pages/Intermediatecare. aspx (accessed July 2011).

British Geriatric Society Website for intermediate care: http://www.bgs.org.uk (accessed July 2011).

Medical day care

The medical day care unit (MDU) provides care for patients that require medical treatment/investigations on a day stay basis who will then be discharged home once their care is complete. If there are complications they may be admitted to a ward. Some of these units are nurse led and run by advanced nurses who are able to prescribe and have

specialist physical assessment skills and advanced knowledge in specialist areas, depending on the area. Examples of some of the treatments that you might see in day care are the following:

- Blood and platelet transfusions.
- Cancer treatments such as chemotherapy.
- Urological investigations.
- Cardioversion – a medical procedure by which an abnormally fast heart rate or cardiac arrhythmia is converted to a normal rhythm, using electricity or drugs.
- Food and allergy testing.
- Bronchoscopy – a technique of visualising the inside of the airways for diagnostic and therapeutic purposes. An instrument (bronchoscope) is inserted into the airways, usually through the nose or mouth or, occasionally, through a tracheostomy.
- Gastroscopy – a test to look inside the oesophagus, stomach and duodenum.
- Colonoscopy – a test to assess the colon (large intestine).

 Activity

Find out what medical investigations are common within your allocated medical day care placement and what body systems they affect. Find out about the nursing care that they may need pre- and post-investigation to help you prepare to meet your learning outcomes once you begin your placement.

Out-patient department

As a student, you may spend some time in placement in the out-patient department, an area of the hospital attended for booked appointments with health professionals of a particular specialty. Patients will often attend this department as part of their patient journey, either pre-or post-discharge from another setting. The out-patient department is a very varied placement where you will meet patients with many different conditions. Patients are referred to specific out-patient departments by their GP or by their consultant on discharge from a medical ward/acute admissions unit, intermediate care or virtual ward. Other patients may self-refer to independent sector departments if they hold private health insurance. There are many learning opportunities in ambulatory care for example, and the aim is for the student to gain an insight into nursing the ambulant patient and participate in the delivery of care to a wide range of patients of all ages. Placements are varied and can include a variety of clinics, such as dermatology, diabetes and chest clinics.

 Activity

How might you be able to help patients mobilise within the out-patient department?

What aspects of health and safety might you need to consider for patients accessing the area?

You will be able to meet some of the key domains for the NMC within the out-patient department, including interpersonal skills and communication. You will need to communicate with many patients each day from a variety of multicultural backgrounds. Some patients may have additional barriers to communication such as deafness or confusion. Many patients are anxious about their appointments and the diagnosis that they might hear, and clinics can over run.

There will also be opportunities to help with wound care and dressings and this can help you to assess and make clinical decisions under supervision (NMC 2010).

◑ Reflection point

Imagine what it must feel like to be waiting and anxious for the outcome of your appointment. What communication skills do you think you will need within the out-patient department?

Learning opportunities in a vascular clinic

You will also have the opportunity to learn about some of the following:
- The effects of ill health and the skin.
- Methods of assessing and caring for wounds, e.g. leg ulcers and abdominal post-operative wounds.
- The use of Doppler measurements and compression bandaging in the prevention and treatment of leg ulcers.
- The roles of the tissue viability and vascular nurse practitioners as a resource and support to patients and carers.
- The importance of aseptic technique.
- The selection and use of various types of dressings used; the treatment of wounds.
- How to carry out dressings under supervision.

Learning opportunities within a diabetes clinic

Within diabetes clinics you may be able to experience the following:
- Blood glucose monitoring.
- Consultant consultations.
- Assessment of care/patient education.
- Chiropody/podiatry consultation.
- Dietician consultation.
- Feet examination – monofilament test.
- Height check.
- Urinalysis.
- Visual acuity.
- Weight check.

Learning opportunities in dermatology

Here are some of the procedures seen by students in the dermatology clinic:

- Iontophoresis (or electromotive drug administration (EMDA)): a technique using a small electric charge to deliver a medicine or other chemical through the skin. It is basically an injection without the needle.
- Phototherapy or light therapy: exposure to light using a variety of devices prescribed by a clinician for a certain amount of time and, in some cases, at certain times of the day. Often used to treat psoriasis.
- Photochemotherapy: used to eradicate premalignant and early-stage cancer.
- Biopsy: the removal of a sample of tissue from the body for examination.
- Nurse-led eczema clinics.
- Bandaging:
  - four-layer bandaging: a compression bandage used in the treatment of venous leg ulcers
  - paste bandage dressing: contains topical medication commonly used for the treatment of eczema and leg ulcers.
- Clinic consultations.
- Patch testing: to determine if a specific substance causes allergic inflammation of the skin.
- Bathing.
- Applying moisturisers.
- Showers.
- Wet wraps: widely used for the treatment of children with eczema.
- Scabies treatments.
- Scalp treatments.

Genitourinary medicine/ sexual health unit

You may find yourself in a placement that provides a comprehensive sexual health service for both men and women. All services are confidential and free and service users can

be under 16 years of age. The units specialise in the treatment of all sexually transmitted infections, including human immunodeficiency virus (HIV) and related infections. They provide a walk-in-and-wait service and departments can be very busy. You will care for patients from all ethnic groups, thus a wide variety of clinical conditions are encountered. Specialist appointment-based clinics can involve male and female survivors of sexual assault, erectile dysfunction, male and female psychosexual problems, treponemal syphilis serology, herpes, hepatitis and warts clinics. The clinics also offer hepatitis A and B screening and vaccinations, emergency contraception and special sessions/advice for gay men. Often psychologists and health advisors will also hold sessions within the clinic and health promotion and health education are very evident within the environments (please refer to the glossary for definitions).

Human immunodeficiency virus services are also included with walk-in emergency HIV services and HIV in pregnancy services, and clinical nurse and midwifery specialists often run nurse-led clinics. Pharmacists provide advice and adherence information to patients and work closely with the team. There is often research nurses and some clinical trials run within these departments.

Patients presenting to the unit will be referred by:
- the individual
- GPs, A&E and NHS walk-in centres
- women's services (antenatal clinic/ termination of pregnancy) and family planning services
- local schools, colleges, universities and youth centres
- the police
- other consultants and wards.

Sexual health units are committed to the following:
- The promotion of sexual health and the prevention of sexually transmitted infections, including HIV and AIDS, and associated psychosocial problems.

- Integrated multidisciplinary team working to provide prompt, sensitive and wide-ranging responses to clinical and psychosocial problems with an emphasis on patient empowerment and continuity of care.
- Provision of a sympathetic, confidential and non-judgemental environment in which to deliver care for out-patient and emergency cases.
- Providing and maintaining a high standard of clinical, health advisory and nursing care by assessing, planning, implementing and evaluating care given to genitourinary and HIV/AIDS patients.
- Maintaining a sexual health service that is open access to ensure that emergency cases are seen on that day or at the next available clinic.
- Introduction of new ways of working combined with rapid referral protocols to ensure that improvements are seen in patient clinical outcomes and waiting times.
- Providing for flexibility of use and allowing for changes in the organisation of clinical, nursing and health advisory work.
- Building realistic and practical partnerships for fluent provision of patient care across all sectors, with shared objectives and vision.
- Providing a suitable clinical setting for the conduct of high-quality research and teaching.

Some of the learning opportunities within sexual health units include the following:

- Getting a patient ready for examination (communication with the patient, maintaining the patient's comfort, privacy and dignity).
- Setting up the female trolley (being able to identify screening equipment and understand its use).
- Setting up the male trolley (being able to identify screening equipment and understand its use).
- Practising universal precautions and safe disposal of equipment.

- Urine testing and identifying abnormal results.
- Doing basic clinical observations (blood pressure, temperature, weight, etc.).
- Basic knowledge of staining slides and microscopy work.
- Identifying and describing basic routine blood screening and equipment used for HIV-positive patients.

 Activity

Give 10 examples of sexually transmitted infections.

 Activity

A 14-year-old girl comes into the clinic requesting emergency contraception:
1. What are the issues involved?
2. Who will need to see her?
3. What is the follow-up care?

Websites that might help you:

http://www.nhs.uk/LiveWell/TeenGirls/Pages/teengirlshome.aspx (accessed July 2011).

http://www.rcn.org.uk/__data/assets/pdf_file/0005/78665/002772.pdf (accessed July 2011).

Within placement learning pathways there are many learning opportunities. This chapter has so far outlined some of the learning opportunities within the out-patient areas and sexual health clinics to help you see that there are vast amounts that you can learn in every practice placement experience, either as a substantial placement of 4 weeks or more or as part of a hub and spoke placement.

Sometimes it is difficult to understand how the learning opportunities can link to your learning outcomes within your field-specific competencies (NMC 2010).

The next section of this chapter aims to help you link those learning opportunities with some of your generic competencies.

Linking your learning opportunities with your NMC learning outcomes

There are four NMC Domains in the new NMC Standards regardless of your field of nursing practice:
1. Professional Values.
2. Communication and Interpersonal Skills.
3. Nursing Practice and Decision Making.
4. Leadership, Management and Team Working.

Within the above medical placements there are learning opportunities that meet all of the above domains.

Sometimes when you are caring for your patients, you may meet some aspects of all of the domains. For example, if you are a first-year student within any of the medical placements above, you will be undertaking observations of vital signs in a patient's home, a clinic or a ward. While undertaking this skill, you will be incorporating professional values, communication and interpersonal skills and nursing practice and decision making. As a third-year student nurse, you may be looking after a caseload of patients whereby leadership, management and team working may also be incorporated.

On your medical placements, introducing yourself to patients might seem a very 'common sense' thing to do, but how you come over in that initial 'meet and greet' can determine the relationship and interaction to follow. You might meet some patients only for the duration of their clinic appointment and look after other patients for a substantial amount of time within a virtual ward, intermediate care environment or acute medical ward. The NMC Domains, and therefore your learning outcomes, will focus on incorporating your communication skills and your professional values. How you

introduce yourself in a professional capacity should be different from how you would do this socially. Think about what the public expects of you as a student nurse within a medical placement?

As a second- or third-year student nurse, you may find yourself in a more acute environment such as a high-dependency medical ward or acute admissions ward. One of the NMC Competencies for adult pre-registration student nurses is (NMC 2010, p. 6):

> *Adult nurses must safely use a range of diagnostic clinical skills, complemented by existing and developing technology, to assess the nursing care of individuals undergoing therapeutic or clinical interventions.*

Within these acute environments you will easily see how to meet this competency, however you could just as easily relate this to your placement within medical day care or the virtual ward. In medical day care you might be nursing a patient requiring an endoscopy who will require you to care for them pre- and post-procedure. Advanced nursing roles such as the nurse endoscopist and upper and lower gastrointestinal nurses exist and are a great learning resource demonstrating advanced practice within these areas. Within the virtual ward you will be able to use diagnostic skills with patients that you meet and will be able to observe the community matron and nurse specialists demonstrating very advanced diagnostic skills within their case management.

All of the medical placements provide learning opportunities that can be linked to the activities of daily living and Table 2.1 can help you understand how you could meet them across the placement learning pathway.

Here is a real experience of a student nurse in her final placement of her adult nursing programme:

> *First, I would like to say confidence comes with knowledge. When I started*

Table 2.1 Applied learning opportunities: activities of daily living

Personal safety and comfort	Infection control; aseptic technique Barrier and reverse barrier nursing Safe drug administration Maintaining patient comfort
Communication	Helping patients with speech problems Maintaining rapport with patients and relatives Documentation skills Nurse to nurse handover Interdisciplinary liaison
Breathing	Monitoring patients with breathing difficulties Positioning patients with breathing difficulties Administering prescribed oxygen Liaising with physiotherapists and respiratory nurse specialists
Eating and drinking	Assisting patient with meals Assisting patients with swallowing problems Nutritional support/nasogastric feeding Percutaneous endoscopic gastrostomy (PEG) feeding Intravenous hydration
Personal hygiene and dressing	Assisting patients with washing and dressing Promoting self-care Maintaining dignity, taking cognisance of cultural beliefs
Mobilising	Manual handling – lifting and moving patients safely Using hoists and pat slides
Elimination	Assisting with bedpan/commode/toilet Caring for urinary catheters Managing the incontinent patient Monitoring urine output Administering suppositories and enemas
Maintaining body temperature	Helping reduce elevated temperature Maintaining normal body temperature
Dignity and sexuality	Respecting patient choice – allowing the patient to dress as he/she chooses Respecting and being non-judgemental regarding personal choice, beliefs and sexual orientation
Working and playing	Helping the patient to pursue his/her interests within the constraints of illness
Sleeping	Promoting sleep and a restful atmosphere
Dying	Helping the patient to have a peaceful and dignified death

my nurse training, I did not have any idea of what was expected from me in a clinical environment. I followed my mentor throughout the shift and sometimes felt like they got annoyed by me following them. Gradually I developed observation skills which I had already learnt during my lectures at the university. I then thought that was all I could do in a placement area. Every time I came on duty I would make beds, assist patients with bathing and feeding and follow my mentor when doing drug rounds.

Summary

This chapter has explored the various medical placements and specific learning experiences that you might encounter, however it is also important for you to focus on general expectations in relation to what is expected by the university and the programme that you are undertaking. The next chapter will consider the preparation for your placement, including the practicalities and expectations of your university, the placement and you.

References

Department of Health, 2004. the NHS Improvement Plan: putting people at the heart of public services. DH, London.

Department of Health, 2010. Intermediate care: halfway home. Updated guidance for NHS and local authorities circular. DH, London.

Lewis, G., 2010. Predictive modeling in action: how 'virtual wards' help high-risk patients receive hospital care at home. Commonwealth Fund, New York. Online. Available at: http://kingsfund. koha-ptfs.eu/cgi-bin/koha/opac-detail. pl?biblionumber=95848 (accessed July 2011).

Nursing and Midwifery Council, 2010. Standards for pre-registration nursing education. NMC, London.

Further reading

Department of Health, 2010. Ready to go? Planning the discharge of patients. DH, London.

Howatson-Jones, L., Ellis, P., 2008. Outpatients, day surgery and ambulatory care. Wiley–Blackwell, Oxford.

Linsley, P., Kane, R., Owen, S., 2011. Nursing for public health. Oxford University Press, Oxford (has an excellent chapter on sexual health).

Websites

Asthma UK: http://www.asthma.org.uk.

British Lung Foundation: http://www.lunguk.org.

British Thoracic Society: http://www.brit-thoracic.org.uk.

Global Initiative for Obstructive Pulmonary Disease: http://www.goldcopd.com.

National Institute for Health and Clinical Excellence guidelines: http://www.nice.org.uk.

Thorax. (journal): http://thorax.bmj.com/.

3 Preparation for placement learning

- To understand what you need to do to prepare for placement
- To understand who is available for support while on placement
- To begin to identify some learning opportunities in different placements

Introduction

You are now aware of what a medical ward is and how it works but what can you do in preparation for your medical ward placement? This chapter aims to give you some tips and preparation activities to ensure that you start your medical ward placement feeling confident and ready to learn. Remember that your practice learning opportunities make up 50% of your nurse training programme and you need to recognise the importance and value of this learning opportunity. You are an adult learner and there will be an expectation that you take personal responsibility for directing your own learning and making the best use of the learning opportunities available. You may worry that the medical ward may not be the right place for you to achieve the learning

outcomes, however let us reassure you – care is always taken to place students in wards that allow them to meet their learning outcomes and placements are linked very closely to your curriculum.

Student reflection

The first day I started practice I had not much confidence at all. I thought 'how can I do this and help a patient?' I put myself in the mindset of a role as a nurse and this mindset helped me a lot throughout my time on practice, but I also talked to my mentor about my concerns and worries and they gave me some guidance and then, in time, my confidence grew and I was able to perform to the best of my abilities.

(Emma Hankin, first-year student nurse)

During your practice placement, your learning outcomes will be assessed by a registered nurse who is a qualified mentor who has undertaken a specific course that is recognised by the Nursing and Midwifery Council (NMC). Sometimes a team of mentors will support you and this may also include co-mentors or associate mentors who have not undertaken the recognised mentor course but are expected to contribute to your learning.

There are a number of aspects that you should consider when preparing for your placement:

- Practicalities.
- Professional practice and behaviour expected.
- Policies.
- The roles and responsibilities of those who can support you during your practice experience.

Practicalities

First of all, when you find out the name of the ward and the location, the Website at your university will probably have placement profile information. This may contain information about the ward, who to contact, phone numbers, shift times and general advice. Do they advise any special preparation activities? It is important to contact the ward at least 2 weeks before your placement to ensure that you know when to start and, even better, if you can arrange to visit the ward before you start (Sharples 2009).

Once you find out the shift times, you need to think about the practicalities of getting to your placement on weekdays and weekends and for the inevitable early starts and late finishes. For example, what are the transport links like and is there parking available for students? You may care for someone at home such as a relative or a child and need to make arrangements for this while you are on placement. It is important to clarify what the expectations of you are regarding attendance in placement and you will find this information in your student handbook. In some universities you will be expected to work the shifts that the ward staff works, and in other placements this might be more flexible.

If you are a more senior student, you may need to work some night shifts or weekends to cover the expectations of your professional body for registration. Ward managers will need to know if you have any special off duty requests so that they can ensure you are allocated to an appropriate mentor who can work with you for the required amount of time to facilitate learning and assessment in practice. Even though you are supernumerary, nursing is fundamentally a practical job and you can only learn with hands-on practice and will need to be there for patient handover to ensure you are fully informed of the patient caseloads.

The university will probably have an identified lecturer who will link with your ward and it is important that you know how to contact this person and the times and dates that they visit the ward. It is also important to consider whether you have any learning needs that require discussion prior to your placement to enable the ward staff to support you appropriately. You will need to find out if there is a planned induction or welcome meeting that you need to attend and if there is a student notice board somewhere locally or centrally within the hospital. The ward will want to keep you safe while you are in your placement and you need to inform them of any adjustments or risk assessments that need to be carried out. For example, if you are pregnant you will be able to achieve your learning outcomes but will need a risk assessment outlining any adjustments required.

If this is your first placement, this is a good time to look through your learning outcomes and consider what your priorities might be and if you have any transferable skills that you can bring to the placement. If this is not your first placement, you should look at the feedback you received from your mentors in your last placement, focusing on areas of strength and areas for development, and consider what your learning objectives are for this ward.

Student reflection

> *My first placement was an experience that I will never forget, but before my first day of placement I prepared myself by watching the clinical skills DVD, reading the clinical skills book, reading the biology and anatomy books and also reading the lecture notes from previous lectures.*
>
> (Emma Hankin, first-year student nurse)

 Activity

Log on to your university Website and find out about your placement. Consider the practicalities involved using the questions in Box 3.1.

Box 3.1 What are the practicalities of this placement?

Look up the ward profile on the student Website:

1. Is there any information about your learning outcomes for this placement on the student Website?
2. Who can be your mentor? If you are a final placement student you will need a sign off mentor (NMC 2008b).
3. What shifts does the ward work?
4. What shifts do you need to work to meet the university's expectations.
5. Do you have any special off duty requests?
6. How do you get to the placement – what are the transport links like?
7. Is there a lecturer from the university who links with the placement?
8. Is there an induction planned?
9. Do you have any learning needs that require discussion with the placement before you arrive?
10. What were the strengths and areas for development highlighted in your previous placement?
11. Do you have transferable skills?
12. What do you want to achieve in this placement?
13. What is the uniform policy?
14. Who do you inform at the university if you are sick or absent from placement?
15. Do you need to make arrangements to see your personal tutor while you are on placement?
16. Are there any university lectures, exams or assignments that you need to plan into your time?
17. Have you attended all the mandatory training at the university prior to your placement?
18. Are you pregnant? If so, have your read the university maternity policy and understand that you will require a risk assessment?

Professional standards and behaviour

As a student nurse you will not only be expected to develop clinical skills but also a certain level of professional attitude and behaviour (Parker 2009). These attributes will be assessed as part of your course and your mentors in the clinical environment will play a key part in your assessment in this area.

A Website worth looking at is:

NMC Guidance (NMC 2009): http://www.nmc-uk.org/Documents/ Guidance/NMC-Guidance-on-professional- conduct-for-nursing-and-midwifery- students.pdf (accessed July 2011).

It is expected that, as a student nurse, you will act in a professional manner at all times. This means not just within the clinical area but in public places as well. It is essential that people feel they can trust nurses, and any behaviour which may damage the respect and credibility of the profession in the eyes of the general public could be detrimental to how safe patients feel when they are admitted to hospital (Levett-Jones & Bourgeois 2009). This may sound daunting but there is plenty of guidance and support available to help you. This chapter aims to help you understand what is expected of you and how to use the support of your mentors in the clinical area to help you develop your professional behaviour.

Good health, good character and fitness to practise

The NMC sets out what they expect from student nurses in their *Guidance on Professional Conduct for Nursing and Midwifery Students* (NMC 2009). At the end of your nursing course your university is required to inform the NMC that you have not only met the educational and clinical requirements of your course but also that you are in good health and are of good character. It is essential that you read this and adhere to it, and discuss it with your mentor at the start of your placement learning experience.

What does good health mean? It means that you are capable of safe and effective practice without supervision. It does not mean the absence of any disability or health condition.

What does good character mean? It is based on your conduct, behaviour and attitude. It takes account of any convictions and cautions you may have that may bring the profession into disrepute.

Both of these elements are required for you to be deemed fit to practise and join the nursing register.

The areas of concern highlighted in Box 3.2 are also cited by the NMC as aspects of your personal life that may influence your ability to be judged as having good health and good character.

(●) Reflection point

1. What do members of the public think when they see a nurse in uniform smoking a cigarette in a public place?
2. What do they think about a nurse doing their shopping in the local supermarket in their uniform?
3. What do they think when they overhear nurses giggling and laughing about their patients?

Box 3.2 Aspects of your personal life that may influence your ability to be judged as having good health and character

- Aggressive, violent or threatening behaviour.
- Cheating or plagiarising.
- Criminal conviction or caution.
- Dishonesty, e.g. misrepresentation of qualifications, fraudulent CV.
- Drug or alcohol misuse.
- Health concerns, e.g. putting others at risk by not seeking help for medical problems or not recognising own limitations.
- Persistent inappropriate attitude or behaviour.
- Unprofessional behaviour, e.g. breach of confidentiality.

Reflection point

Now that you have read about behaviour that is not acceptable for a nurse to display, list the positive attributes and behaviours you would expect to see in a nurse and consider how you can ensure that these are displayed in your personal and professional life.

The NMC Code (2008a) in the UK is a set of strict standards that registered nurses must adhere to. The sooner you become familiar with these, the easier it will be to ensure that your practice and behaviour are meeting the standards required for registration. Other countries will have similar guidance and standards, so ensure you are familiar with the requirements of the country you are registering in.

Accountability

Accountability is a word you may hear your mentor and other registered nurses use. It is integral to nursing practice and, although the level of accountability expected of you as

a student differs from that which will be expected of you as a registered nurse, it is important that you understand what it means to you and to your practice.

Accountability can be described as (Thompson et al 2006, p. 84):

> The ability to give account of one's actions, in particular to give a coherent, rational and ethical justification for what one has done.

Registered nurses are accountable in four ways:
1. To their profession.
2. To their employer.
3. To the patient.
4. To the law.

Professional accountability

The NMC Code (2008a) states that:

> As a professional, you are personally accountable for actions and omissions in your practice and must always be able to justify your decisions.

Your mentors are accountable for passing or failing you – they need to be able to justify their decisions. At the heart of their decision will be patient safety. Patients have expectations of nurses – that we are registered, educated to a certain level, keep up to date and that we will not harm them. Patients do not expect us to know everything but they expect us to acknowledge when we cannot do something competently and to seek assistance and advice if we are ever unsure.

In our daily lives we have expectations of other registered practitioners. For example, if a gas fire is not working we would only employ someone who is a registered up-to-date gas fitter to come and fix it, as anyone else could harm us and our families.

So what should patients expect from a registered nurse? This is a good starting point:
- To feel safe.
- To be pain free.
- To be clean and dry.
- To feel like a real person.
- To feel cared for.
- To know who is in charge.
- To know who is looking after them each shift.
- To know when the shift changes.
- To know what's happening to them and when.
- To feel respected.
- That care is evidence-based.
- That nurses work to policies/guidelines.
- That nurses are not afraid to challenge poor practice.
- That nurses work in a team for their benefit.
- That nurses monitor the standards of care ensuring quality, safety and efficiency.

The roles and responsibilities of those who can support you doing your medical practice placement

The mentor

During your practice placement, your learning outcomes will be assessed by a registered nurse who is a qualified mentor who has undertaken a specific course that is

recognised by the NMC (NMC 2008b). The mentor who assesses you must be registered within the same field of practice as you and have attended a mentor update within the last year. The placement holds registers of mentors and their updates and is expected to be able to produce this evidence for the NMC. Each mentor also has a triennial review to ensure that they are meeting the NMC Standards and a record of this is kept by each placement. Your curriculum documentation will often have a section that requires the mentor to print and sign their name, year of registered mentor course and the last update they attended to ensure the validity of your assessments.

You are expected to work with your mentor for 40% of your placement time and this must be evident through the duty roster (NMC 2008b, 2011). Your mentor may work weekends, nights, 7.5-hour or 12.5-hour shifts and your allocated duties should follow this. Mentors will also have annual leave and study days themselves, so sometimes this will be difficult to achieve and you may be allocated more than one mentor. Sometimes a team of mentors will support you and this may also include co-mentors or associate mentors who have not undertaken the recognised mentor course but are expected to contribute to your learning (NMC 2008a). Associate or co-mentors are registered nurses who you will often work with and learn from, and they will often provide feedback on your performance to your main mentor. They may do this verbally or by writing in your record of achievement page, for example in a mentor comment page. However, they will not be able to assess you until they have undertaken the recognised mentor course.

The sign-off mentor

The role of the sign-off mentor is to 'sign off' that a student has met all of the NMC Standards and Competencies at the end of their NMC pre-registration nurse programme for entry to the register. The sign-off mentor has completed the NMC mentor course but has been further assessed against the NMC Standards for Learning and Assessment in Practice (NMC 2008b) and has met the criteria to be a sign-off mentor. The sign-off mentor in your final placement will assess and supervise your learning but will also be making judgements based on decisions of other mentors who have supervised you earlier in your final year. It is important that you make sure that there is sufficient evidence from other mentors to allow your sign-off mentor to be satisfied that you have been assessed sufficiently within your recent placements. The sign-off mentor will only sign you off as proficient if they are satisfied that you are fit to practise and for purpose and safe to practise as they hold that responsibility and accountability. The NMC (2010) emphasises the requirement for a record of achievement for each student which documents comments from mentors and is passed from one placement to another. This record of achievement is shared with academic staff, and if there are any concerns in practice, there is an expectation that the placement mentors and academic staff from the university will work in partnership to address these.

A useful resource for mentoring and mentors is: http://www.rcn.org.uk/__data/assets/pdf_file/0008/78677/002797.pdf (accessed July 2011).

The practice experience/ education facilitator or practice experience manager

At the end of the 1990s the role of the practice experience/education facilitator or practice experience manager was developed to support the increasing numbers of students in practice (Department of Health 1999, United Kingdom Central Council for Nursing, Midwifery and Health Visiting (UKCC; now the NMC) 1999). These roles have many titles within organisations, but for the purposes of this chapter will be called the practice education facilitator. The role of the practice education facilitator is to provide a quality learning environment for students which involves supporting them in their practice placements and preparing and facilitating mentors to assess the students. The practice education facilitator also links with the university and will spend time meeting with programme leaders, personal tutors, placement units and link lecturers to ensure that the quality of learning is sustained.

The practice education facilitator will often provide inductions, evaluations, workshops, organise teaching for you and your mentors and, in partnership with the university, undertake educational audits of the environments within which you are placed to ensure and enhance the quality of placement learning (Lauder et al 2008).

A Website you might like to visit:

Nursing and midwifery in Scotland: being fit for practice. The report of the Evaluation of Fitness For Practice Pre-Registration Nursing and Midwifery Curricula Project 2008: http://www.nes.scot.nhs.uk/media/6962/ffpfinalreportsept082.pdf (accessed July 2011).

The link lecturer

The role of the link lecturer is to ensure that there are strong links between the university and the placement and to support students and mentors in these areas. For the majority of their role, a link lecturer will continue to teach and have responsibilities at the university, however one aspect of their job will be to link with a number of areas within organisations. Link lecturers will often work closely with the practice education facilitator to support students and mentors within their placements. Some organisations have lecturer/practitioner roles which are 50:50 practice/lecturer roles employed by the NHS 50% of the time and the university 50% of the time.

 Activity

Log on to your university Website and find out the practice education facilitator and the link lecturer for your area. Write down their names and contact details and any visiting dates that they have put on the Website.

The personal tutor

When you join university you will be given a personal tutor normally for the duration of your training who will play a key role in supporting your progression throughout. They keep all of your records for your training and will monitor your progress and attendance throughout the course. They will book appointments to see you regularly throughout your programme, and you should contact them if you have any issues or worries as they have a key role in providing pastoral support for you and will be the person that can refer you to other agencies if you need help. Universities normally have an outline of the role of the personal tutor and these can differ from one university to another.

 Activity

Make an appointment to see your personal tutor and ask them what their role is, what they expect from you and what you can expect from them.

Meetings with your mentors/sign-off mentors

Within each of your placements you should have three meetings with your mentors:

1. An initial meeting – this should occur within your first week of placement.
2. An interim meeting – this should occur midway through your placement.
3. An endpoint meeting – this should occur at the end of your placement.

See Table 3.1 for what should occur within these meetings.

Student reflection

Every time I came on duty I would make beds, assist patients bathing and feeding and following my mentor when doing drug rounds. I thought that was not enough and wanted to do something more challenging than that. I gradually developed a skill of learning by negotiation. I put my objectives in writing so that when I am on duty I would show my mentor and ask if it was possible to follow my objectives. This helped me to achieve my objectives in time. I would sit down with my mentor and discuss how my objectives would be met. I learnt that we can learn through various ways like observing someone doing something or by practically doing it.

(Patricia Moyo, third-year student nurse)

It is important to remember to inform your mentor of any adjustments that you require during your practice learning experience. You may have learning needs, for example dyslexia, dyspraxia or dyscalculia, that you have shared with your personal tutor at university to ensure that adjustments and support are offered for your academic work. Remember that you continue to learn within your placement and it is important that your mentors are aware so that they can make reasonable adjustments in practice to ensure that you receive the support you require. The practice experience facilitator will be working closely with the university and will be able to provide further support to you and the mentor.

The following Website can help: http://www.rcn.org.uk/__data/assets/pdf_file/0003/333534/003835.pdf (accessed July 2011).

Table 3.1 An example of what should occur within your three meetings with your mentor

	Initial	Progress	Evaluation
Timing	During the first week	Midway through the placement	During the final week
Objectives	To work on forming the mentoring relationship	To maintain and monitor the learning experience	To review progress and the objectives set earlier
Content	Ward layout Ward profile Learning resources Introduction to staff (nurses and the multidisciplinary team) Health and safety (including emergency) procedures Set learning objectives Discuss aspects of assessment documents Identify specific learning opportunities Identify special skills that need developing Discuss and arrange dates for future meetings Where will you meet? When will you meet?	Acknowledge achievement of learning goals Set new goals Seek further learning opportunities Identify barriers to learning Discuss how to overcome barriers Identify how their experience is helping meet objectives Identify clinical skills they have developed Explore their role in the team	Review assessment documents Discuss assessment decisions Personal reflection of experience Analysis of any significant incidents Ensure documentation completed

This is a Royal College of Nursing (2010) publication which has been developed for students as well as qualified nurses and others. in particular, it is a supportive publication which would be reassuring for any student with any of these three learning difficulties to negotiate assistance both before and during placement.

Practice assessment decisions

An area that can be confusing to students is who can assess them in practice. The standards introduce a flexible approach to the assessment of practice learning, and Table 3.2 summarises who is required to make assessment decisions at various stages of the programme.

 Activity

Consider Table 3.2 and where you are in your nurse programme. Look at your learning outcomes together with your medical placement learning opportunities to understand who could possibly assess and help you to meet these outcomes.

Table 3.2 Assessment decisions at various stages

Throughout each part of the programme	At the first progression point	At the second progression point	For entry to the register
A registered nurse mentor or, where decisions are transferable across professions, an appropriate registered professional who has been suitably prepared	Normally a mentor who is a registered nurse from any of the four fields of practice	A mentor who is a registered nurse from any of the four fields of practice	A sign-off mentor who is a registered nurse from the same field of practice as that which the student intends to enter

(NMC 2011)

As a senior student, you will be working alongside junior students. The NMC expects all nurses to mentor junior colleagues and it is important for you to adopt this role as you prepare to be a registered nurse (NMC 2008b,2010):

All nurses must continue their professional development, supporting the professional and personal development of others, demonstrating leadership, reflective practice, supervision, quality improvement and teaching skills.
(NMC 2010)

Combined with this, there is an expectation that the student nurse will progress to registered nurse with the ability to display leadership, management and team working (NMC 2010). You will find that a more junior student will often come to you before they will approach a registered nurse. It is important that you role model professional behaviour, are approachable and refer anything that you are unsure of. You will find that your knowledge base is required to be up-to-date in your final year of training and registered nurses will find it useful if you share any new knowledge or information.

When you are a registered nurse you will find that nurses often become link nurses for specialist areas, for example tissue viability, continence and infection. They will attend meetings run by clinical nurse specialists and they will have an obligation to share any new knowledge with their colleagues for practice to remain evidence-based, enabling patients to receive the best care possible.

As teaching will be a learning outcome for you, it is important that you speak to your mentor about how you can achieve this on the medical ward. Your mentor has undertaken a formal NMC recognised qualification to prepare to support learning and assessment within practice and should be able to help you develop your teaching skills. In your university modules in the final year, it is normal to find mentorship and teaching others as one of the main topics in preparation for you to make the transition from student to registered nurse.

Your mentor will understand where there will be opportunities to teach more junior colleagues and will support you with this. Your mentor may be able to suggest some areas for development that staff have identified. You may feel a lack of confidence and worry that you don't know enough to teach, however with adequate preparation and support from your mentor you should be able to achieve this. It may help you to think about students who have taught you in your first year and how knowledgeable they seemed. You could speak to junior colleagues and explain that you would like to undertake a teaching session and ask if there is anything they are struggling with or would like to learn.

Teaching within practice can take place formally or informally. Sometimes teaching is opportunistic and unplanned. For example, you might be handing over a group of patients and a junior colleague asks you what a term means, for example COPD. You might be planning discharge and someone might ask you why the patient needs a district nurse. Often junior students will be unclear about the plans of care for patients and will often struggle with nursing models and care planning.

Learning often takes place during professional discussions. For example, as you discuss patients with the multidisciplinary team, there are opportunities to clarify and reflect in and on care. Learning is not always formal or planned and it is important to take time at the end of the day to think about what you have learnt. You can document this in your reflective diary/journal.

When undertaking a formal teaching session for a few junior colleagues, ask your mentor how she plans her teaching? You will find examples of teaching plans within many books/articles, and once you have decided what to teach it is helpful to plan your teaching. Planning is an essential component for effective teaching (Fry et al 2001) and provides a clear framework even when the process is informal:

- It is important to consider where teaching can take place – most wards have an area where meetings take place and you may be able to book this space for your teaching.

- Make sure that you find out what is available – is there a white board, flip chart, does the ward have a laptop and projector? Your mentor will be able to help you with this.

- Is your session practical (e.g. taking manual blood pressure) and does the ward have enough sphygmomanometers and stethoscopes available?

- Think about the timing of your teaching and the knowledge level of your students. Do you want this to be an interactive session and do you want to assess their knowledge base at the beginning of the session? Sometimes a quiz can help with this. For example, do the students know the normal values for blood pressure?

- What is the aim of your teaching? Set specific objectives. What will they learn and what will they do? How will you evaluate what they have learnt? What resources do you need?

◈ Activity

Take time to share your ideas with your mentor and listen to their advice. Try to ensure that your mentor observes your teaching and take time to reflect on your mentor's feedback. Your link lecturer may also be able to help you – remember that you have a lot of support. Ensure that this becomes one of your objectives.

Transferable skills

Whether this is your first ever placement or one of your final placements, you will have a wealth of transferable skills – skills you have acquired elsewhere that can be utilised in your new placement. It is worth spending some time thinking about what these skills may be before you commence your placement.

This will give you an opportunity to reflect on your previous experiences and strengths and help build your confidence when starting in a new placement area.

It is not always easy to identify what your transferable skills may be, and this section aims to help you identify those relevant to your medical placement and give you some guidance as to how you can put them into practice.

Communication skills

Your communication skills will be wide ranging and probably quite advanced, even at an early stage in your training. They are the cornerstone of good nursing practice and you would not have been selected for your course if you had not already shown you had the potential to be a good communicator. They will be included within your learning outcomes as communication and interpersonal skills are a key NMC competency domain (NMC 2010). They are also part of the NMC Competencies for entry to the register and form part of the essential skills clusters (NMC 2010), whatever field of practice you are in.

> Graduate nurses must have 'presence' demonstrated through the energy and quality of their interaction. They must communicate safely and effectively with individuals and groups of all ages, using a variety of complex skills and interventions including communication technologies. Communication must be characterised at all times by respect for the individual differences, care, compassion and dignity.
>
> (NMC 2010)

Reflection point

Make a list of all the situations in your day-to-day life that require you to exercise your communication skills.

You may have thought of some of the following:

- Using the telephone to give information, make enquiries, confirm arrangements.
- Giving instructions to others, your children.
- Listening to the views, worries and concerns of family and friends.
- Making small talk with strangers, neighbours.
- Judging the mood of others from their body language, tone of voice.
- Asking questions to find out information from strangers, family and friends.
- Dealing with members of the public in current or previous jobs.
- Difficult situations such as conflict, bereavement.

Reflection point

Now consider how your communication skills in each of these situations could be of benefit on your medical placement.

All of your communication skills will be of benefit to you on your placement. Telephone skills are essential and you will be expected to be able to answer the telephone as soon as you commence your first shift. It won't matter if you aren't able to answer the query on the other end of the line, but being able to answer politely and transfer the call and a message to someone who is able to help is essential. Being able to listen effectively to patients and other members of staff is vital if you are to carry out your duties well, and the ability to ask questions if you are not clear about instructions or information will be expected of you.

An awareness of your own body language and the ability to interpret that of others is very important, especially as patients may not always feel they are able to talk honestly about their feelings when they are feeling vulnerable. An ability to pick up on subtle non-verbal cues will be a skill you develop throughout your training, but even from your first placement you will have some ability to judge the mood and feelings of others as we are attuned to do this with our own family and friends. Have confidence that your communication skills are already in the process of developing and the time you spend on the medical ward will be invaluable in continuing this process.

 Activity

> Identify an area of your communication skills that needs particular development and include this in your learning objectives for the placement. Your mentor and other staff on the ward will be well placed to help you develop these skills.

Managing information

From the moment you step onto the ward you will find yourself bombarded with information. This may include the nursing handover at the start of the shift, giving you vital information about the patients you will be caring for; it may be instructions and advice from staff on where you will be working and what will be expected of you. Also, as mentioned before, it may be information given directly to you from patients, relatives or other members of the team that needs to be communicated to others. Whatever this information is, you need to be able to manage it appropriately and use it to get the best out of your placement.

 Activity

> It is your first day on your medical ward placement and within the first hour of your shift you have been given the following information:

> - Name and role of all the staff on duty.
> - Ward layout and location of emergency equipment.
> - The name of your mentor and when they will be on duty.
> - Name, age, diagnosis and progress update for 26 patients.
> - Instructions from the nurse in charge as to which patients you will be looking after, who you will be working with and what you will be expected to do.
> - Requests for pain relief from two patients.
> - A telephone call from a relative wanting to know how their loved one is.
>
> Consider what your strategies would be for managing all of this information.

There are a number of different skills you will employ to manage the information given to you and many of them will come naturally to you. The situation in the activity above may seem daunting to some but you are probably used to managing this amount of information in your everyday life.

 Reflection point

> Think about how often you are juggling information in your day-to-day life:
> - Appointments you need to keep.
> - Times and places that children, family members and friends need to be picked up or dropped off.
> - Important dates, birthdays, anniversaries.
> - Shopping lists.
> - Directions to places you are visiting.
>
> How do you usually manage these sorts of information?

A common way to manage information – especially that which is important or unfamiliar to us – is to write it down. This will be an essential strategy to use on your medical placement. Different placement areas will have different policies on what patient information may be written down for your personal use, so it is important that you are familiar with local policy and procedures regarding this. A working understanding of the confidentiality policy of your placement area and the Data Protection Act is also necessary.

Information such as your shift patterns, meetings with your mentor and other study sessions you need to attend while on placement can all be written down and kept somewhere safely, as this sort of information is not necessary for you to remember at all times. Information pertaining to the patients you are looking after, requests from patients and messages or instructions from others will need to be close at hand on your shift and possibly dealt with immediately. Again, don't be afraid of writing down the seemingly small things as well as those that seem very important, as having the information to hand when someone asks for it will give you confidence.

Think carefully about where you write things down and how. Lots of scraps of paper with different bits of information on may only make you more confused, although, if you write everything in the same place (in a notebook for example) and this becomes mislaid, you have lost all your important information. Probably a combination of the two is the better option. Use a notebook for things you may want to reflect on or use later, and use separate pieces of paper for messages to be passed on or information that can be discarded appropriately after use. You must be careful what you write down to ensure that a patient cannot be identified, in case you ever misplace it, to protect patient confidentiality (NMC 2009).

Find out how confidential waste is managed in your placement area so you can dispose of anything with patient details on in the right manner.

As you become more confident and familiar with your medical placement and as you proceed through your training, the way you manage information will change as managing previously unfamiliar information becomes the norm. Managing information such as blood test results and vital signs can be difficult unless you have a good understanding of how these things are measured and what the normal value ranges are. Similarly the names of conditions being experienced and investigations your patients may need may be very unfamiliar. It is worth doing some revision on the sorts of conditions you are likely to meet on the medical ward to prepare yourself and build your confidence when handling this kind of information (see Ch. 1 for suggestion on what to revise).

Another challenge will be ensuring that any information you pass on or is passed to you can be understood. For this, it is essential that you are able to make clear written notes that both you and others will be able to understand later on. Abbreviations are useful when you are taking down a lot of information in a short amount of time, but be sure that you will remember what you meant later on. Try to avoid the use of abbreviations when passing on information to others as they can often mean different things to different people. If you have been taught abbreviations in a previous placement, check that they mean the same thing in your medical placement, as different specialties will often use the same abbreviation to mean different things. If the person giving you information is using abbreviations, don't be afraid to stop and ask them what they mean – they will assume you understand if you don't say anything.

Technology

Nursing practice is becoming increasingly reliant on technology as a way of sharing information and monitoring the progress of a patient's condition. You no doubt will already have at least basic computer skills and considerable experience using a range of electronic equipment at home. All of these skills will be invaluable to you on your placement. Your placement organiser will probably arrange for you to have training and access to the computer systems used locally, but you will need to ask your mentor to guide you in the most appropriate use of these systems in your placement area. If you have already been on a placement within the same hospital or institution, then your transferable skills in this area will be considerably greater and you may even be able to use your knowledge to support students who are on their first placements.

Other pieces of equipment do vary though, so even if you are working in the same hospital as your previous placement, the equipment being used may be different or the same piece of equipment may be being used in a different way. Ensure you ask your mentor about which equipment you need to be trained to use.

Caring for patients

Providing direct care to patients is the essential business of nursing but can also be the most daunting when you commence a new placement and especially your first placement. You will have many transferable skills in this area that you probably don't even realise you have.

If this is your first placement then a good rule of thumb is to think about how you would want to be cared for if you were a patient in hospital. When providing personal care such as help with washing, dressing or toileting, then protecting your patient's dignity is the most important thing you can do and all the other necessary skills will soon follow. Asking your patient what

they would like you to help with is the best way to start and be guided by them at all times if they are able to tell you.

If you have had previous placements in other areas then this may be an area you feel considerably more confident in. This placement may then be an opportunity for you to develop your skills in this area, such as enhancing your assessment skills when helping with personal care and teaching junior students.

Many clinical skills are also taught in a simulated environment such as a skills lab prior to commencing a placement. This will enhance your confidence and competency in such situations as helping to provide direct care to patients, moving and handling, resuscitation, bed making, taking vital signs and many more.

The routine on a medical placement is likely to be different to that of other specialties, so ensure you ask your mentor about the routine and what is seen as priority on the ward. For example, some wards may record the patients' vital signs before breakfast; other places will record them at 10 a.m. if they had been recorded at 6 a.m. by the night shift. Understanding the routine of the medical placement will help you use your transferable skills to the best of your ability.

Local knowledge and information

If you live in or close to the area of the hospital you are placed in then your knowledge of the local environment and population will be very useful when seeking to understand the problems faced by many of your patients. It will also serve as a talking point to break the ice when meeting patients for the first time. Having an awareness of the demography of your local population, prominent cultures, religions and languages and socioeconomic status is an important starting point in providing direct care to your patients, ensuring you have a greater understanding of their problems and can ensure they are treated with dignity and respect. If you speak any of the languages used in your local area then this will be a skill you may often be called upon to use.

If you don't know the local area well, there are plenty of ways to find this out. Talk to other students or friends who may know the area better. Your university tutors and placement organiser will have a good knowledge of the hospital and the area it is situated in.

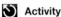 **Activity**

When you meet your mentor, prepare to ask a few questions about the local population that you think might help you. A quick search on the Internet will take you to many local community and local government Websites which will also give you an insight into the population you are caring for.

Summary

Throughout your placement you will continue to gain skills that you will be able to take with you to your next placement and on through your career in nursing. You wouldn't be undertaking your nursing training if you didn't already have the beginnings of the essential skills required to be a good nurse, so be confident in yourself and the skills you have gained from all aspects of your life and don't be afraid to ask questions!

References

Department of Health, 1999. Making a Difference. Strengthening the nursing, midwifery and health visiting contribution to health and healthcare. Department of health, London.

Fry, H., Ketteridge, S., Marshall, S., 2001. A handbook for teaching & learning in higher education : enhancing academic practice. Kogan Page, London.

Lauder, W., Holland, K., Roxburgh, M., et al., 2008. Measuring competence, self reported competence and self-efficacy in preregistration students. Nursing Standard 22, 35–44.

Levett- Jones, T., Bourgeois, S., 2009. The Clinical Placement A Nursing survival guide, 2nd ed. Elsevier, London.

Nursing and Midwifery Council, 2008a. The code: standards of conduct, performance and ethics for nurses and midwives. NMC, London.

Nursing and Midwifery Council, 2008b. Supporting assessment and learning in practice. NMC, London.

Nursing and Midwifery Council, 2009. Guidance on professional conduct for nursing and midwifery students. NMC, London.

Nursing and Midwifery Council, 2010. Standards for pre-registration nursing education. NMC, London.

Nursing and Midwifery Council, 2011. Advice and supporting information for implementing NMC standards for pre-registration nursing education. NMC, London.

Parker, P., 2009. Why should we assess in practice? J. Nursing Management 17, 559–569.

Royal College of Nursing, 2010. Dyslexia, dyspraxia and dyscalculia: a toolkit for nursing staff. RCN, London.

Sharples, K., 2009. Learning to learn in practice: a guide for nursing students. Transforming nursing practice. Learning Matters, Exeter.

Thompson, I.E., Melia, K.M., Boyd, K.M., et al., 2006. Nursing ethics, 5th ed. Churchill Livingstone, Edinburgh.

United Kingdom Central Council for Nursing, Midwifery and Health Visiting, 1999. Peach report. UKCC Commission for Nursing and Midwifery and Education fitness for practice. UKCC, London.

Further reading

Ball, M.J., 2010. Nursing informatics: where caring and technology meet, 4th ed. Springer, New York.

Benbow, W., Jordan, G., 2009. A handbook for student nurses: introducing key issues relevant for practice. Reflect Press, Exeter.

Burton, R., Ormrod, G., 2011. Nursing: transition to professional practice. Oxford University Press, Oxford.

Holloway, I., Wheeler, S., 2010. Qualitative research in nursing and health care, third ed. Wiley–Blackwell, Oxford.

Nursing and Midwifery Council, 2011. Annex 1. Confirmation of resources to support achievement of intended programme outcomes. NMC, London. Online. Available at: http://www.nmc-uk.org/Documents/Circulars/2011Circulars/nmcCircular03_2011_Annexe1-Confirmation-of-resources.pdf (accessed July 2011).

Peate, I., 2005. Compendium of clinical skills for student nurses. Whurr, London.

Richardson, R. (Ed.), 2008. Clinical skills for student nurses: theory, practice and reflection. Reflect Press, Exeter.

Roberts, D., 2010. How you will learn in practice. In: Hart, S. (Ed.), Nursing: study and placement learning skills. Oxford University Press, Oxford.

Roberts, P.M., Priest, H., 2010. Healthcare research: a handbook for students and practitioners. Wiley–Blackwell, Oxford.

Websites

http://www.nmc-uk.org/Students/Guidance-for-students/ (accessed July 2011).

http://www.nmc-uk.org/Students/Good-Health-and-Good-Character-for-students-nurses-and-midwives/ (accessed July 2011).

There are a number of helpful publications for student nurses at the Royal College of Nursing Website which would be helpful to read prior to undertaking any clinical placement experience:

Helping students get the best from their practice placements (2004: reprinted with amendments in 2006). Please keep in mind when reading it that the NMC have now amended their standards for pre-registration nursing education (NMC 2010): http://www.rcn.org.uk/development/publications/publicationsA-Z?78808_result_page=H#H (accessed July 2011).

An ageing population: education and practice preparation for nursing students learning to work with older people. A resource pack for nursing students (RCN 2008). A very useful publication based on a research project which will help students understand the specific needs of older people in any healthcare setting: http://www.rcn.org.uk/__data/assets/pdf_file/0005/149558/003222.pdf (accessed July 2011).

Benchmarks for children's orthopaedic nursing care. RCN guidance (RCN 2007). An excellent publication relating to children's nursing care in an orthopaedic context which also has sections relating to surgical nursing, pre- and post-operative care: http://www.rcn.org.uk/__data/assets/pdf_file/0007/115486/003209.pdf (accessed July 2011).

Dignity in health care for people with learning disabilities (RCN 2010). Another excellent publication offering examples of best practice in caring for people with learning disabilities in various healthcare settings, including being in hospital: http://www.rcn.org.uk/__data/assets/pdf_file/0010/296209/003553.pdf (accessed July 2011).

Dyslexia, dyspraxia and dyscalculia: a toolkit for nursing staff (2010). This is a publication which has been developed for students as well as qualified nurses and others. It is a particularly supportive one which would be reassuring for any student with any of these learning difficulties to negotiate assistance, both before and during placement: http://www.rcn.org.uk/__data/assets/pdf_file/0003/333534/003835.pdf (accessed July 2011).

Section 2. Placement learning opportunities

4 The patient journey within medical placements

CHAPTER AIMS

- To understand the complex and broad nature of medical learning pathways and their journey through the healthcare system
- To identify the learning opportunities within this journey
- To link this to some of the national changes within healthcare provision

Introduction

It is important to think about your practice learning pathways and how these can truly reflect the journey your patients are taking. Health care is changing rapidly and it is essential that you are knowledgeable and competent at the point of registration to care for a patient wherever they are within their healthcare journey. Practice learning opportunities should, where possible, reflect local and national care delivery approaches including care pathways (Nursing and Midwifery Council (NMC) 2010a). This might mean that while you are on placement you could move between the community, social care, voluntary sector, non-NHS sector and acute hospital to

follow a patient though their journey. Or it could be for you to gain an understanding of the healthcare journey that some of your patients might experience.

This chapter aims to provide you with some examples of patient journeys and how these can translate into practice learning. It will also provide you with an introduction to the key documents you should be familiar with and how they may impact on your practice and the practice of those around you. It will look at clinical policies and guidelines as well as professional guidelines, such as those produced by the NMC, that you should be adhering to as a student nurse.

The broad nature of medical learning pathways and their journey through the healthcare system

Some of your practice learning pathways will be 4 weeks, with others being up to 12 weeks or longer. It is important that you discuss your placement needs and expectations with your mentor. Your mentor will be used to assessing students within their area and will be able to discuss the possible practice learning pathway placements that you may wish to negotiate.

The welcome pack and information on your university Website will also help to prepare you for what to expect from this placement. Most mentors have established effective working relationships with other members of the multidisciplinary team across the patient journey and some may have planned your experience to ensure that your placement learning truly reflects the experience of the patient journey. There are many learning opportunities and experiences of the patient pathway that you may wish to negotiate with your mentor.

Stroke unit

A patient who has suffered a stroke will come into contact with a number of the multidisciplinary team. The patient will spend some time in the acute phase of their condition and then some time rehabilitating. Personnel involved in their care might include a psychologist, speech and language therapist, physiotherapist, occupational therapist and doctors. There may also be voluntary groups for carers and patients that you could explore and spend time with. Table 4.1 provides an example of a typical week in the life of a patient following a stroke that you might experience on an 8-week placement.

The learning opportunities within this 8-week placement are vast and really allow you to gain knowledge and understanding of the patient journey and experience. The bespoke 1-day placements with the the psychologist, etc., may already be arranged for you by your mentor or there may be an expectation that you, as an adult learner, will arrange these bespoke days. However, you can discuss this with your mentor during your initial meeting. To meet your learning outcomes in such a placement, you would need to negotiate and discuss with your mentor how you could evidence what you have learnt within all of your experiences, and when you would meet up for your midpoint and endpoint meetings to discuss your learning. The teams work closely together and there will be space within your record of achievement/practice curriculum documentation to allow for comments from other nurses and healthcare professionals to document what you have achieved and experienced within your 1-day and 8-week placements (NMC 2010a).

 Activity

> Look at your curriculum documentation and the learning outcomes for your placement and think about what you could negotiate with your mentor, now that you are aware of some of the placement opportunities, to ensure that you maximise your learning.

Table 4.1 Example of an 8-week placement: the patient experience and interprofessional working (negotiated with the mentor)

	Day 1	Day 2	Day 3	Day 4	Day 5	Day 6	Day 7
	Stroke ward for 8 weeks	Physio-therapist and the gym	Nurse consultant for stroke or research nurse	Occupa-tional therapist	Community stroke team	Speech and language therapist	Goal setting meeting with the multi-disciplinary team	Psycho-logist

Acute medical admissions unit

You could also be placed on an acute medical admissions unit which would look very different from a stroke unit, however the same principles might apply. Your patient may come in from the accident and emergency (A&E) department and you may find it helpful to spend some time there to understand how the department works and what your patient might have experienced. Your patients may be transferred to other departments and it will be helpful to discuss this with your mentor to determine where else you might need to spend some of your placement time. Some patients may be discharged home with a care package and others may go to a general medical ward or high-dependency unit. Other members of the multidisciplinary team will be involved and, again, you can find this out from your mentor. Table 4.2 gives an example of acute medical admissions unit placement opportunities.

Virtual ward

You may find that your placement base is on a virtual ward. The term 'virtual ward' may mean nothing to you and you may worry that you may be disadvantaged or undertaking simulated practice when other members of your cohorts appear to be in more technical or acute placements.

Virtual wards were discussed in Chapter 2 but here is a brief outline. Virtual wards provide support in the community for people with complex medical and social needs. People are cared for by a team of staff as they would be in hospital, however there is no physical building. The virtual ward aims to provide multidisciplinary case management, to prevent admission to secondary care (acute hospital wards) and to enhance the communication for all those involved in the care. The patient is at the centre of the care. There are different models for virtual wards with some being nurse led and others GP led. The patients that you will care for during your virtual ward placement will still require nursing care and interprofessional team working, which will be coordinated by a community matron. There will be liaison with the acute hospital and some teams will work across the acute and community journey of the patients.

For a 4-week learning pathway on a virtual ward, the weeks might be set out as in Table 4.3. For every practice learning pathway you will be provided with a mentor and, as can be seen in Table 4.3, there could be a variety of nurses who might be assigned as your mentor. It could be the community matron, the district nurse or one of the more specialist nurses.

During this placement your mentor can directly or indirectly supervise you (NMC 2008a) and how this will occur will be negotiated during your inital meeting. Within the virtual ward, teams of healthcare professionals will work closely together and a team approach may be taken to ensure that your mentor has all the evidence required to assess you. You should ensure, when you are working with another healthcare professional, that what you have experienced and achieved are documented. Other members of the healthcare team that

Table 4.2 An example of acute medical admissions unit placement opportunities

	Day 1	Day 2	Day 3	Day 4	Day 5	Day 6
Acute medical admissions unit for 8 weeks	Clinical nurse specialist for diabetes	A&E	Discharge coordinator	Physio-therapist	District nurse	Social worker

Table 4.3 An example of a 4-week placement on a virtual ward

Week 1	Week 2	Week 3	Week 4
Community matron	District nursing team	Variety of set days with physiotherapist, psychologist, pharmacist, social worker and occupational therapist	Days with the respiratory early discharge team who will visit patients within the acute hospital as well as at home

you spend time with should have been suitably prepared to ensure they are familiar with your learning needs and their role in contributing to your assessment (NMC 2010a).

6-week medical investigations ward placement

The medical investigations ward may also be called the medical day care unit and provides care for patients who require medical treatment/investigations on a day stay basis who will then be discharged home once their care is complete. Care is often provided on a day case basis and there are now more medical day care units within NHS and non-NHS hospitals.

As a student, after discussion with other students, you may consider that you feel disappointed about not going somewhere more acute and may feel disadvantaged. Do not worry – medical day care is a fabulous experience and you will be able to follow the patient journey from pre-admission to discharge. You will be able to experience the care of the patient pre-procedure, peri-procedure and post-procedure for a number of conditions. Medical day care is often multifaceted with several specialties running alongside each other. It may also be part of the journey for patients who are admitted to acute medical admissions, high-dependency and general wards. You may have the opportunity to follow them back to their ward base and be able to understand their journey. Other patients will be admitted from nursing homes, intermediate care and out-patient departments. Table 4.4 shows an example of how a 6-week placement could look in medical day care.

Table 4.4 An example of how a 6-week placement could look in medical day care

Week 1	Week 2	Week 3	Week 4	Week 5	Week 6
Medical investigations ward	Medical investiga-tions ward	Out-patient department and pre-admission nurse	Clinical nurse specialists for haematology, endoscopy, diabetes, urology, uppper GI and lower GI	Procedure room	Medical investigations ward

GI, gastrointestinal

12-week placement on a general medical ward

Of course, placements can be longer, and a 12–14 week placement is not uncommon within any year of your programme regardless of your field of practice. Longer placements can be really useful in allowing your learning to become much deeper and sustained. Table 4.5 shows an example of a 12-week placement. In this example, you could spend 6 weeks on a general medical ward and then spend 1 or 2 weeks within the specialist clinic environment linked to that ward or spend time with a variety of clincial nurse specialists that your patient may encounter during their journey.

Spending some time with the discharge coordinator can be eye opening and you may begin to understand how vital early discharge planning is and the impact on the patient, carers and organisation if this does not run smoothly. If you can spend some time within a community area that your patients are commonly discharged to, you will be begin to broaden your understanding of the patient journey outside of acute hospital admission. It will help you to understand what information the practitioners require to look after your patient within the community and highlight the resources available there.

The above practice placement pathways are just examples, but hopefully have allowed you to think about the possible learning opportunities when placed on a medical ward, day care or virtual ward.

Some mentors may use the hub and spoke model of placing students, where the placement is considered the hub and all the spokes relate to who the patient might come into contact with and where during their stay in your placement. The spokes also represent learning opportunities and possible experiences that you as a student could benefit from. The examples given in Figures 4.1 and 4.2 look at some hub and spoke models for respiratory and HIV wards.

 Tip

When you speak with your patients, try to find out about their journey so far. How long have they been unwell, who have they seen so far and what phase of their journey are they in?

For example, a patient may be admitted to the ward with liver failure due to excess alcohol intake/addiction. So far, the patient may have encountered the following throughout the health journey:

Table 4.5 A 12-week placement in a general medical ward

Weeks 1 and 2	Week 3	Week 4	Week 5	Weeks 6 and 7	Week 8	Week 9	Week 10–12
General medical ward	Genitourinary medicine clinic	General medical ward	Spend time with bed managers and discharge coordinator	Virtual ward	General medical ward	Spend time with clinical nurse specialists – tissue viablity, diabetes, etc.	General medical ward

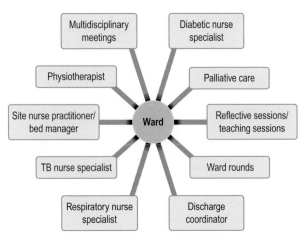

Fig 4.1 Hub and spoke model in practice if you are placed on a medical ward specialising in respiratory medicine

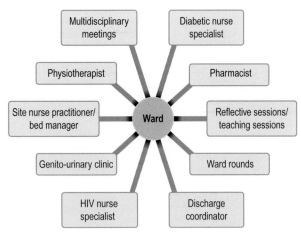

Fig 4.2 Hub and spoke model in practice if you are placed on a medical ward where patients with HIV/AIDS are cared for

- Drug and alccohol dependency clinic.
- Doctors including the GP, A&E doctors, consultant physicians in the out-patient department and ward departments and a psychiatrist within the drug and alcohol dependency clinic and in an acute ward stay.
- Psychologist.
- Counsellor.
- Social worker.
- Adult nurse and mental health nurse.
- Physiotherapist.

This patient has spent time in clinics, wards, day care units and more acute departments.

Keeping up with the changing healthcare service

As you move through your training you will no doubt learn or hear about the seemingly constant changes in the structure, organisation and management of the healthcare system in which you are working. These changes in structure, organisation and management impact on the patient journey as they will affect the commissioning and procurement of resources for patients. Such changes are often not felt directly by staff on the frontline but they have an indirect influence on care through the formation of policy and guidance.

You may feel far removed from the policy makers and politicians who set the guidance, standards and benchmarks by which we provide care services. You may even feel that they have little or no relevance to your day-to-day life as a student nurse. But the reality is that all the care you will observe or take part in is related to a guideline, policy, standard or benchmark that has been set either locally, based on national guidance, or directly by a governing body such as the Department of Health, Care Quality Commission or Nursing and Midwifery Council.

One of the competencies from the NMC leadership management and team working

You may find it helpful to look up the following Websites which outline the 'High Impact Actions' for nursing and the Commissioning for Quality and Innovation targets:

http://www.institute.nhs.uk/building_ capability/general/aims (accessed July 2011).

http://www.miltonkeynes.nhs.uk/assets/_ managed/editor/file/QMK/Quality% 20improvements/Monitoring/ UsingtheCQUINframework_1.pdf (accessed July 2011).

http://www.cqc.org.uk (accessed July 2011).

(NMC 2010a) incorporates the need the nurses to be able to manage the care of their patients:

> *across their health care journey recognising when to communicate with and refer to other professionals to deliver positive outcomes and smooth effective transition between services and, where possible, to secure their preferred place of care.*

One aspect of demonstrating leadership as a nurse requires you to be politically astute and aware of the culture and context of the healthcare system that you work in.

Activity

The following Website can help you understand the journey of the NHS since 1948 and has a couple of informative videos:

http://www.nhs.uk/NHSEngland/ theNHS/NHShistory (accessed July 2011).

Now look at the BBC Website to see the latest news regarding the NHS and consider how the new White Paper (Department of Health (DH) 2010a) could affect patients' journeys in the future:

http://www.bbc.co.uk/search/nhs (accessed July 2011).

This is considered one of the most radical changes to health care since 1948. How does it affect the organisations that you are placed in?

Once you have looked at these Websites, you will understand that there may be other providers such as private health firms and social enterprises that may be involved with the patient journey and this could affect who you are communicating with and referring patients to. What is important is that you recognise that changes in the structure, organisation and management of the healthcare system will continue to occur throughout your career which you need to be aware of if you are going to lead, manage and work within teams as a nurse for the benefit of your patients.

Understanding some of the key policy documents related to your placement area will give you an insight into the culture and context of the organisation and why certain things are done in a certain way, why staff monitor or regularly audit aspects of their care and the pressures that staff are working under.

Local policy and guidance

Each care institution will have its own set of policies and guidance that staff must adhere to. These will range from operational issues, such as management of a major incident or a uniform policy, to health and safety policies and clinical guidelines. These policies or guidelines are usually produced by the department/ clinician responsible or specialist in that area. They aim to translate national policy, legal frameworks and evidence-based practice into a usable document that will apply specifically to the area you are working in. It is important that you are aware of these local policies and guidelines as you will be expected to adhere to them while you are working in that area (see Box 4.1).

National guidance and policy

Government departments, such as the Department of Health, regularly produce policies and guidance which aim to ensure that care services provided are of an equal standard across the country. As their guidance and policy are required to reach a wide range of care providers, they can often be very broad and may require a more

---

Box 4.1 Local policies

Where to find local policies

■ Look on the trust intranet or internal Web pages.

■ Ask ward staff – there may be a folder of policies on the ward.

What to look for

■ Think of policies that apply specifically to you – uniform, health and safety, fire, moving and handling.

■ Think of policies or guidelines that may be associated with the clinical area you are working in – infection control, wound management, slips, trips and falls.

■ Think of clinical procedures that are common in the clinical area – insertion of a nasogastric tube, care of a chest drain.

---

specific local version to be created in individual institutions.

Having an understanding of current national policy and guidance around health care is essential for nurses. It provides the background to understanding why we practise health care in the way we do, what the constraints on that care are and what the government and the public feel should be care priorities. In the UK, the public is increasingly being consulted on priorities in care and this is subsequently being reflected in policy (see Box 4.2).

You will no doubt hear nursing staff, particularly ward managers and matrons, talking about auditing aspects of the care they are providing. This is often the method trusts will use to monitor standards of care and ensure that they are meeting the guidance, targets and benchmarks set by government policy. Some of these audit results have to be reported directly to the Health Protection Agency, for example infection control rates of MRSA and *Clostridium difficile* (see http://www.hpa.org.uk/infections (accessed July 2011)).

As there is a plethora of policy and guidance nationally, it is difficult to know where to start and how to determine which is the most useful for you to be aware of. To begin with, it is good to be aware of any policies that are specifically aimed at nursing care as these are the ones that are most likely to impact on your day-to-day practice (see Box 4.3).

The next set of policies or guidelines you might like to look for should be based on any national priorities in care (see Box 4.4). These are often issues that are very topical so if you are unsure what they may be, think back to any recent media stories that have made newspaper headlines or aspects of health care that have been discussed on television news programmes, for example dignity issues and infection control issues. Also ask your colleagues, mentor and tutors what they think the priorities in health care are at the moment and then try searching with these terms on the DH Website or other healthcare Websites.

Box 4.2 Where to find national policies and guidance in the UK

- http://www.dh.gov.uk – this is the Department of Health Website which contains all policies and guidance issued by the Department of Health, health service circulars and the Chief Nursing Officer bulletin which also contains useful information about new policy and guidance.
- http://www.nice.org.uk/ – the National Institute for Health and Clinical Excellence is an independent organisation that produces clinical guidelines based on best available evidence.
- http://www.institute.nhs.uk – the NHS Institute for Innovation and Improvement supports the NHS by promoting tools and news ways of working that improve care and the patient experience.

Box 4.3 Examples of nursing policy in the UK

Essence of Care (DH 2010b)

Essence of Care is a set of benchmarks and a toolkit aimed at helping nurses get the 'basics of care' right. The benchmarks include: continence; communication; personal and oral hygiene; food and nutrition; pressure ulcers; privacy and dignity; record keeping; principles of self-care; safety of clients with mental health needs; and promoting the healthcare environment.

High Impact Actions for Nursing and Midwifery (Institute for Innovation and Improvement 2009)

This document contains eight high-impact actions that have the potential to improve quality, the patient experience and reduce cost in the NHS. They are to be driven by nurses and midwives. The eight high-impact actions concern: pressure ulcers; falls; nutrition; promoting normal birth; end of life care; reducing sickness absence in the NHS; improved discharge; and urinary tract infections.

Box 4.4 Examples of policy based on care priorities in the UK

Dignity in Care (DH 2010c)

This is a set of resources including best practice frameworks, guidance and toolkits to help organisations drive up dignity in care and can be found at: http://www.dignityincare.org.uk/ (accessed July 2011).

Saving Lives (DH 2007)

This is a toolkit for organisations to help implement the Code of Practice for Prevention and Control of Healthcare-Associated Infections which is a legal requirement for trusts. It includes care bundles and guidance to direct the care of: central and peripheral venous catheters; renal catheters; urinary catheters; reducing surgical site infections; ventilated patients; MRSA; *Clostridium difficile*; antimicrobial prescribing; and blood cultures.

Finally you may want to look at policies or guidelines that specifically target the clinical area you are working in (see Box 4.5). You could do this by searching healthcare Websites, such as those of the DH or National Institute for Health and Clinical Excellence (NICE), with the specialty you are working in (e.g. cardiac care, respiratory) or speak to the nurses working in your area, especially senior nurses and specialist nurses. They should be able to direct you to the most current and appropriate policies and guidelines for the clinical area. Governing bodies such as

---

Box 4.5 Examples of specifically targeted policies/guidance in the UK

National service frameworks (NSFs)

These frameworks set out standards of care and treatment in a number of specialties and aim to ensure that, wherever patients receive care for these conditions, the service and care they receive is equitable and based on best practice. There are NSFs for older people, long-term conditions, renal, mental health, coronary heart disease, stroke, diabetes, primary care and children and maternity services. Progress towards achieving these standards is measured regularly and then standards are reviewed as necessary. They can be accessed via the DH Website.

NICE guidelines

These guidelines often target the treatment and care of a specific condition (e.g. urinary incontinence, back pain) or they may focus on the more general services needed for a particular condition (e.g. dementia). These guidelines are evidence-based and reflect cost-effectiveness of the treatments recommended. Again, they are to ensure that individuals receive the same diagnostic care and treatment wherever they receive services.

---

the NMC and trade unions such as the Royal College of Nursing (RCN) also often produce guidance in caring for specific groups of patients so a search of their Websites will be useful. (See the list of Websites at the end of the chapter.)

Professional guidance

As a student nurse, you are bound by some extent to the same codes of conduct and practice that registered nurses will be. Developing a working understanding of how these apply to you now will help as you progress through your training and stand you in good stead when you become a

registered nurse. The Website of your governing body, the NMC in the UK, will be the best place to start. Look specifically for any guidance that applies to student nurses but also read those that concern general standards of professional behaviour and areas of care that you may be involved in such as documentation and administration of drugs (see Box 4.6).

Translating policy to practice

As you read the policies and guidance that are applicable to you and the clinical area you are placed in, in some cases it will be obvious how you can apply them to your practice. In other cases, you may be left feeling none the wiser

---

Box 4.6 Nursing and Midwifery Council guidance in the UK

■ The code (2008a).
■ Standards for medicines management (2008b).
■ Guidance on professional conduct for nursing and midwifery students (2009a).
■ Record keeping: guidance for nurses and midwives (2009b).
■ Good health and good character: guidance for students, nurses and midwives (2010b).

Box 4.7 Checklist

- Who wrote the policy and who was it aimed at?
- Is the policy a legal requirement, mandatory, statutory or contractual requirement – does it have to be done?
- Is the policy or guidance based on referenced evidence-based care?
- What benefits would this policy have for you and/or your patients?
- Break the policy down into manageable parts, e.g. one standard or quality measure at a time.
- Do nurses have a part to play in achieving each standard or quality measure? Think about nurses in other clinical areas and the community too.
- What is it that nurses need to do to ensure this is achieved? Could you play a part in this?
- Look to see if this is happening in your clinical area. If so, ask your mentor about it, get involved in an audit or monitoring of standards of care.

 Activity

Consider your patient's journey

Identify a suitable patient with your mentor and then undertake the following.

Speak with one of your patients on your placement and ask them about their experiences of health care and what that healthcare journey has been like for them. Consider the following points:

1. Where are they in their journey – pre-admission, acute admission, rehabilitation, discharge, follow up, etc.?
2. How do they feel about their care?
3. Can they identify the healthcare professional involved in their care?
4. Who do they feel is leading their care?
5. What is their understanding of their goals for care and treatment?
6. Do they feel that all the professionals involved in their care communicate effectively with them?
7. When looking at patient documentation, electronically and written, are the goals of the patient's care clear?
8. Have they any carers?
9. What research has influenced the care they have received?
10. What national and local policies and practice guidelines have influenced their journey?

about what is expected of you or even if it applies to your practice at all. The checklist in Box 4.7 may help you to summarise what you have read and begin to see how it could influence your practice and that of those around you.

Summary

This chapter has encouraged you to think about your practice learning pathways and how these can truly reflect the journey your patients are taking. It has given you some examples of patient journeys and how these can translate into practice learning. You have been prompted to think about constant changes in the structure, organisation and management of the healthcare system in which you are working, to understand the impact on the patient experience and the need for you to keep up to date.

References

Department of Health, 2007. Saving lives: reducing infection, delivering clean and safe care. DH, London. Online. Available at: http://www.dh.gov.uk/en/Publicationsandstatistics/Publications/PublicationsPolicyAndGuidance/DH_124265 (accessed July 2011).

Department of Health, 2010a. Equity and excellence. Liberating the NHS. DH, London. Online. Available at: http://www.dh.gov.uk/en/Publicationsandstatistics/Publications/PublicationsPolicyAndGuidance/DH_117353 (accessed July 2011).

Department of Health, 2010b. Essence of care. DH, London. Online. Available at: http://www.dh.gov.uk/en/Publicationsandstatistics/Publications/PublicationsPolicyAndGuidance/DH_119969 (accessed July 2011).

Department of Health, 2010c. Dignity in care. DH, London. Online. Available at: http://www.dhcarenetworks.org.uk/dignityincare/ (accessed July 2011).

Institute for Innovation and Improvement, 2009. High impact actions for nursing and midwifery. Online. Available at: http://www.institute.nhs.uk/building_capability/general/aims/ (accessed July 2011).

Nursing and Midwifery Council, 2008a. The code: standards of conduct, performance and ethics for nurses and midwives. NMC, London.

Nursing and Midwifery Council, 2008b. Standards for medicines management. NMC, London.

Nursing and Midwifery Council, 2009a. Guidance on professional conduct for nursing and midwifery students. NMC, London.

Nursing and Midwifery Council, 2009b. Record keeping: guidance for nurses and midwives. NMC, London.

Nursing and Midwifery Council, 2010a. Standards for pre-registration nursing education. NMC, London.

Nursing and Midwifery Council, 2010b. Good health and good character: guidance for students, nurses and midwives.

Further reading

Best, C., Hitchings, H., 2010. Day case gastrostomy placement for patients in the community. British Journal of Community Nursing 15 (6), 272–278.

Department of Health, 2005. The national service framework for long-term conditions. DH, London.

Department of Health, 2007. Saving lives: reducing infection, delivering clean and safe care. DH, London. Online. Available at: http://www.dh.gov.uk/en/Publicationsandstatistics/Publications/PublicationsPolicyAndGuidance/DH_078134.

Department of Health, 2010. Ready to go? Planning the discharge and the transfer of patients from hospital and intermediate care. DH, London.

Glasper, A., 2010. Can high-impact nursing actions result in enhanced patient care? British Journal of Nursing 5 (6), 1056–1057.

Kempshall, N., 2010. The care of patients with complex long-term conditions. British Journal of Community Nursing 15 (4), 181–187.

Levett-Jones, T., Bourgeois, S., 2009. The clinical placement. A nursing survival guide, 2nd ed. Baillière Tindall, Edinburgh.

Lawlor, P., 2009. Referring patients with complex problems to community matrons. Primary Health Care 19 (1), 122–124.

Mellor, S., 2009. Managing dysphagia in practice. Journal of Community Nursing 23 (8), 10–13.

O'Leary, K., Thompson, J., Landler, M., 2010. Patterns of nurse–physician communication and agreement on the plan of care. Quality and Safety in Healthcare 19 (3), 195–199.

Shirley, M.R., 2008. Nursing practice models for acute and critical care: an overview of care delivery models. Critical Care Nursing Clinics of North America 20 (44), 365–373.

Snoddon, J., 2010. Case management of long-term conditions: principles and practice for nurses. Wiley–Blackwell, Oxford.

Vaughan, B., Lathlean, J., 1999. King's Fund, London.

Websites

Institute for Innovation and Improvement: http://www.institute.nhs.uk.

National Institute for Health and Clinical Excellence: http://www.nice.org.uk.

Royal College of Nursing: http://www.rcn.org.uk.

Nursing and Midwifery Council:

http://www.nmc-uk.org/Students/Good-health-and-good-character-Guidance-for-students-nurses-and-midwives/.

http://www.nmc-uk.org/Students/Guidance-for-students/.

http://www.nmc-uk.org/Documents/Guidance/NMCandYou-September-2010.PDF.

http://www.nmc-uk.org.

5

Nursing practice: admission and beyond

- To understand the admission process and rationale for information required on admission

- To understand how admission influences the care planning process

- To be able to explore the role of the nurse and other professionals within the admission process

- To be able to identify learning opportunities from the admission process

- To understand the importance of infection control within the admission process and throughout the care of a medical patient

Introduction

This chapter aims to prepare you for what may be your first contact with a patient on your medical placement – their admission. It will describe the admission process and help you to identify how you can be involved in the admission process and meet your learning outcomes, whether you are in your first year

or your final placement prior to joining the register. It will also cover some important aspects of infection control which need to be addressed on admission and throughout your patient's journey.

Admitting a patient is an opportunity to be involved at the start of the care planning process and the preparations you made in Chapter 1 will enable you to now put this knowledge into practice. This chapter will also form the basis for the following chapters on risk assessment and the assessment of patients' vital signs and changing health status, which are often an integral part of a patient's admission as well as their ongoing care.

Depending on where your placement learning experience is, your patients could be admitted from a number of different areas.

If you are placed on a medical admission unit, the majority of your patients will come from the accident and emergency (A&E). There may also be an arrangement with local GPs that patients can be referred to the on-call medical team and admitted directly to the admissions unit rather than go through A&E.

On a medical ward, your patients may be admitted from a number of different areas. Most will come from the admissions unit or directly from A&E if there isn't an admissions unit in your hospital. Some patients may be admitted directly from the out-patient department if the doctor feels they are unwell and need to stay in hospital for treatment or investigations.

Other patients may have been day patients in a medical investigations unit, for example for an endoscopy, and are too unwell to be discharged home the same day. They may also be transferred from another ward if their needs will be better met in your placement area. This might be because the nature of their medical problem is the specialty of your ward or they have specialist needs, for example a need for barrier nursing for infection control reasons and your ward has a single room available.

In an intermediate care or virtual ward setting, your patient could be transferred to you from a medical ward or they may be admitted from home following an assessment from their GP or community matron.

Admitting a patient requires a specific set of skills including communication, patient assessment, documentation, prioritising and delegating. You are likely to have competencies and/or learning outcomes associated with all of these skills. The competencies from the Nursing and Midwifery Council (NMC; 2010a) Domains – Professional Values, Communication and Interpersonal Skills, Nursing Practice and Decision Making – will all be particularly relevant to patient admission.

◑ Activity

Speak to your mentor and find out all the different places your patients are likely to be admitted from. Maybe you could visit some of these areas or arrange to spend some time in them if they are not already a part of your placement learning experience (see Ch. 4 for examples of a patient's journey).

Depending on where you are placed, a patient being admitted to your area may have been in another area of the hospital for a few days already, but other patients may have only been in hospital for a few hours before they get to you.

◑ Reflection point

Imagine how it may feel for a patient when they are admitted to hospital in an emergency. What sort of emotions and anxieties might they have? If you have a friend or family member who has been a patient in hospital, ask if they would be happy to tell you about how it felt.

Now think how it might feel to be moving from one area, such as the admissions unit, to another area, such as a hospital ward. What could you do to make the process easier for the patient?

Think of all the different areas of a hospital a patient may move between – A&E, out-patient clinic, ward, X-ray department – and how a patient may feel moving from one area to another often within a short space of time.

The admission process

A certain amount of information will have been collected about your patient in the department they started their journey in. Usually this will consist of at least their:

- – name
- – date of birth
- – address details
- – contact details for next of kin
- – GP details.

A member of staff from the area your patient is being admitted from will accompany the patient and 'handover' their care to you. The handover in this case is when the nurse from the area transferring the patient to you hands over or communicates verbally all the information they have about the patient, their plan of care and treatment required so that you can continue to provide care to the patient.

The handover process is vital in ensuring that all the necessary information about the patient is communicated to the receiving nurse, so that the transfer of care happens as smoothly as possible. (For more information about handover and skills required to hand over successfully, see Ch. 8.)

 Activity

Discuss with your mentor how you can be involved in the handover of a patient being admitted to your area. Think about the information you are likely to need to know in order to provide care for your patient and then, when you have the opportunity to be involved in receiving a handover, listen to how this information is communicated and subsequently recorded.

When taking handover from the nurse transferring the patient, you will need to know the following:
• Why the patient was admitted and when.
• The medical team caring for the patient and contact number.
• A provisional diagnosis.
• What the patient has been told about their provisional diagnosis.
• Infection control status.
• Vital signs on transfer and frequency of monitoring.
• Nursing interventions required, e.g. wound care, fluid balance monitoring, blood sugar monitoring.
• Treatment given prior to transfer.
• Planned treatment and/or investigations.
• Results of any investigations so far.

• Problems identified so far, e.g. pain, incontinence, pressure ulcers, and interventions required.
• Estimated date of discharge.
• Social circumstances of the patient.
• Any referrals that have been made, e.g. specialist team/nurse, social worker, physiotherapist.
• Patient's next of kin and whether they have been informed of admission.

Chapter 8 includes more information about the different types of nursing handover and their importance.

Orientating your patient to the ward is extremely important. Informing them of the ward name and their whereabouts in the hospital can help to reassure them and help them to inform any relatives or friends that may call them wishing to visit. Knowing the ward routine, the location of toilets, bathrooms, where they can store their personal belongings and how to call for the nurse are all essential for the patient to know to help them feel in control of their situation.

Once your patient is settled into their bed and orientated to the ward, you will need to prioritise their needs accordingly. If the patient has been transferred from another setting within the same hospital or organisation, some of their assessments and care planning may already have been completed. If this is the case it is essential that you check all of this and make yourself familiar with the patient's care plans and ensure that they are still relevant.

For many patients you will need to begin with a full assessment to inform your care planning.

You may find that the documentation used when admitting a patient will be arranged to fit with a particular nursing model, for example Roper, Logan and Tierney's (2000) 'activities of daily living'. It is vital that completing such documentation is not seen as merely a paper exercise but as an essential opportunity to learn about your patient, their actual and perceived needs and an opportunity to start to plan their care.

Activity

> Refresh your memory about the nursing process discussed in Chapter 1 and reflect on how this happens within your placement area. Which members of staff assess patients, when and how is care planned and implemented and how often is it evaluated? Find out where all of the patients' assessments are documented and familiarise yourself with the paperwork used in your placement area.

Patient assessment

Your initial assessment of your patient needs to inform yourself and your colleagues of the patient's actual and potential problems and the plan of care to address these problems. The assessment will also help to determine your priorities in caring for your patient. Your assessment will often include all or some of the following, depending on your placement area:

- Confirming patient details, e.g. date of birth, GP, next of kin.
- Vital signs.
- Assessment of needs based on a nursing model, e.g. activities of daily living.
- Physical assessment of skin condition, mobility, wound condition.
- Risk assessments, e.g. falls risk, pressure ulcer risk, malnutrition risk.
- Collection and testing of specimens, e.g. urine sample, stool sample, MRSA swabs, wound swabs.
- Measurement of the patient's weight, height and calculation of body mass index.

Assessment of vital signs and risk assessment will be covered in detail in Chapters 6 and 7. This section will focus on the assessment of your patients' needs and care planning.

The initial assessment of your patient can be quite lengthy so it is important that you plan for this to take place when there is sufficient time. For example, if meals are about to be served it may be appropriate to complete some of the assessments, such as measuring vital signs and taking any details about dietary needs and assistance required with eating and drinking, before the meal is served and then complete the remaining assessments afterwards. Also, if your patient is in pain or requires urgent treatment or intervention, this should take priority along with checking of vital signs and confirming their personal details.

In some circumstances your patient will not be able to take part in the assessment. They may be confused and unable to understand or answer your questions or they may be unconscious or too drowsy. They may also be very unstable and too unwell to hold a full conversation. When this is the case, it is important that you complete all the physical assessments, checking of vital signs, collection of swabs and specimens, etc., with your patient and then use other sources to complete the nursing needs part of your assessment.

Your placement area is likely to have a standardised set of questions to ask which

 Activity

> Speak to your mentor and identify an opportunity to observe or take part in a patient assessment. Find out which aspects of assessment above are carried out in your placement area and which nursing model is used to structure the assessment. Read up on this model to refresh your memory.

Activity

Consider how you may find out information about your patient's abilities and needs if they are not able to tell you themselves.

Some of the possible sources of information to help complete your assessment will be:

■ Talking to family, friends, carers of your patient.

■ Transfer documents or a phone call to the care home your patient lives in.

■ Information already recorded in the medical/nursing notes from the patient or family.

■ Previous admissions and assessments made which are filed in the patient's notes.

■ Contacting social services or care agencies if the patient is in receipt of a care package at home.

■ Contacting the patient's GP – this will be particularly useful if you have any queries about previous medical conditions, medications, etc.

form the basis of the patient's nursing needs assessment. Appendix 4 in Holland et al (2008) has questions to consider during the assessment stage of care planning based on the activities of daily living model.

Care planning

In Chapter 1, the nursing process was introduced as a systematic way of assessing, planning, implementing and evaluating nursing care (see Habermann & Uys 2005). This same process is reflected in care planning.

Nursing care plans are paper or electronic documents used to help direct the care we give to patients, detailing what the patient's actual or potential problems are, the goals we are aiming for and the care required to achieve these goals. Every organisation will have a slightly different system with regards to how they produce their care plans, where they store them and how they record their evaluation of them.

When you arrive in your placement area, speak to your mentor about the system used and take some time to familiarise yourself

with the paperwork used. Some examples of nursing care plan documents can be found in Holland et al (2008). Most care planning documents will have space to document the patient's actual or potential problems and then the nursing actions required to care for the patient. The date of review and evaluation will also be recorded on the care plan.

Standardised care plans which are preprinted for a specific condition are used in some areas. They have the advantage of reducing the time required to write the care plan and also ensure that the standard of care received by all patients with a similar condition is the same. But they don't allow for individual variation and not all patients will have the same needs, even if they have the same medical problem. Consequently, if you are using standardised care plans, it is important that you take the time to individualise them as appropriate to meet your patient's needs.

The alternative to standardised care plans are hand-written ones that are developed specifically for an individual patient. They can be tailored to meet the specific needs of the patient and address all of the needs your patient may have. It is essential, though, that such care plans are evidence-based and written by a nurse who understands not only the condition of patients but also the patients themselves.

Ideally care plans should be written in conjunction with the patient, but this will not always be possible depending on the condition of the patient. Some patients will be too unwell to take part and others may not wish too. It is important that, even if the patient is not involved in planning their care, you try to establish how involved they want to be in their overall treatment plan: for example, do they want to know what investigations are planned and why? For some patients, knowing all the details will help to relieve their anxieties, but for others it may cause more distress and they would rather only know when there are definite results to be given or decisions to be made.

 Reflection point

Think about why patients may or may not want to be involved in their care. What might influence their decisions to be involved or not? Consider the influence of a patient's cultural or spiritual beliefs, age, family or home circumstances.

Infection prevention and control in your medical placement

The infection control status of your patient is an important aspect of the handover you receive when the patient is admitted as it may affect the physical environment your

Case history 5.1 A patient with a chest infection

Ian is a 68-year-old man with chronic obstructive pulmonary disease (COPD). He lives alone and has a carer once a day to help him wash and dress. His daughter visits daily to help him prepare meals. He has long-term oxygen therapy at home and rarely leaves the house – when he does he requires a wheelchair. He has developed an infective exacerbation of his COPD and his GP sent him to A&E yesterday as he was not responding to oral antibiotics. He has been admitted to hospital and transferred to your ward.

Ian is breathless, his respiratory rate is 28 breaths/min and he is unable to speak in full sentences. His oxygen saturations are 92% on 2 litres of oxygen. Ian speaks English and understands why he is in hospital. He is currently receiving intravenous antibiotics to treat his chest infection and intravenous fluids as his breathlessness is reducing his ability to drink adequately and his increased respiratory rate means his insensible fluid loss is increased.

 Activity

Imagine you are assessing Ian using the Roper, Logan and Tierney model.

1. Which activities of daily living do you think he will require assistance to maintain at the moment?
2. What do you think his actual and potential problems may be?
3. Try to write a care plan for each of these problems and consider how you would evaluate whether Ian has met the goals set in his care plans.

(See page 82 for answers.)

patient is placed in. For example, if you are placed on a ward and your patient has an infection that could be passed on to other patients, they may need to be nursed in a single room. You also need to know what precautions you may need to take to protect yourself and your patient.

Infection control will be an essential aspect of any placement area you are working in. It also forms a large part of the Essential Skills Clusters (NMC 2010b) which contain competencies you must achieve at all levels throughout your training in infection prevention and control. At entry level to the register it will be expected that:

- You can identify and take effective measures to prevent and control infection in accordance with local and national policy.
- You can maintain effective standard infection control precautions and apply and adapt these to the needs and limitations in all environments.
- You can provide effective nursing interventions when someone has an infectious disease including the use of standard isolation techniques.
- You can fully comply with hygiene, uniform and dress codes in order to limit, prevent and control infection.
- You can safely apply the principles of asepsis when performing invasive procedures and be competent in aseptic technique in a variety of settings.
- You can act, in a variety of environments including the home care setting, to reduce risk when handling waste, including sharps, contaminated linen and when dealing with spillages of blood and other body fluids.

Most organisations will have a policy or procedure regarding how information about infection control is communicated, to ensure that those who need to know the infection control status of a patient are able to obtain the information easily, but at the

 Activity

Look at the competencies you have for your medical placement and identify which ones are related to infection control. As you work through this section, try to identify how you may achieve these and then discuss this with your mentor.

same time ensuring the confidentiality of such sensitive information. Consequently, you need to be careful about where you are physically in the placement area when discussing infection control issues as you may not want other patients or relatives to overhear such sensitive information.

 Activity

Speak to your mentor about the infection control policies and procedures in the organisation you are placed in and where you can access these. Take some time to make yourself familiar with them and find out about the procedure for transferring a patient between areas and admitting a patient that has an infection control need.

You are likely to have received lectures about infection control and may have been assessed in the classroom or simulation sessions on hand hygiene or adhering to other important aspects of infection control, for example aseptic wound dressing techniques.

Now that you have commenced your medical placement you will begin to realise that infection control principles are continually being applied. It is important to understand why infection control is so high on the agenda.

Activity

What have you heard about in the media concerning infection control and health care? Look at the following Website to read some of the high-profile media stories of recent years:

http://www.bbc.co.uk/search/news/infection_control (accessed July 2011).

Consider how your patients may feel if they are coming into hospital for the first time and have heard or read some of the media stories about infection control. Look around your placement environment; are there any posters or leaflets that may reassure patients that infection control is a priority for staff? Is there anything you could do to reassure your patients?

Reducing healthcare-associated infections

In 2007 the Department of Health introduced 'Saving Lives', a programme to reduce healthcare-associated infections through a series of high-impact interventions. High-impact interventions relate to key clinical procedures or care processes where the risk of infection could be reduced if the procedure or process is performed correctly. Each high-impact intervention is presented as a 'care bundle' or a set of clinical actions that can be adapted to the care environment, whether it is a hospital ward or department or a nursing home. The aim is to ensure consistency of care across care environments and to provide tools for organisations to measure through audit of their practice (see Box 5.1).

The aim of the high-impact interventions is to provide safe care, reduce healthcare-associated infections and to ensure that care is not just measurable but that clinical staff can receive rapid feedback regarding their

 Activity

Spend some time looking at the NHS 'Clean, Safe, Care' Website, familiarising yourself with the high-impact intervention care bundles and the evidence base for each one:

http://www.clean-safe-care.nhs.uk (accessed July 2011).

care in these specific areas to ensure that they are aware of any changes they might need to make to meet the standards within the interventions.

 Activity

Consider which of the high-impact interventions would apply to your placement area. Speak to your mentor about how these interventions are audited in the organisation. If possible, arrange to take part in one of the audits.

Box 5.1 High-impact intervention care bundles and their aims

- Central venous catheter care bundle: to reduce the incidence of catheter-related bloodstream infection.
- Peripheral venous cannula care bundle: to reduce the incidence of peripheral intravenous cannula infections.
- Renal haemodialysis catheter care bundle: to reduce the incidence of renal dialysis catheter-related bloodstream infection.

Box 5.1 High-impact intervention care bundles and their aims—cont'd

- Care bundle to prevent surgical site infection: to reduce the incidence and consequences of surgical site infection.
- Care bundle to prevent ventilation-associated pneumonia: to reduce the incidence of ventilation-associated pneumonia.
- Urinary catheter care bundle: to reduce the incidence of urinary tract infections related to short-term and long-term indwelling urethral catheters.
- Care bundle to reduce the risk from *Clostridium difficile*: to reduce the risk of infection from, and the presence of, *C. difficile* by outlining guidance for prevention and management.
- Care bundle to improve the cleaning and decontamination of clinical equipment: to improve the cleanliness and decontamination of near-patient equipment, to help reduce the risk of healthcare-associated infection and cross-contamination, to embed the importance of cleaning into the everyday work routine of the ward, to improve patient confidence.
- Antimicrobial prescribing care bundle: to outline an approach to safe and rational antimicrobial prescribing in the healthcare setting and a method of auditing it.
- Reducing the risk of infections in chronic wounds care bundle: to reduce the risk and incidence of chronic wound infections and chronic wound-related bloodstream infections.
- Enteral feeding care bundle: to reduce the risk of infection associated with enteral feeding.
- Taking blood cultures: a summary of best practice.

Infection control teams

Every organisation has an infection control team and the size of the team will depend on how large the organisation is. Most infection control teams will incorporate a doctor and infection control nurses whose roles are to provide advice to medical teams caring for patients with infectious diseases, advice on the nursing care of patients with infectious diseases and the precautions needed to prevent the spread of infection to other patients. Education and training of all staff within the organisation and ensuring that the organisation meets requirements set by the Department of Health will also be a large part of their role. Many medical placement areas will also have a permanent member of nursing staff who has responsibility to work closely with the infection control team and this nurse is often called a link nurse. It is the duty of the link nurse to disseminate information and teaching to the rest of the ward staff to ensure that quality and safety of care of patients remains up to date and effective.

Activity

Find out who is in the infection control team in your placement? Does your ward/area have a registered nurse who has responsibility for infection control? Find out if it is possible for you to spend a day with the infection control team.

Infection prevention and control throughout the medical patient's journey

Most medical wards comprise of bays and side rooms which are utilised in a variety of ways depending on the client group. On a medical ward there will be some patients who will require isolation due to infection; this is usually called barrier nursing. If a patient is being nursed in a side room because they have an infection that could be transmitted to another patient, you will see a notice on the outside of the door. This acts as a warning but also will provide information about what protective equipment you should be wearing when entering the room. It is standard for the equipment to be provided by the entrance of the room. The notice will not have a diagnosis but will outline the types of precautions that need to be taken prior to entering the room. The type of isolation required will be dependent on the organism that is causing the infection and its method of transmission. See Wilson's *Infection Control in Clinical Practice* (2006) for information on common types of infection, their method of transmission and isolation precautions required in the clinical setting.

If a patient is discharged home from the room, special cleaning will be required before another patient can be looked after in that room. Please check with your mentor to make sure that you know how equipment should be cleaned.

The conditions in Box 5.2 are ones you are likely to come across on your medical placement and would often require the patient to be barrier nursed.

Many patients are screened for MRSA on admission to hospital and this may be something you are required to do during your initial patient assessment. It is usually patients who are thought to be most at risk of having MRSA (i.e. those who have been in hospital in the last 12 months and those who live in care homes) who are screened.

 Activity

Find out what the local policy and procedures are for MRSA screening. Which patients are screened and when? What happens to the patient while you are waiting for MRSA swab results?

Ask your mentor to show you how to take swabs for MRSA and identify an opportunity where you will be able to do this. Find out how to label the swabs correctly and the correct procedure for sending them to the laboratory.

The following link will take you to a tutorial and video demonstration in talking a nose swab for MRSA:

http://www.cetl.org.uk/learning/MRSA_swab_technique/player.html (accessed July 2011).

Hand hygiene is one of the core principles of infection control and the most effective way of preventing the spread of infections such as MRSA and *C. difficile*. We are used to washing our hands if they look dirty, before we eat or after we have been to the toilet but we may not always be washing our hands effectively. According to the Essential Skills Clusters (NMC, 2010b), demonstrating effective hand hygiene is a competency that must be achieved by your first progression point.

Watch the following video clip demonstrating the six-step hand hygiene technique and then spend some time practising it for yourself:

http://www.youtube.com/watch?v=vYwypSLiaTU (accessed July 2011).

Health professionals are now encouraged to use alcohol-based hand gels to decontaminate their hands before and after

Box 5.2 Commonly encountered infections in a medical placement area

Clostridium difficile

C. difficile is an anaerobic, Gram-positive bacterium and patients usually suffer from foul-smelling diarrhoea containing blood/mucus, fever, leucocytosis and abdominal pain following antibiotic therapy. The condition is mild and a full recovery is usual, however older patients may become seriously ill (Damani 2003). To diagnose this condition, faecal specimens are sent to the laboratory. *C. difficile* produces spores that cannot be disinfected using alcohol gel and, therefore, soap and water must be used. Any patient with *C. difficile* should be isolated and personal protective equipment should be worn inside the room by staff and visitors and removed before leaving the room to prevent contamination outside of the room. Hospitals will have policies and care bundles for this condition and you need to ensure that you are aware of these.

Tuberculosis

Tuberculosis is an infection caused by *Mycobacterium tuberculosis* and is usually a pulmonary disease, however it can occur in other organs but this is rare. Tuberculosis is an airborne disease and you should follow the precautions for airborne diseases in your local policy. The patient will be isolated in a side room that has effective ventilation for this condition and you will need to wear a special mask when you enter the room. It is important that you wear the identified masks correctly and ask staff to teach you the correct technique. The treatment for this condition lasts months and patients are usually looked after by a community-based team in their own home. This community team will work closely with the patients when they require admission to an acute medial ward.

Methicillin-resistant *Staphylococcus aureus* (MRSA)

MRSA is a condition that is well publicised in the news and may cause you some concern. *Staphylococcus aureus* is common in skin and tissue infection and many healthy people carry it in their nose, throat and skin. The problem arises when the *S. aureus* is resistant to most commonly used antibiotics and requires the use of intravenous antibiotics. When MRSA is diagnosed, the infection control team will advise the doctors to prescribe the correct antibiotic (Damani 2003). Every hospital will have a policy for screening patients for MRSA and you need to make yourself aware of the policy. The screening for MRSA involves swabs being taken from the patient's throat, nose and perineum and sent to microbiology. There will be protocols for treatment and you will need to ensure that you ask your mentor about these.

each patient activity. In hospitals, most beds have a holder with hand gel at the end of the bed. You will also see them on the walls in most departments. Some nurses will carry around a small bottle of gel attached to their uniform. It is also common practice to see hand gel at entrances to wards and departments to encourage relatives and visitors to clean their hands before coming in.

Alcohol-based gels will not kill all bacteria though, and if your hands are visibly dirty you should always wash them with soap and water. Alcohol-based gels are not effective against *C. Difficile* or norovirus, so if your patient has diarrhoea or vomiting you must always wash your hands following the six-step technique with soap and water.

The World Health Organisation (2009) has created a resource called 'Five moments' which details the five moments during your care of a patient that require your hands to be cleaned. The resource can be accessed via the Infection Prevention Society Website: http://www.ips.uk.net (accessed July 2011). Also read the article by Sax et al (2007) which describes the rationale behind the five moments.

From your classroom-based simulation and lectures you will start to have an understanding of the standard precautions to take and practices that you must adopt when coming into contact with a patient's blood or body fluids. These practices should be used all of the time.

Aseptic technique

There will be opportunities to practise your aseptic technique within your medical placement and competencies associated with aseptic technique are aligned with your second progression point (Essential Skills Clusters; NMC 2010b). There are many procedures

which require the principles of asepsis – cannula care, wound dressings and insertion of a urinary catheter, to name a few.

 Activity

> Discuss with your mentor the opportunities within your placement for using aseptic technique and identify appropriate opportunities for you to observe and/or be involved in these.

If you are a first-year student, you may feel nervous about undertaking an aseptic technique (e.g. for a wound dressing) and it is important that you are knowledgeable about the procedure and have had opportunities to observe this in practice. You will need to undertake an aseptic technique under the direct supervision of a registered nurse. Before you undertake the procedure, ensure that you have read the plan of care and gained the patient's consent.

Watch the tutorial at the following link demonstrating and explaining the rationale behind an aseptic dressing technique:
http://www.cetl.org.uk/learning/aseptic-dressing-technique/player.html (accessed July 2011).

 Activity

> Take some time to find out where personal protective equipment (e.g. gloves, aprons, goggles) are stored on the ward. Also familiarise yourself with the sluice and equipment used to collect specimens and the procedures for disposing of blood and body fluids within your placement area. Look at Rennie-Meyer (2007) for information on how to use personal protective equipment and management of waste.

Reflection point

Reflect on an aseptic procedure that you have been able to undertake. Ask your mentor for feedback on how you did. What aspects of the technique did you find difficult and are there opportunities for you to practise this in a simulated environment at the university or with your mentor or practice experience facilitator?

Infection control affects every part of a medical patient's journey and it should factor into everything you do for your patients.

 Activity

You may find that you need to revise some of your learning about infectious diseases and prevention of infection in hospital – now would be a good time to do this. Even as a registered nurse you will be required to undertake annual training in infection control to keep you up to date with current practice.

The e-learning resources at http://www.corelearningunit.nhs.uk (accessed July 2011) are used by many trusts as mandatory update training and contain two short courses on infection prevention. They can be accessed by students. You are required to register the first time you access the site and will need to select the health authority and trust you are working in.

You may be unsure of some of the diagnoses that you encounter and therefore you may not understand how infections are transmitted. It is really important that you ask questions about a patient's diagnosis – remember, no question is silly. It is important that you keep yourself and the patient safe on the ward.

Time management, prioritising and delegation

Throughout the admission process and your initial patient assessment you will be identifying a number of needs your patient has, but you may not be able, or be the most appropriate person, to meet all of these needs. First, it is important to identify the other members of the team that should be involved in your patient's admission and assessment.

 Activity

Look back to the 'who's who' in Chapter 1 and try to identify which members of staff might be involved in the admission of a patient to your placement area.

Other healthcare professionals such as physiotherapists, occupational therapists and speech language therapists may be involved in making an initial assessment of the patient on admission if the primary problem the patient has relates to their specialty. For other patients it will be the responsibility of the nurses and doctors admitting the patient to make a referral to the appropriate therapist or specialist nurse when it is identified that they can help to meet a patient's needs.

There will also be other members of the nursing team you are working in who will help you to meet the needs of your patient,

---

> ### ◑ Activity
>
> Speak to your mentor and find out what the referral process is to different
> specialists within your placement area – how do you refer, when do you refer? Discuss
> with your mentor how you can become involved in making a referral for one of your
> patients.

both during admission and your initial
assessment and throughout care.

As you progress through your training
towards registration as a nurse, your learning
outcomes will increasingly incorporate
skills such as time management, prioritising
and delegation. For example, the Essential
Skills Clusters for Nurses (NMC 2010b) state
that at entry level to the register you will
need to be able to demonstrate that you
can do the following:

- Act autonomously and take
  responsibility for collaborative
  assessment and planning of care delivery
  with the person, their carers and their
  family.
- Work within the context of a
  multiprofessional team and work
  collaboratively with other agencies
  when needed to enhance the care
  of people, communities and
  populations.
- Refer to specialists when required.
- Prioritise the needs of groups of people
  and individuals in order to provide care
  effectively and efficiently.
- Take an effective role within the team
  adopting the leadership role when
  appropriate.
- Act as an effective role model in decision
  making, taking action and supporting
  others.
- Work within the requirements of
  the code (NMC 2008) in delegating
  care and when care is delegated
  to you.
- Take responsibility and be accountable
  for delegating care to others.
- Prepare support and supervise those to
  whom care has been delegated.

- Recognise and address deficits in
  knowledge and skill in yourself and others
  and take appropriate action.

Your learning outcomes or competencies
may require you to demonstrate that you are
able to competently manage a caseload of
patients under the supervision of a
registered nurse. You will progress towards
this by starting out managing one aspect of a
patient's care, managing the care of one
patient throughout your shift and so on
until you are confident and competent in
managing a larger caseload. Your mentor
will support you to progress to this level.
Managing the care of one patient or a
group of patients will require planning
your time effectively and this is not
always an easy skill.

A good place to start may be discussing
the following with your mentor:

- What your experiences of time
  management are – do you have any
  transferable skills?
- What, if any, strategies you employ to
  manage your time.
- How your mentor manages their time.
  It is a good idea to ask more than
  one mentor or registered nurse as
  different strategies work for different
  individuals.

> ### ◑ Reflection point
>
> Think about a shift where you felt that
> everything ran smoothly, was organised
> and patient care was of a high standard.
> What strategies did the registered nurse
> use to ensure that this occurred? What
> can you learn from this?

You will probably have reflected that some of the factors contributing to this shift running well included the following:

- Good communication and information sharing between all team members.
- Work was prioritised appropriately.
- Work was delegated among the team appropriately.
- Everyone in the team knew their roles and what was expected of them.
- Effective leadership from the nurse in charge.

Prioritising care is an important skill to learn, and as you progress through your training you will have the opportunity to observe many registered nurses and care assistants prioritising their care. This is a skill you can practise before you are required to lead a team or manage the care of a number of patients.

Your patients can also help you in prioritising care. For example, if you are assisting a group of patients in their personal care in the morning, some of them may be ready to get washed and dressed while others may prefer to stay in bed a little longer or have a bath or shower later in the day. By establishing what your patients want to do alongside what you have established as your clinical priorities (e.g. a patient being discharged home or going to another department for an investigation), you can begin to prioritise your care appropriately. It is important to keep your patients informed as you prioritise care. If they would like you to assist them right away but you have another patient that takes clinical priority, it will help the patient who needs to wait if they understand why you can't assist them right away and how long it is likely to be before someone can assist them.

Delegation can be very difficult as a student nurse but a good starting point is to think about how you would like to be asked to do something. Would you like someone to ask you politely and give you a rationale for what they are asking you to do?

 Activity

Once you have received the handover for a group of patients, take a few minutes to think about the priorities for these patients and then talk this through with your mentor and explain what you think the priorities for the shift should be. Your mentor can then discuss this with you and provide the rationale for anything they may have prioritised differently.

When you are prioritising, consider the following:

1. What is a high and low priority?

2. How urgent is the task? Does something need to be done about this now?

3. How important is it? Do I need to do this myself or can I delegate this to someone else?

 Activity

Think about role models that you respect and how they delegate. Ask your mentor how they learnt to delegate and about the strategies they employ.

☑ **Tip**

Top tips to consider when delegating:
- Be clear yourself about the task you wish to delegate.
- Is the person you are delegating to competent to do this task?
- Is the task a routine part of their role or is this something they wouldn't usually do?
- How long will this task take?
- What other tasks is this person already doing?
- Be specific when telling the person what you want them to do.
- Keep checking with them that they are happy to continue.
- Ask them to report back to you when they have finished and agree a review time.
- Always check and follow up something you delegate.
- Remember to thank the person for doing the task.

🖎 **Activity**

Prioritising and delegating

Imagine that your mentor is supervising you in managing a group of patients on a medical ward. You are in effect the team leader for the shift. She has agreed that you can delegate work to her and the care assistant working with you. You are on an early shift and have the following patients to care for:
- A 55-year-old male patient with *C. difficile* being nursed in a side room.
- A female patient with COPD who is due to be discharged home today. Transport has been booked to take her home and home oxygen has been arranged. The doctors need to complete a discharge summary for her GP letter and the nursing team need to make a district nurse referral. Her husband is waiting for her at home.
- A 35-year-old female with diabetes mellitus who is due insulin before breakfast.
- A 56-year-old female with dyspnoea booked for a bronchoscopy at some point today.
- A 44-year-old female who has had unstable vital signs overnight and has a high early-warning score.
- A 60-year-old female with a chest infection who has been stable overnight and is waiting to be reviewed by the respiratory team.

It is now 8.30 a.m., breakfast is being served and patients are starting to get up and wash and dress for the day. The morning medicines still need to be administered. Consider the following:

1. Think of the needs of each patient. Which patients will require attention as a priority?
2. Is there any more information you will need in order to prioritise your care?
3. Which patients could you delegate to the care assistant working with you?
4. What priority will you give to meeting the needs of each patient and who of the three of you is the best person to meet those needs?

(See page 86 for answers.)

Summary

The admission of a patient is a great opportunity to begin using your nursing skills and knowledge, in particular your communication and assessment skills. As you progress through your training, your skills in managing time and your workload will also increase and you will find that your competencies and learning outcomes will start to reflect this. This chapter has given you the basis for a patient assessment on admission which should help you to identify both possible learning outcomes and learning opportunities while on your medical placement. Developing your knowledge and skills in infection control will be a set of skills that are transferable to all of your other placements and your medical placement is a good place to start to develop these skills. By now you should be able to identify where your learning needs are in relation to infection control and be working with your mentor in order to meet these.

References

Damani, N., 2003. Manual of infection control procedures, 2nd ed. Cambridge University Press, Cambridge.

Department of Health, 2007. Saving lives: reducing infection, delivering clean and safe care. DH, London.

Habermann, M., Uys, L.R., 2005. The nursing process: a global concept. Churchill Livingstone, Edinburgh.

Holland, K., Jenkins, J., Solomon, J., et al., 2008. Applying the Roper, Logan, Tierney model in practice, 2nd ed. Churchill Livingstone, Edinburgh.

Nursing and Midwifery Council, 2008. The code: standards of conduct, performance and ethics for nurses and midwives. NMC, London.

Nursing and Midwifery Council, 2010a. Standards for pre-registration nursing education. NMC, London.

Nursing and Midwifery Council, 2010b. Essential skills clusters. NMC, London.

Rennie-Meyer, K., 2007. Preventing the spread of infection. In: Brooker, C., Waugh, A. (Eds.), Foundations of nursing practice. Mosby, Edinburgh.

Roper, N., Logan, W., Tierney, A., 2000. The Roper–Logan–Tierney model of nursing. Churchill Livingstone, Edinburgh.

Sax, H., Allegranzi, B., Uckay, I., et al., 2007. 'My five moments for hand hygiene': a user-centred design approach to understand, train, monitor and report hand hygiene. Journal of Hospital Infections 67, 9–21.

Wilson, J., 2006. Infection control in clinical practice. Baillière Tindall, Edinburgh.

World Health Organization, 2009. WHO guidelines on hand hygiene in healthcare. WHO, Geneva.

Further reading

Brooker, C., Waugh, A., 2007. Foundations of nursing practice. Mosby, Edinburgh.

Childs, L.L., Coles, L., Marjoram, B., 2009. Essential skills clusters for nurses: theory for practice. Wiley–Blackwell, Chichester.

Department of Health, 2003. Winning ways: working together to reduce healthcare infection in England. The Stationery Office, London.

Dingwall, L., 2010. Personal hygiene care. Wiley–Blackwell, Chichester.

Fraise, A.P., Bradley, C., Ayliffe, G.A.J., 2009. Ayliffe's control of healthcare-associated infection: a practical handbook, 5th ed. Hodder Arnold, London.

Gould, D., Brooker, C., 2008. Infection prevention and control, 2nd ed. Palgrave Macmillan, Basingstoke.

Hewison, A., 2004. Management for nurses and health professionals: theory into practice. Blackwell Science, Oxford.

Mallik, M., Hall, C., Howard, D., 2004. Nursing knowledge and practice, 3rd ed. Elsevier, Edinburgh.

National Patient Safety Agency, 2004. Ready, steady, go! The full guide to implementing the cleanyourhands campaign in your trust. National Patient Safety Agency, London.

Smith, B., 2010. Infection control. Student nurse survival guide. Pearson Education, Harlow.

Thomas, V., 2011. Fundamental aspects of infection prevention and control. Quay, London.

Websites

Centre for Excellence in Teaching and Learning – contains video tutorials of a variety of clinical skills aimed at student nurses: http://www.cetl.org.uk (accessed July 2011).

NHS Core Learning Unit – contains e-learning modules on infection prevention: http://www.corelearningunit. nhs.uk (accessed July 2011).

Answers

Case history 5.1: a patient with a chest infection

Care plans for some of the problems you may have identified for Ian
- Ian is breathless due to his long-term condition exacerbated by a chest infection.
- Ian's mobility is reduced due to his breathlessness and his long-term condition.
- Ian has difficulty communicating due to his breathlessness.
- Ian has a reduced appetite and is dehydrated.
- Ian may have difficulty getting to the toilet due to his breathlessness.
- Ian may require assistance with personal hygiene due to his breathlessness.
- Ian is at risk of developing a fever due to his chest infection.

Ian's nursing care plans

Problem: Ian is breathless due to his long-term condition exacerbated by a chest infection.

Goal: To restore normal breathing pattern.

Nursing action	Rationale
Administer prescribed oxygen at 2 L	Oxygen is a drug Its potency in treating hypoxia is often underestimated and, if given inappropriately, is lethal
Help Ian to understand why oxygen therapy is important for him	To ensure concordance with therapy and reduce any anxieties Ian may have
Encourage Ian to sit upright for lung expansion, in a comfortable position with support and pillows	Making use of his full lung capacity will aid breathing
Monitor and document Ian's observations of his vital signs	To promptly identify any deterioration in his condition
Observe for cyanosis	Cyanosis is a sign of poor oxygen perfusion and will signify a deterioration in his condition

Continued

Nursing action	Rationale
Administer any medication as prescribed and keep Ian fully informed	To optimise treatment of chest infection and ensure that Ian knows what medication he is taking and why
Ask Ian to provide a sputum specimen for culture and sensitivity and explain why this is important and provide tissues and a sputum pot	To identify type of bacterial infection and start appropriate antibiotic therapy
Place Ian's call bell within easy reach	Ian's mobility will be restricted due to his breathlessness so he will require assistance with some activities of daily living. Ian may also be anxious and will be reassured if he can summon help quickly
Refer Ian to the physiotherapist	Chest physiotherapy will help Ian to clear his chest of secretions and expectorate Gently mobilising with assistance when he can will help his recovery
Inform the nurse in charge or doctor of any change in Ian's condition	To ensure prompt attention if there is a deterioration in Ian's condition

Problem: Ian's mobility is reduced due to his breathlessness and his long-term condition.

Goal: For Ian to be able to mobilise as well as he could prior to his chest infection.

Nursing action	Rationale
Ensure all Ian's personal belongings are close at hand	To enable Ian to be as independent as possible without needing to mobilise
Ensure his nurse call bell is within reach at all times	To allow Ian to call for assistance when he needs it and reduce anxiety
When Ian is able to, establish his baseline mobility – how far does he usually need to walk at home?	To enable realistic goal setting
Refer to physiotherapist	To improve mobility once well enough
Encourage Ian to mobilise as he feels able to, with assistance	To maintain his independence and encourage mobility as his condition improves
Monitor Ian's pressure areas on a regular basis and discuss pressure-relieving techniques with Ian	To prevent complications of immobility and early identification of any skin/tissue damage

Problem: Ian has difficulty communicating due to his breathlessness.

Goal: To ensure Ian's needs are met while he is finding it difficult to communicate.

Nursing action	Rationale
Ensure Ian's nurse call bell is within reach at all times	To allow Ian to call for assistance when he needs it and reduce anxiety
Give full explanations to Ian about what is happening and why	To reduce the number of questions Ian will need to ask
When talking to Ian, use closed questions and limit the number of questions asked to those that are essential	To reduce the amount of information that Ian needs to give
Gain Ian's consent to ask a person close to him for information about his previous abilities, etc., if he is unable to give such information	To enable you to plan Ian's care and goals without Ian needing to undergo a lengthy assessment

Problem: Ian has a reduced appetite and is dehydrated.

Goal: For Ian to have adequate fluid and dietary intake.

Nursing action	Rationale
Maintain strict food and fluid balance monitoring Inform Ian about this and provide Ian with the rationale	To allow prompt identification of a reduced food and fluid intake and an imbalance in intake/output To enable sharing of information with other team members, e.g. dietician
Ensure a malnutrition risk assessment (e.g. MUST) has been undertaken and referral to dietician as appropriate	To identify whether Ian is malnourished or at risk of malnourishment and referral for specialist advice from dietician and supplements or fortified meals as needed
Encourage Ian to eat and drink, finding out his likes and dislikes and times of the day he would usually eat or drink	If Ian does not feel like eating or drinking you could encourage him with small amounts of foods that he likes and at regular intervals rather than set mealtimes
Monitor and document Ian's observations of his vital signs	To identify promptly any deterioration in Ian's condition, e.g. hypovolaemia

Continued

Nursing action	Rationale
Inform the nurse in charge or doctor if Ian's diet or fluid intake are below the normal limits	To allow prompt treatment of any complications
Administer intravenous therapy as prescribed and ensure that a cannula care plan is in place for this	To treat dehydration and prevent complications associated with an intravenous cannula
Keep Ian informed of his condition	To reduce anxiety and enhance concordance with treatment

MUST, malnutrition universal screening tool

Problem: Ian may have difficulty getting to the toilet due to his breathlessness.

Goal: To ensure Ian is able to use the toilet when he needs to.

Nursing action	Rationale
Ensure his nurse call bell is within reach at all times and is responded to promptly	To allow Ian to call for assistance when he needs the toilet
If Ian is happy to use a urinal bottle to pass urine, ensure one is within reach at all times and is removed promptly when he has used it	To allow Ian to pass urine at his bedside to conserve energy
Assist Ian to the bathroom to use the toilet when necessary, using a wheelchair to take him to and from the toilet and portable oxygen	To allow Ian to use the toilet in private within the limits of his mobility and breathlessness

Problem: Ian may require assistance with personal hygiene due to his breathlessness.

Goal: To assist Ian to manage his personal hygiene until is able to do so independently.

Nursing action	Rationale
Offer Ian assistance to wash by his bedside or with portable oxygen in the bathroom if he prefers	To maintain Ian's privacy and dignity and allow him a choice about how to meet his needs
Encourage Ian to do what he can for himself and offer assistance with anything he is unable to manage	To maintain Ian's independence while ensuring his needs are met

Continued

Nursing action	Rationale
Ensure all the items he requires for washing and dressing are within reach	To enable Ian to be independent
Offer Ian the opportunity to meet his personal hygiene needs at any time during the day, when he feels he has the energy to	To help Ian conserve his energy and allow him a choice about when his needs are met

Problem: Ian is at risk of developing a fever due to his chest infection.

Goal: For Ian's temperature to be maintained within normal parameters.

Nursing action	Rationale
Monitor Ian's vital signs at least 4 hourly, including temperature	To allow early detection and treatment of a fever
Administer antipyretic medication as prescribed	To treat and prevent the development of a fever
Use non-pharmacological methods of cooling as appropriate, e.g. electric fan, minimal bedding, loose clothing	To help reduce Ian's temperature and ensure he is comfortable
Assist Ian to meet his personal hygiene needs as required	To keep Ian comfortable
Monitor Ian's fluid intake and output and encourage his oral fluid intake	To allow early detection and treatment of dehydration

Activity: prioritising and delegating

These are some of the things you may have considered when prioritising and delegating the care of your six patients:

- Your first priority would need to be the 44-year-old female patient who has been unstable overnight. It would be recommended that you review the patient with your mentor to determine her immediate needs and call for support from the medical team as necessary. This will then determine a large part of your workload for the shift.
- Your 35-year-old female patient requiring insulin before breakfast is also a priority as breakfast is currently being served. This could be delegated to your mentor or another registered nurse while you are meeting the needs of your first patient.
- You could ask the care assistant working with you to check on your patient in the side room to ensure they are comfortable and to check that the other four patients are managing with their breakfast.
- The next priority is for the medication to be administered. This could be delegated to your mentor.

- The care assistant could help to ensure that your patient being discharged is ready to go while you complete the district nurse referral and ensure her doctor completes the discharge summary.
- You could then assist your patient who is due to have a bronchoscopy to ensure she is prepared for when the porters arrive.
- Either you or your mentor will need to accompany the respiratory team when they arrive to assess your patient with a chest infection to ensure you are aware of her treatment plan.
- You should be liaising frequently with your mentor and the care assistant working with you to keep updated on the progress of your six patients. For example, has your patient with *C. difficile* had any episodes of diarrhoea and is he maintaining his fluid balance? What are the vital signs of all of your patients?

6

Assessment of risk and the medical patient

CHAPTER AIMS

- To understand why risk assessments are important for medical patients
- To identify the risk assessments undertaken in the placement learning pathways throughout the patient journey
- To begin to understand the nursing actions taken when a risk is identified to ensure patient safety
- To understand the term 'vulnerable adult' and be able to identify patients who are vulnerable
- To understand safeguarding adult procedures and the use of the Mental Capacity Act in your placement area
- To understand what constitutes abuse
- To understand the needs of a patient with learning disabilities in your placement area

Introduction

Life is full of risks and we are constantly making risk assessments for ourselves without realising it. Each time you get into a car to drive, you are unconsciously making an assessment of risk: is it safe to drive to my destination, do I have the skills and knowledge to drive, will I be tired, is the weather good, do I have an alternative way of getting to my destination? Making these sorts of risk assessments for ourselves becomes a part of life that we rarely spend any time thinking about.

Patients with a medical health problem may be at risk in a number of ways, such as the risk of developing a pressure ulcer, of falling, of abuse. Part of your role as the nurse caring for a medical patient is to assess their risk and plan their care accordingly. These risks will apply in any setting the medical patient is in, so risk assessment will be an essential skill to learn wherever your placement learning experience may be.

Within your curriculum you will have a number of competencies and/or learning outcomes around risk assessment and safeguarding. This chapter aims to help you identify the essential knowledge and skills required to meet these learning outcomes and be able to identify opportunities within your medical placement to do this. The Essential Skills Clusters (Nursing and Midwifery Council (NMC) 2010a) include competencies around risk assessment and safeguarding vulnerable adults, organisational aspects of care, infection prevention and control and nutrition and fluid management.

The NMC (2010b) Domain 'Professional Values' is relevant to risk assessment and safeguarding. For example, the competencies include the following:

- You must understand and apply current laws relating to the care of adults and, where appropriate, children and young people. This includes safeguarding vulnerable individuals, including during end of life care.
- You must practise in a holistic, non-judgemental, caring and sensitive manner that supports social inclusion and recognises and respects diversity and the beliefs, rights and wishes of individuals of all ages, groups and communities. Where necessary, you must challenge inequality, discrimination or exclusion from access to care.
- You must support and promote the health, wellbeing, comfort, dignity and rights of individuals, groups, communities and populations whose lives are affected by transition, disability, mental capacity, ill health, distress, disease, ageing or death. You must understand how these can affect the care and health promotion of people from different communities.

There are also aspects of the domain 'nursing practice and decision making' that apply to risk assessment and safeguarding. For example, the competencies include the following:

- You must work closely with individuals, groups and carers, using a range of skills to carry out comprehensive, systematic and holistic assessments. These must take into account current and previous physical, social, cultural, psychological, spiritual, genetic and environmental factors that may be relevant to the individual and their families.
- You must know the limitations and known hazards in the use of a range of technical nursing skills, activities, interventions, treatments, medical devices and equipment. This must include safe application and evaluation of the outcome in a variety of care settings, including complex, technical, diverse environments, to provide effective person-centred care for people of all ages and backgrounds. Interventions will include safe medicines management, wound management, pain relief and infection prevention and control. You must report any concerns through appropriate channels and modify the plan of care to maintain safe practice.
- You must know when a person of any age is at risk and in a vulnerable situation in any environment and in need of extra support and protection. You must also act to safeguard them against abuse of any kind.

What is risk assessment?

Risk assessments are a way of identifying potential problems your patient may have so that actions can be put into place to prevent these risks occurring. For example, if you identify that your patient is at risk of falls, you can put into place a plan of care to reduce their risk of falling.

 Activity

Speak to your mentor and find out which risk assessments are carried out within your placement learning experience on a regular basis. If you can get copies of these, it is a good idea to take them away with you and familiarise yourself with them.

Were you surprised at the number of risk assessments that are carried out?

Now find out when and how often these assessments are carried out. Are they carried out on all patients or are there criteria to decide who gets the risk assessment? If so, find out what these criteria are.

It is also worth asking whether the risk assessment is locally driven or a nationally driven assessment. For example, is it linked to national best practice guidelines such as those developed by the National Institute for Health and Clinical Excellence: http://www.nice.org.uk/ (accessed July 2011)?

Most of the risk assessments you will have found will be standardised instruments that have been locally or nationally validated. The validity (that it measures what it sets out to measure) and reliability (that it consistently measures what it sets out to measure) of a tool is important as it helps you to know that the results of the risk assessment can be relied upon.

 Activity

If you are not sure whether the risk assessment tools you are using on your medical placement have been validated, try searching for the tool on the Internet.

Enter the name of the tool into a search engine and see if any author names or articles are in the results. These should be articles published in peer review journals that describe how the tool was developed and how it was validated.

If you cannot find the tool you are using, speak to your mentor as it may be a locally developed tool which has been validated locally and not published.

Examples of risk assessment tools

The following are examples of the kind of risk assessments you may find and some of the validated tools that are in use:

- Falls risk assessment, e.g. Morse (1997), STRATiFY (Oliver et al 1998).
- Bed rail assessment, e.g. National Patient Safety Agency (NPSA; 2007a) tools.

- Pressure ulcer risk assessment, e.g. Waterlow (2005), Norton et al (1962).
- Malnutrition risk assessment, e.g. Malnutrition Universal Screening Tool (British Association for Parenteral and Enteral Nutrition (BAPEN) 2008).
- Manual handling.
- Infection control, e.g. Visual Infusion Phlebitis score (Jackson 1998) to detect signs of phlebitis.
- Early warning scores to detect patient deterioration, e.g. Modified Early Warning score (Stenhouse et al 1999).

Different risk assessment tools will apply at different stages of your patients' journey. Some of them will be common across all stages of the journey (Box 6.1).

Some risk assessments are tied to statutes, for example manual handling. You should have received training in moving and handling patients before you commenced your clinical placement, and some of you may have found that you were not able to commence your placement until this was completed. Check with your university to find out their requirements and provision of manual handling training.

How are risk assessment tools developed?

The assessments are often based on evidence-based factors that contribute towards a certain risk. These factors are then given a numerical value which will give a total value at the end of the assessment and this helps you to decide the level of risk your patient is at.

It is important that you understand why certain factors put some people at an increased risk. Spending some time looking at a tool and working out how risk factors are determined is a useful exercise. Look at the Waterlow score (Waterlow 2005) in Figure 6.1 for assessing risk of developing pressure ulcers. Think about each category of risk and why such factors contribute to

---

> **Box 6.1** Examples of risk assessment across the patient journey
>
> **In the community – virtual ward, intermediate care, at home, in a care home**
>
> - Pressure ulcer risk assessment.
> - Falls risk assessment.
> - Moving and handling risk assessment (if they have carers looking after them).
> - Bed rail assessment.
> - Malnutrition assessment.
>
> **In the medical investigations or day unit or out-patient department**
>
> - Infection control, e.g. phlebitis score.
> - Early warning score (if undergoing a procedure).
> - Moving and handling risk assessment.
> - Falls risk assessment (to enable staff to plan care that may be needed at home).
> - Malnutrition risk assessment (to enable staff to plan care that may be needed at home).
>
> **On a medical ward or medical admissions ward**
>
> - Pressure ulcer risk assessment.
> - Falls risk assessment.
> - Moving and handling risk assessment.
> - Bed rail assessment.
> - Malnutrition assessment.
> - Infection control, e.g. phlebitis score.
> - Early warning score.

the development of pressure ulcers – you will need to think back to anatomy and physiology. Table 6.1 describes what each of the categories for risk within the Waterlow score mean.

But risk assessment is not just about completing a risk assessment form. You must know what actions to take depending on the results of the assessment. Many widely used forms will have guidance about how to interpret the results and the actions you need to take, but these may not always be obvious if you have not used the tools before. Again, ask your mentor about this and do some reading around the tool to help you understand its significance to your patient.

It is also important to know the limitation of the risk assessment you are carrying out. You must always use you clinical judgement as well as the risk assessment. If the tool is telling you there is no need for concern, but your clinical judgement is telling you otherwise, then always follow your judgement and take whatever action is necessary to safeguard your patient.

The popularity of risk assessment tools also changes and new evidence may show that some well used tools are not as useful as they have been. Examples of this are falls risk assessment tools. Recent evidence has shown that they are not absolutely necessary

Waterlow pressure ulcer prevention/treatment policy						
Ring scores in table, add total. More than 1 score/category can be used						

Build/weight for height		Skin type Visual risk areas		Sex/Age		
Average	0	Healthy	0	Male	1	
BMI = 20–24.9		Tissue paper	1	Female	2	
Above average	1	Dry	1	14–49	1	
BMI = 25–29.9		Oedematous	1	50–64	2	
Obese	2	Clammy, pyrexia	1	65–74	3	
BMI > 30		Discoloured	2	75–80	4	
Below average	3	Grade 1		81+	5	
BMI < 20		Broken/spots	3			
BMI = Wt(kg)/Ht(m)^2		Grade 2–4				

Continence		Mobility	
Complete/catheterised	0	Fully	0
Urine incontinence	1	Restless/fidgety	1
Faecal incontinence	2	Apathetic	2
Urinary and faecal incontinence	3	Restricted	3
		Bedbound e.g. Traction	4
		Chairbound e.g. wheelchair	5

Score
10+ at risk
15+ high risk
20+ very high risk

Fig 6.1 Waterlow score (Printed with permission of Judy Waterlow MBE SRN RCNT: www.judy-waterlow.co.uk)

Continued

Fig 6.1—cont'd

Waterlow pressure ulcer prevention/treatment policy *(continued)*

Malnutrition screening tool (MST) *(nutrition vol.15, no. 6 1999, Australia)*

A – Has patient lost weight recently

Yes .... – go to b

No .... – go to c

Unsure .. – go to c and score 2

B – Weight loss score

0.5 – 5kg	1
5 – 10kg	2
10 – 15kg	3
>15kg	4
Unsure	2

C – Patient eating poorly or lack of appetite

'No' score – 0   'Yes' score – 1

Nutrition score
If > 2 refer for nutrition assessment/intervention

Special risks

Tissue malnutrition		Neurological deficit		
Terminal cachexia	8	Diabetes, MS, CVA	4–6	
Multiple organ failure	8	Motor/sensory	4–6	
Single organ failure .... (resp. renal, cardiac)	5	Paraplegia (max of 6)	4–6	
		Major surgery or trauma		
Peripheral vascular .... disease	5	Orthopaedic/spinal	5	
Anaemia (Hb < 8)	2	On table > 2 hrs	5	
Smoking	1	On table > 6 hrs	8	

Medication – cytotoxics, long term/high dose steroids, anti-inflammatory (max of 4)

*scores can be discounted after 48 hours provided patient is recovering normally

© J Waterlow 1985 revised 2005*
Obtainable from The Nook, Stoke road, Henlade Taunton TA3 5LX
*the 2005 revision incorporates the research undertaken by Queensland Health.
www.judy-waterlow.co.uk

Table 6.1 The categories for risk within the Waterlow score

Risk factor	How it contributes to pressure ulcer development
Build/weight for height	Being overweight restricts your mobility and consequently your ability to relieve the pressure on parts of your body when sitting or lying down. Being underweight reduces the subcutaneous fat that protects your bony prominences from increased pressure
Skin type	If skin is dry it is much more likely to crack and damage easily. Tissue paper skin is thin and more easily damaged. Skin that is stretched over oedematous areas is also thinner and more easily damaged. Oedema will also reduce the blood supply to the skin surface. Discoloration is a sign that damage has already occurred. Skin that is clammy or damp is more susceptible to friction and shearing forces
Sex/age	Skin loses its elasticity as it ages and a reduction in blood supply to the skin surface means that it will take longer to heal
Continence	Wet and soiled skin from incontinence can become easily excoriated, increasing risk of skin breakdown. It also makes the skin more susceptible to friction and shearing forces
Mobility	The less able a person is to move, the less able they are to relieve pressure when sitting or lying down
Tissue malnutrition	There are many conditions that contribute to a reduced perfusion and blood flow to tissues and reduced overall mobility of the patient. These will all increase the risk of skin breakdown and delay healing
Neurological deficit	A condition that results in a sensory deficit will mean the person is unable to fully feel pressure or pain and therefore will not change position to reduce pressure
Major surgery or trauma	The prolonged period of immobility associated with major surgery or trauma increases the risk of pressure damage
Medication	Medication that reduces the body's own inflammatory response will affect the skin's ability to heal
Nutrition	Being underweight, having significant weight loss and a poor appetite all contribute to an increased risk of acute illness and immobility and a reduced ability of the skin to heal

in the prevention of falls for patients in hospital and that an assessment of modified risk factors should always be carried out with or without a numerical risk assessment (NPSA 2007b).

You may have considered that Mrs Kalra (see case history 6.1) would need a nutritional risk assessment as she is not eating and drinking well at present. As her mobility is reduced, she would require a manual handling risk assessment to determine the safest way for staff to help her mobilise, reducing the risk of injury both to Mrs Kalra and nursing staff. She may also be at risk of falls due to her confusion, dehydration and poor mobility so a falls risk

---

Case history 6.1

Mrs Kalra is a 73-year-old lady who lives locally with her family who are her main carers and are very supportive. Over the last 10 days they have found it increasingly difficult to manage her daily needs. She has become weaker, is not eating and drinking so well and her mobility has decreased. She has also had some urinary incontinence on occasions. Mrs Kalra has a past medical history of osteoarthritis in her hips, which she takes regular analgesia for, and she has Alzheimer's disease. Her ability to speak English has reduced as her Alzheimer's disease has progressed. She now speaks mainly in her first language, Gujarati.

Her family called the community matron who, after assessing her, feels she should be admitted to the local intermediate care unit for intravenous fluids. She has also developed a grade 2 pressure ulcer on her sacrum as a result of her reduced mobility in the last few days.

Activity

Imagine you are the nurse admitting Mrs Kalra at the intermediate care unit. Which risk assessments would you carry out and why?

Using the Roper, Logan and Tierney (2000) model of activities of daily living (introduced in Ch. 1), identify which activities Mrs Kalra will require assistance to meet. Construct a care plan detailing the nursing actions you would take to meet each of these activities of daily living.

(See page 104 for answers.)

---

assessment would be necessary. She already has a grade 2 pressure ulcer and her reduced mobility and oral intake will put her at risk of developing further pressure ulcers, so a pressure ulcer risk assessment would be required to help guide your management of her pressure ulcer risk. She is about to commence intravenous fluids, so her intravenous cannula site would require regular assessment for early detection of phlebitis or other complications.

One major consideration in your assessment and management of the risks that Mrs Kalra may face is her limited ability to understand and speak English. You will need to consider the best way to communicate with Mrs Kalra. Initially this may be with the help of a bilingual advocate or a member of her family, but on a daily basis you may need to rely heavily on visual prompts and cues. You will also need to get detailed information from her family about her usual routine, likes and dislikes as this is an important aspect of delivering person-centred care for a person with dementia.

Use this opportunity to improve your knowledge about caring for people with dementia in a hospital/intermediate care setting. The following two articles by Dewing describe some of the challenges of caring for people with dementia in an acute setting and an intermediate care setting along with suggestions about how nursing care for such patients can be improved.

Dewing J (2001) Care for older people with dementia in acute hospital settings. Nursing Older People 13(3):18–20.
Dewing J (2003) Rehabilitation for older people with dementia. Nursing Standard 18(6):42–48.

The Alzheimer's Society has produced a document 'This is me' aimed at gaining as much information as possible about a person with dementia to ensure the care they receive is person centred. It can be accessed at:

http://www.alzheimers.org.uk/ countingthecost (accessed July 2011).

Protecting from harm – safeguarding adults

Some risks, as described in the first part of this chapter, are known risks that we can assess and have strategies in place to prevent. Some of the other risks that make your patients vulnerable are not as obvious but can have devastating consequences.

All patients may be vulnerable despite their age, diagnosis or social situation. The experience of being unwell and adapting to a care environment for any patient is often very frightening. This, coupled with the fact that a power balance exists between health professionals and patients, means that some patients are reluctant to question the decisions made by health professionals and are even less likely to complain or raise concerns if the care they are receiving is below standard, especially if they are dependent on the health professionals caring for them to maintain their wellbeing, for example washing and dressing, toileting, helping with eating and drinking and pain control.

A vulnerable adult is defined as someone over the age of 18:

> who is or may be in need of community care services by reason of mental or other disability, age or illness; and who is or may be unable to take care of him or herself, or unable to protect him or herself against significant harm or exploitation.
>
> (Department of Health (DH) 2000)

It is an important role of the nurse and everybody working in a healthcare environment to be aware of the kinds of abuse that patients may be suffering, or are vulnerable to, and to act in order to safeguard that person.

The NMC (2010c) states that 'Safeguarding is part of everyday nursing and midwifery practice in whatever setting it takes place' and that 'you should have the skills to confidently recognise and effectively manage situations where you suspect a person in your care is at risk of harm, abuse or neglect, including poor practice'.

As a student nurse, you may feel uneasy and not so confident about raising concerns over possible abuse of vulnerable adults. If the abuse has taken place outside of the care environment you are placed in, for example in the person's own home or care home, then each local authority will have a procedure in place to report the concern.

🔖 Activity

Find out what the safeguarding adult procedures are in your placement area. Is there a policy you should be aware of? Is there a lead person to contact if you have concerns? Talk to your mentor about the support available and how you would go about raising an alert if you felt it was necessary.

Make yourself familiar with the national guidance as well – *No Secrets: Guidance on Developing and Implementing Multi-agency Policies and Procedures to Protect Vulnerable Adults from Abuse* – available to download from the Department of Health Website (search for 'No Secrets'):
http://www.dh.gov.uk (accessed July 2011).

If you are concerned that practice within your placement area is poor and may constitute abuse, it is also essential that you raise your concerns appropriately. The NMC provides guidance for this in *Raising and Escalating Concerns* (NMC 2010d) and, specifically for students, states that you should:

- inform your mentor, tutor or lecturer immediately if you believe that you, a colleague or anyone else may be putting someone at risk of harm
- seek help immediately from an appropriately qualified professional if someone for whom you are providing care has suffered harm for any reason
- seek help from your mentor, tutor or lecturer if people indicate that they are unhappy about their care or treatment.

Types of abuse

There are seven broad categories of abuse:

1. Physical, e.g. slapping, kicking, punching, restraint and inappropriate use of medication (for example, to sedate a person).
2. Psychological, e.g. emotional abuse, threats of harm or abandonment, humiliation, blaming, intimidation, coercion, isolation, verbal abuse, controlling, deprivation of contact.
3. Sexual abuse, e.g. rape, sexual assault, sexual acts that have not been consented to or where the person could not consent or was pressured into consenting.
4. Financial abuse, e.g. fraud, exploitation, theft, misuse of or pressure in connection to property, benefits or possessions.
5. Neglect and acts of omission, e.g. ignoring medical or health needs, withholding adequate food, drink, medication, heating, etc., failing to provide access to health and social care services.
6. Discriminatory abuse, e.g. racism, sexism, ageism, based on disability, other forms of harassment or slurs.
7. Institutional abuse, e.g. abuse that occurs in prisons, hospitals, schools, care homes, such as restrictive routines, inappropriate, or a lack of, policy and procedures, poor management.

Activity

Go to the NMC Website and look at the safeguarding resources there: http://www.nmc-uk.org/Nurses-and-midwives/safeguarding/ (accessed July 2011). Watch the three short films showing safeguarding vulnerable adults from different perspectives:

- The first concerns an older man living in a care home and shows how his dignity is compromised and his needs neglected as they get him ready for breakfast.
- The second concerns a young woman attending an antenatal clinic with her husband. The midwife identifies bruising on the woman's arms but is unsure of how to deal with this as the lady does not speak English and her husband answers all questions for her.
- The third concerns a young woman with a learning disability in hospital who is clearly distressed when her mother comes to visit. The mother speaks to the nurse about her concerns but is not listened to.

Spend some time reflecting on how you would respond if you were the nurse caring for these patients.

Abuse can occur in any setting. It may occur in the patient's own home or a day centre or other facility that they visit. It may also occur in a hospital or long-term care setting. The perpetrator of abuse can also be anyone – it may be a relative, a friend or a carer, or it could be a health professional in hospital. Therefore, you need not only to be aware of signs of abuse that could have happened before the patient was admitted, but also be alert to any situations that may arise while they in are hospital, in particular acts of omission or neglect. Examples of this type of abuse in a healthcare setting could be prescribed medications not being given, assistance not being provided in a dignified way to wash and dress, not addressing toileting needs, assistance not being given to eat and drink.

 Activity

Looking at the seven types of abuse above, what signs might you look out for that would indicate abuse was taking place?

Look at the following Website from Action on Elder Abuse for some information about the signs of abuse:

http://www.elderabuse.org.uk/About%20Abuse/What_is_abuse%20define.htm (accessed July 2011).

Talk to your mentor about vulnerable adults they have looked after. How did they identify issues of abuse and how did they deal with it? Think especially about how you talk to the patient you suspect is being abused. This is a difficult topic to discuss and needs to be addressed sensitively. Your mentor may have experience of this or will know who the best person to contact is in these situations.

The Mental Capacity Act

The Mental Capacity Act 2005 (DH 2005) (an Act of Parliament in the UK) provides a legal framework for acting or making decisions on the behalf of those who lack the capacity to make the decision themselves. It provides clear guidance on how to assess capacity, document it and make decisions that are in the best interests of the person concerned. As a nurse, you are likely to be involved in helping to assess the capacity of patients with regard to some of the decisions they need to make, therefore it is important that you make yourself familiar with the Act and how to apply it in your practice. The NMC Code (2008) states that:

> You must be aware of the legislation regarding mental capacity, ensuring that people who lack capacity remain at the centre of decision making and are fully safeguarded.

You may find the following Website useful, as it not only explains what the Mental Capacity Act is but includes guidance and tools on assessing mental capacity:

http://www.amcat.org.uk/ (accessed July 2011).

Caring for the patient with learning disabilities

Recently in the UK there has been considerable concern about the care that people with learning disabilities receive when they are admitted to hospital with acute medical problems. The number of people with learning disabilities is set to increase over the next decade (to see the latest statistics and information regarding adults with learning disabilities in the UK,

Case history 6.2

Mr Gray is a 56-year-old man admitted to your medical ward with dehydration. He is malnourished and cachexic. He has a history of alcohol abuse and a psychiatric history of schizophrenia. He lives alone in a one-bedroom flat.

1. Would you call Mr Gray a vulnerable adult? If so, why? What are your initial concerns about Mr Gray?

   While you are assessing Mr Gray and asking him about how he manages his activities of daily living, he tells you that he gives his bank card to a friend who withdraws money from his account and does his food shopping for him. He also tells you that his friend sleeps in the only bedroom of the flat and that he sleeps on the sofa in the living room.

2. Would you be concerned that he is at risk of abuse? If so, what kind of abuse? What would you do with this information?

   The trust lead for safeguarding adults comes to see Mr Gray and carries out a Mental Capacity Act assessment to see if he has the capacity to decide whether or not his friend should have access to his money. He finds that Mr Gray does have capacity. He is also able to contact the friend, who tells the safeguarding lead that he does do the shopping for Mr Gray and that he cooks and leaves food for Mr Gray to eat but he often doesn't eat it.

3. If Mr Gray is to be discharged, what actions do you think would be necessary to safeguard him at home?

   In this case you would initially be concerned that Mr Gray is being financially abused and neglected by his friend who has control over his money and his ability to get food. But as the case is looked into further, Mr Gray has the capacity to decide who has his money and buys him food and also whether or not he eats it. He is clearly a vulnerable adult though, and a referral to social services to provide him with some support at home, if he is willing to accept this, would be important.

---

go to http://www.learningdisabilities.org.uk). This means that you are very likely to have patients who also have a learning disability on a medical placement.

Two high-profile reports identified the problems adults with learning disabilities face when they are admitted to hospital and these included not receiving acceptable standards of basic care and, in some instances, people being denied health care and treatment because they had a learning disability. You can access both of these reports online:

- *Death by Indifference* – published by MENCAP (2007): http://www.mencap.org.uk/node/5863 (accessed July 2011).

 Activity

Your placement organisation is likely to have a local policy or strategy about caring for people with learning disabilities and may have access to an acute liaison nurse, who will be a learning disability nurse, or team based in the hospital to provide support to people with learning disabilities, their carers and staff when they are admitted to hospital. Ask your mentor about what is available in your organisation and how to access support if you need it.

- *Six Lives* – a report of the Parliamentary and Health Service Ombudsman (2009): http://www.ombudsman.org.uk (accessed July 2011).

There are some basic principles of care that will help you to support a patient with learning disabilities during you medical placement:

- Find out as much as you can about the person – some of this information will come from the patient, but you will need to talk to their carer or relatives to get more information.
- Find out about their usual routine at home – what they like to eat or drink, what helps them relax, what makes them anxious, etc.
- See if they have a hospital passport – an individualised document that contains all the important information you need to know about the person you are caring for.
- Always tell the person what you are doing and why.
- Think about your communication style and adjust it to meet the needs of the person you are caring for.
- Pay particular attention to ensuring that the person is eating and drinking well and having their toileting and personal care needs met.
- The person may also have a Health Action Plan – a plan detailing the actions, services and support the person needs to maintain their health. It is an individualised document and will have been produced in conjunction with the person. For more information on Health Action Plans, see Health Action Planning and Health Facilitation for People with Learning Disabilities: good practice guidance: http://www.dh.gov.uk (accessed July 2011).
- Always seek specialist advice if you are not sure – your mentor will know who to contact and how.

The following guidance from the Royal College of Nursing (RCN) will also help to increase your knowledge and confidence in caring for a person with learning disabilities:

Royal College of Nursing (2007) Meeting the health needs of people with learning disabilities. RCN, London.

Royal College of Nursing (2010) Dignity in health care for people with learning disabilities. RCN, London.

Summary

Assessment of risk and safeguarding adults are important aspects of a nurse's role. They will not only guide and inform the care you give, in the case of risk assessments, but will also ensure the safety and wellbeing of your patients, alerting you to their changing healthcare needs. This chapter aims to equip you with the basic knowledge you need to identify when and which risk assessments are necessary and how they consequently help to form a plan of care. As you become more experienced, risk assessment will become a natural part of your day-to-day nursing care, whichever setting you are working in. The risk assessment skills you develop throughout your medical placement will be useful to you in many different clinical settings.

Safeguarding vulnerable adults is often a difficult aspect of caring for patients with medical needs, but as you progress through your training you will develop confidence in identifying and acting upon situations where a patient may be at risk of abuse or being abused. Until you feel confident about this, do not be afraid to raise a concern even if you are not sure about it. Speak to your mentor or any of the registered nurses you are working with. They would rather you raise a concern that turns out to be nothing than ignore some information that may be crucial to the safety of your patient.

Case history 6.3

Louise is a 36-year-old woman with severe learning disabilities. She has very little verbal communication and is only able to make sounds to express how she feels. She lives in a community home with three other people with learning disabilities and they receive 24-hour care from trained carers. She has a past medical history of epilepsy and has been admitted via the accident and emergency department to the medical admissions unit following a seizure.

1. Would you call Louise a vulnerable adult? If so, why? Do you have any initial concerns about Louise?

   When you are helping to wash and change Louise she is very resistant and screams continually. You stop what you are doing and wait for her mother to visit. She is calmer when her mother is present and it is easier to help her wash and dress. But she still screams every time you touch her left arm. Over the next couple of days, significant bruising appears on her left arm and an X-ray confirms that she has fractured her humerus. Louise's mother is very concerned as she was not informed by the carers at her home that Louise had fallen or had any kind of accident.

2. Are you concerned that she is at risk of abuse? If so, what kind of abuse? What would you do with this information?

   The lead for safeguarding adults raises a safeguarding alert about her care at home and this is subsequently investigated by an independent person. The findings of the investigation were that one of the other people with learning disabilities who shares the home with Louise had pushed her over which had resulted in the fracture, and a review of their care needs took place.

   Louise is a vulnerable adult and, although there were no initial concerns about her care at home, an unexplained injury should always be investigated. You would have been right to suspect she might have been being physically abused.

   It is important in a situation like this that an alert is raised by the trust and that it is investigated independently. Louise would stay in hospital or move to another place of safety while this takes place, not return to her home, until the investigation and any subsequent action to reduce her risk of being abused has taken place.

References

British Association for Parenteral and Enteral Nutrition, 2008. Malnutrition Universal Screening Tool. BAPEN, Redditch. Online. Available at: http://www.bapen.org.uk/must_itself.html (accessed July 2011).

Department of Health, 2000. No secrets: guidance on developing and implementing multi-agency policies and procedures to protect vulnerable adults from abuse. Department of Health & Home Office, London.

Department of Health, 2005. The Mental Capacity Act. Office of the Public Guardian, London.

Jackson, A., 1998. Infection control: a battle in vein infusion phlebitis. Nursing Times 94 (4), 68–71.

Morse, J.M., 1997. Preventing patient falls, first ed. Sage, Thousand Oaks, California.

Nursing and Midwifery Council, 2008. The code: standards of conduct, performance and ethics for nurses and midwives. NMC, London.

Nursing and Midwifery Council, 2010a. Essential skills clusters. NMC, London.

Nursing and Midwifery Council, 2010b. Standards for pre-registration nursing education. NMC, London.

Nursing and Midwifery Council, 2010c. Safeguarding adults. NMC, London. Online. Available at: http://www.nmc-uk.org/Nurses-and-midwives/safeguarding/ (accessed July 2011).

Nursing and Midwifery Council, 2010d. Raising and escalating concerns. Guidance for nurses and midwives. NMC, London.

National Patient Safety Agency, 2007a. Resources for reviewing or developing a bed rail policy. NPSA, London.

National Patient Safety Agency, 2007b. Slips, trips and falls in hospital: the third report from the patient safety observatory. NPSA, London.

Norton, D., McLaren, R., Exton-Smith, A.N., 1962. An investigation of geriatric nursing problems in hospital. National Corporation for the Care of Old People, London.

Oliver, D., Britton, M., Seed, P., et al., 1998. A 6 point risk score predicted which elderly patients would fall in hospital. British Medical Journal 315, 1049–1053.

Roper, N., Logan, W., Tierney, A., 2000. The Roper–Logan–Tierney model of nursing. Churchill Livingstone, Edinburgh.

Stenhouse, C., Coates, S., Tivey, M., et al., 1999. Prospective evaluation of a modified Early Warning Score to aid earlier detection of patients developing critical illness on a general surgical ward. British Journal of Anaesthesia 84, 663.

Waterlow, J., 2005. Pressure ulcer risk assessment and prevention. Online. Available at: http://www.judy-waterlow.co.uk/index.htm.

Further reading

Brooker, C., Waugh, A., 2007. Foundations of nursing practice. Mosby, Edinburgh.

Fyson, R., 2009. Independence and learning disabilities: why we must also recognise vulnerability. Journal of Integrated Care 17 (1), 3–8.

Gates, B., 2004. Learning disabilities: toward inclusion, 4th ed. Churchill Livingstone, Edinburgh.

Hewitt, D., 2009. Not just in the Mental Capacity Act: using the law to protect vulnerable adults. Journal of Adult Protection 11 (2), 25–31.

Kydd, A., Duff, T., Raymond Duffy, F.J., 2009. Care and wellbeing of older people. Reflect Press, Devon.

Morgan, A., 2010. Review of safeguarding practice points towards a new culture of transparency. Nursing Older People 22 (1), 6–7.

Websites

The Alzheimer's Society Website has a section dedicated to researchers and professionals which contains many excellent resources including the brain tour, an interactive video describing how the different types of dementia affect the brain: http://www.alzheimers.org.uk (accessed July 2011).

MENCAP, a leading learning disability charity, has a section for professionals with good resources to read and video clips to watch: http://www.mencap.org.uk/ (accessed July 2011) this website contains information on assessing mental capacity including tools to use: http://www.amcat.org.uk/ (last accessed 16.05.11.).

European Pressure Ulcer Advisory Panel: http://www.epuap.org (accessed July 2011).

Answer

Case history 6.1

Mrs Kalra may need assistance with the following activities of living:
• Communication.
• Mobilising.
• Eating and drinking.
• Elimination.

The following are examples of care plans you may have considered for Mrs Kalra:

Problem: Mrs Kalra has limited English which makes it difficult for her to communicate her needs and to fully understand the goals for her treatment. Her ability to communicate may also be affected by her Alzheimer's disease.

Goal: To ensure that Mrs Kalra is able to communicate her needs and understand her treatment as far as possible.

Nursing action	Rationale
Ensure a bilingual advocate is available at the first assessment and as frequently as possible afterwards	To establish a baseline of what Mrs Kalra is able to understand about her reason for admission, problems and treatment plan To enable Mrs K to discuss her condition confidentially and to ensure that she is fully informed
Spend time finding out as much as possible about how Mrs Kalra usually communicates and complete a document such as 'This is Me' (www.alzheimers.org.uk), e.g. how she asks for the toilet, a drink, something to eat, how she expresses herself when in pain, upset, angry	To ensure that the care provided to Mrs Kalra is person centred and that staff are able to communicate with her and understand her needs
Ask the family to translate basic words, e.g. drink, pain, I need the toilet, if Mrs Kalra would understand these	To enhance communication
Allow a family member to stay with Mrs Kalra to reduce her anxiety if they wish to do so	To reduce Mrs Kalra's anxiety levels
Use non-verbal communication to enhance understanding, e.g. pointing to things, gestures	To promote and enhance communication
Ensure time is spent attempting to communicate with Mrs Kalra while her other care needs are being met, e.g. when helping her to wash and dress, at mealtimes, when giving medication	To enable staff to build a rapport with Mrs Kalra which will make understanding her needs and communicating with her much easier

Continued

Nursing action	Rationale
Introduce yourself to Mrs Kalra each time you see her and be prepared to repeat information as many times as necessary	To compensate for Mrs Kalra's memory problems

Problem: Mrs Kalra is not eating or drinking adequately due to her condition.

Goal: For Mrs Kalra to have adequate fluid and dietary intake.

Nursing action	Rationale
Ensure a malnutrition risk assessment is undertaken in the first 24 hours	To determine Mrs Kalra's nutritional status
Maintain strict food and fluid balance monitoring With the help of an advocate, inform Mrs Kalra about this and provide Mrs Kalra with rationale Inform the nurse in charge or doctor if Mrs Kalra's diet or fluid intake are below the normal limits	To ensure that Mrs Kalra receives adequate fluids and nutrition To prevent complications of dehydration To ensure that there is effective communication within the multidisciplinary team
Find out what kinds of foods Mrs Kalra would eat at home and what time she would usually eat Discuss with dietician/kitchen about providing such foods	To provide food and drink which is familiar to Mrs Kalra at familiar times to encourage her oral intake
Encourage Mrs Kalra to drink nutritional supplements in a flavour she likes	High-calorie/high-protein supplements aid recovery and wound healing
Monitor and document Mrs Kalra's observations of her vital signs, including weight	To detect any deterioration/ improvement
Administer intravenous therapy as prescribed and ensure that the cannula site is inspected regularly for signs of phlebitis	To reduce the risk of cannula-associated infection/complications

Problem: Mrs Kalra has a pressure ulcer.

Goal: To heal the wound and to prevent infection.

Nursing action	Rationale
Assess the wound every time it is dressed – size, depth, width and length	To assess deterioration or improvement

Continued

Nursing action	Rationale
Document deterioration/improvement on the wound assessment and review chart	
If wound shows any signs of infection – redness, increased pain, heat, swelling, increased exudates, odour – send wound swab for culture and sensitivity	To detect infection
Aseptically dress the wound with a hydrocolloid dressing	To prevent infection
Consider analgesia prior to dressing changes	To keep Mrs Kalra as comfortable as possible
Weekly Waterlow score	To determine risk
Provide pressure redistribution mattress and cushion	To promote comfort, healing and prevent deterioration
Encourage Mrs Kalra to mobilise – refer to physiotherapist (see mobility care plan)	See mobility care plan
Ensure Mrs Kalra has a high-protein diet (see eating and drinking care plan)	A high-protein diet will enhance wound healing
Liaise with the tissue viability/wound nurse specialist	For specialist advice and best practice

Problem: Mrs Kalra has pain in her hips and from the wound site.

Goal: To relieve the pain.

Nursing action	Rationale
Using a pain assessment tool that is appropriate for a non-English speaking patient and also a person with dementia, assess severity of Mrs Kalra's pain Observe for behavioural changes and non-verbal cues that might indicate she is in pain	To determine the type, intensity and site of the pain using a tool that Mrs Kalra can understand if possible
Administer prescribed analgesia	To reduce the pain
Reassess pain to determine the effectiveness of the analgesia	To assess the effectiveness of the analgesia given
Inform the doctor if Mrs Kalra's pain relief is inadequate, referring to the analgesic ladder	For analgesia to be increased promptly
Assist Mrs Kalra to manage her pain by careful positioning and other non-pharmacological techniques	To increase comfort and reduce pain using culturally appropriate pain relief methods to complement the analgesia

Continued

Nursing action	Rationale
Consider timing the analgesia for wound dressings and physiotherapy	To ensure full benefit of physiotherapy and to ensure comfort during therapy and wound dressings

Problem: Mrs Kalra has reduced mobility due to weakness and pain.

Goal: To maximise Mrs Kalra's mobility.

Nursing action	Rationale
Refer to the physiotherapist and liaise to ensure that Mrs Kalra mobilises safely	For full assessment of mobility problems and provision of walking aids if necessary
Using a bilingual advocate and other communication strategies identified, explain why it is important to mobilise and encourage her to do so as often as she can, e.g. to the toilet	To increase likelihood of Mrs Kalra wanting to mobilise and reduce the chances of her losing the ability to walk
Administer analgesia prior to physiotherapy	To control pain and maximise ability to walk
Complete a falls risk assessment	To address any modifiable risk factors that may contribute to falling
Minimise friction on movement	To reduce the risk of skin breakdown
Ensure that Mrs Kalra does not sit out of bed for more than an hour at a time to prevent further pressure damage	To reduce the risk of further pressure damage

Problem: Mrs Kalra has recently become incontinent of urine.

Goal: To keep Mrs Kalra clean and dry, maintain her dignity and to determine cause.

Nursing action	Rationale
Obtain mid-stream specimen of urine for ward-based urinalysis and to send to the lab for culture and sensitivity	To determine if infection is present and to determine antibiotic sensitivity
If possible, using a bilingual advocate, ask Mrs Kalra about her urinary symptoms Alternatively, her family may be able to provide information	Ongoing treatment and investigation of incontinence will depend on type of incontinence

Continued

Nursing action	Rationale
Complete a bladder diary and a fluid chart for a minimum of 3 days to establish her pattern of incontinence	To assist in creating a regular toileting regime to help maintain continence and ensure adequate fluid intake
Ensure her bed is placed close to the toilet and her walking aid and call bell are at hand	To enable Mrs Kalra to use the toilet in the bathroom in a timely manner
Offer assistance and prompting to use the toilet at regular intervals, according to the bladder diary	To provide a reminder to Mrs Kalra to use the toilet and an opportunity for her to establish a regular voiding routine
Mrs Kalra may need to be shown where the toilet is on a regular basis as a result of her memory problems	
Provide an incontinence pad and fixation pants if necessary	For her dignity to be maintained
Help Mrs Kalra to maintain her hygiene needs	To ensure Mrs Kalra is comfortable, for her dignity to be maintained and reduce risk of skin breakdown

7

Assessment of vital signs and changes in health status

CHAPTER AIMS

- To help the student understand how to assess vital signs and recognise the changes within a patient's physical and mental health status

- To help the student to recognise and respond to the deteriorating patient on a medical placement

- To explore why a patient's health status may change and how this can affect their decision making

Introduction

Wherever you are placed during your medical placement, you will be involved in undertaking observations of patients' vital signs. Whether you are placed within an out-patient department, virtual ward, and medical ward or on medical day care, you will be undertaking physical and mental assessments of your patients from the first year to your final placement.

As students from all fields of nursing, you will have been exposed to simulated practice within the university. However, when you are undertaking observations of patients'

vital signs during your medical placement, you may not find them as easy to perform as you did within simulated practice. Patients vary, and it can be daunting at first as patients are sick and your competence is also being assessed. Remember that your mentor is there to help, guide and supervise you and that you should not undertake any clinical skills alone until your mentor has assessed your competence. This assessment of competence should not be carried out on just one patient but with a variety of patients with differing health problems. Always ask for a rationale. As you progress towards your third year of training you will already be competent in the Essential Skills for years one and two (Nursing and Midwifery Council (NMC) 2010). However, your learning outcomes will be expecting you to demonstrate assessment skills, prioritisation and clinical decision making for a group of patients. Some students find this easier than others to achieve, however, good communication with your mentor regarding your learning needs can really help you to develop in this area.

Observations of vital signs and recognition of changes in your patients' health status will be an essential clinical skill within your learning outcomes regardless of your chosen field of nursing. Undertaking observations of vital signs and recognising changes in patients' health status will incorporate all of the NMC

(2010) Standard Competencies – professional values, communication and interpersonal skills, clinical decision making, and leadership, management and team working. For example, within decision making, part of the standard competency states that: 'decision making must be person-focused, and through a process of critical analysis learning to a range of technical and nursing interventions from basic to the highly complex'.

For communication, the NMC Competency states that nurses 'must communicate safely and effectively with individuals and groups of all ages' (NMC 2010) and you may find that your record of achievement/practice curriculum documentation has mapped the Essential Skills Clusters for care, compassion and communication with the specific competencies within the domains.

When you are undertaking your observations of vital signs, you will behave with professional values, communicate with your patients, make clinical decisions and often need to liaise with multidisciplinary teams (Box 7.1). You will also meet some of the Essential Skills Clusters while undertaking observations of vital signs, for example some of the organisational aspects of care, compassion and communication skills (NMC 2010).

Box 7.1 Some of the specific competencies that you might meet while undertaking observation of vital signs

Field Standard for Competence: Professional Values Domain, Adult:

All nurses must practise confidently according to the NMC (2010) code.
All nurses must recognise the limits of their own competence and knowledge. They must reflect on their own practice and seek advice from, or refer to, other professionals where necessary

Field Standard for Competence: Communication and Interpersonal Skills Domain

All nurses must use a range of communication skills and technologies to support person-centred care and enhance the quality and safety of health care. They must make sure that people receive all the information about their care in a language and manner that is right for them, and that allows them to make informed choices and consent to treatment.

Field Standard for Competence: Nursing Practice and Decision-Making Domain

Adult nurses must be able to carry out accurate health, clinical and nursing assessments across all ages and show the right diagnostic and decision-making skills. They must have the confidence to provide effective adult nursing care in the home, community and in the hospital settings.

Adult nurses must recognise early signs of acute illness in young people, adults and older people and accurately assess and start appropriate and timely management of those at risk of clinical deterioration, who are acutely ill or who need emergency care.

Demonstrating competence

What will your mentor expect to see you doing within the first year of your training and what will the mentor expect to see you doing differently as a more senior student? Hopefully the following will help you and your mentor to match expectations.

Within your first year

Your mentor will expect to see you do the following in your first year:
- Display the professional behaviour and conduct expected of a nurse, for example gaining agreement from the patient first and explaining what needs to be done.
- A competent technique.
- Report abnormalities – you may not understand why a patient has abnormal vital signs but you would be expected to report it.
- To use the early warning score.
- To detect deterioration.
- To document accurately.
- To follow the organisation's policy.

As you progress through your first year you should try to think about the reasons why your patients' vital signs might be outside normal limits and think about the interventions that might help. If you do not know, ask your mentor and discuss the frequency of observations of vital signs, plan of care and evaluation. Also think about how this relates to pathophysiology.

Within your final year

Your mentor will expect to see you do the following in your final year:
- Demonstrate a patient-centred focus.
- Use the early warning score accurately.
- Detect changes and report, recheck, seek guidance.
- Clearly integrate theory and practice.
- Prioritise care.
- Follow policy and role model professional practice behaviour.
- Be able to relate the patient's health problem to the patient, context and specialty, discuss care and articulate the rationale to the mentor.
- Initiate actions and interventions.
- Initiate, evaluate and reassess the plan of care using a structured approach.
- Be confident in communication with the multidisciplinary team.

Reflection point

At this point in your training, what do you think you should know about observations of vital signs? Look at your curriculum documentation for this placement and find out what your learning outcomes are with regard to vital signs and responding to changes in your patients' health status.

You will be expected to assess the physical and mental status of your patient and will be involved in assessing the following:
- Temperature.
- Pulse/heart rate.
- Respiration.
- Oxygen saturation.
- Peak flow.
- Blood pressure (BP).
- Neurological status.

When we perform something very often, it is easy to forget the underlying theory and principles for practice. Here is a quick revision guide to the observations of vital signs that you undertake every day within your medical placements.

Quiz

(Answers on pp 127–133.)

Temperature

7.1 What is it?
7.2 Why do we check it?
7.3 How do we check it?
7.4 What is a normal temperature?
7.5 What does an abnormal temperature mean?

Also see this resource for a demonstration of taking a temperature:
  http://www.cetl.org.uk/learning/temperature-a/player.html (accessed July 2011).

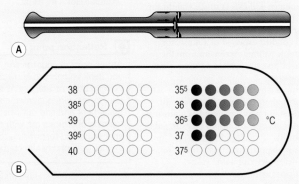

Fig 7.1 (A) Disposable chemical dot thermometer. (B) Recording area of a disposable thermometer (Holland et al 2008, with permission)

7.6 Moira is a 36-year-old lady admitted to the ward with a temperature of 38.5 °C. She complains of pain on inspiration and has had a chesty cough for the last week. How could you help Moira to feel more comfortable and what nursing actions could you undertake?

Pulse

7.7   What is it?
7.8   Why do we check it?
7.9   How do we check it?
7.10 What is a normal pulse rate?
7.11 What does an abnormal rate mean?

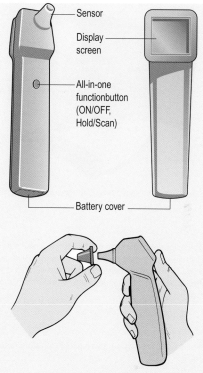

Fig 7.2 Tympanic thermometer (Holland et al 2008, with permission)

Blood pressure

7.12 What is it?
7.13 Why do we check it?
7.14 How do we check it?
7.15 What is a normal BP?
7.16 What does an abnormal BP mean?

Also see these resources for a demonstration of taking BP:

http://www.cetl.org.uk/learning/bpm/player.html (accessed July 2011)
http://www.cetl.org.uk/learning/BP_Korotkoff_sounds/player.html

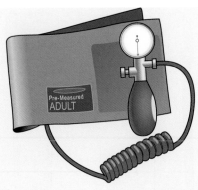

Fig 7.3 Sphygmomanometer used for blood pressure measurement (Jamieson et al 2007, with permission)

7.17 You are undertaking your placement on medical day care and are caring for Mustafa who has just had a gastroscopy. When you take his observations of pulse and BP, you find that he is tachycardic at 110 beats per minute and his BP has decreased to 90/60 mmHg. What are your thoughts? What could be happening to Mustafa? What nursing actions do you need to take to help Mustafa?

Respiration

7.18 What is it?
7.19 What is the difference between type 1 and type 2 respiratory failure?
7.20 Why do we check it?
7.21 How do we check it?
7.22 What is a normal respiratory rate?
7.23 How do you assess a patient's respiratory function?
7.24 What does an abnormal respiratory rate mean?
7.25 Your patient, Henry, is a patient on the virtual ward. He has a long-term health problem of chronic obstructive pulmonary disease (COPD) and when you visit him you notice that he has difficulty speaking in full sentences, has an elevated respiratory rate of 32 breaths per minute and is anxious. What nursing actions could you undertake to help Henry's breathing? Who else might you need to inform?

Pulse oximetry

7.26 What is it?
7.27 Why do we check it?
7.28 How do we check it?
7.29 When might you need to use a pulse oximeter?
7.30 What is normal oxygen saturation?
7.31 What does abnormal oxygen saturation mean?

Peak expiratory flow rate

7.32 What is peak expiratory flow rate?

7.33 Why and how do we check it?

7.34 What is the normal peak flow reading (predicted or expected)?

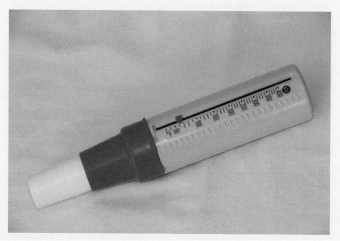

Fig 7.4 Peak flow meter (Kelsey & McEwing 2008, with permission)

7.35 Imran is a 28-year-old man admitted to the acute medical admissions ward with an acute asthma attack. His morning peak flow is 200 L/min, respiratory rate 28/min and saturations 92%. What would your nursing actions be at this point?

Also see this resource for a demonstration of peak flow monitoring:
http://www.youtube.com/watch?v=oHRTiytvuow (accessed July 2011).

Neurological status of your patient

The neurological status of your patient is equally important as an indicator of how well your patient is. One of the simplest ways of monitoring neurological status is by using a simple tool called AVPU:

A – alert.

V – responding to voice.

P – only responding to pain.

U – unresponsive.

Sometimes you may look after a patient for more than one shift and you may find that you notice a change in how alert they are – sometimes this can be quite a subtle change where your patient seems drowsy or there might be a very sudden change to unresponsive. Another tool that is commonly used is the Glasgow Coma Scale

(Fig. 7.5), which comprises of scores for three different measurements – best verbal response, best eye response and best motor response (Brooker & Waugh 2007). The Glasgow Coma Scale takes a lot of practice and it will be helpful for you and your mentor to discuss this in detail when you are caring for a patient who requires this observation, for example a patient who has suddenly become unresponsive or has suffered a cerebral vascular accident.

Within the best motor response, a patient may have a long-term health problem such as a cerebral vascular accident, Parkinson's disease or multiple sclerosis which will mean that they would normally not score 6/6 for that section.

Within the best verbal response, a nurse will be assessing whether a patient is confused, however, this may be a feature of a number of neurological health problems, such as dementia, and therefore the patient would never score 15/15. What is important in this case is that, within your assessment, you establish the cognitive status of your patient when they are well. It is therefore very important that you have the tools, knowledge and skills to detect a deterioration in cognitive status, e.g. delirium.

Delirium

One common syndrome you may come across during your medical placement is delirium. This may also be referred to as acute confusion. Patients suffering from delirium can sometimes be challenging to care for and it can provoke anxiety for you if this is something you have not had much experience with. It is important to remember that delirium is also very distressing for the patient and their relatives and they will need a lot of reassurance during this time. By understanding a little more about what causes delirium and how to prevent and manage it, you may be able to provide some reassurance to both your patient and their relatives.

Delirium can be characterised by 'disturbed consciousness, cognitive function or perception, which has an acute onset and fluctuating course' (National Institute for Health and Clinical Excellence (NICE) 2010).

Although delirium can affect about a quarter of older medical in-patients, it can also affect younger people and some patients will be more at risk of developing delirium than others, for example those who have had a stroke.

Recognising delirium is important and nurses are often those most likely to observe changes in someone's mental state or behaviour, especially if the changes are quite subtle. Delirium is often associated with severe, acute illness and may be a sign that your patient is deteriorating.

Any patient can develop delirium but some are more at risk of developing it than others. Those most at risk are the following:

- People with dementia or other cognitive impairments.
- People with sensory impairments – poor eyesight, poor hearing.
- Those who are immobile/physically frail.
- Patients with dehydration/infection.
- Those with severe illness.

This Website offers excellent explanations about this problem and links to other resources:
http://www.nmhdu.org.uk/our-work/mhep/later-life/lets-respect/ (accessed July 2011).

 Activity

What are the common causes of delirium you might come across in your medical placements?

How would you determine the difference between a chronic cognitive impairment such as dementia and an acute problem like delirium?

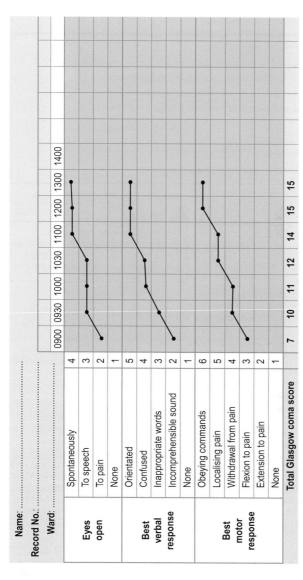

			0900	0930	1000	1030	1100	1200	1300	1400
Eyes open	Spontaneously	4								
	To speech	3								
	To pain	2								
	None	1								
Best verbal response	Orientated	5								
	Confused	4								
	Inappropriate words	3								
	Incomprehensible sound	2								
	None	1								
Best motor response	Obeying commands	6								
	Localising pain	5								
	Withdrawal from pain	4								
	Flexion to pain	3								
	Extension to pain	2								
	None	1								
Total Glasgow coma score			7	10	11	12	14	15	15	

Fig 7.5 Glasgow Coma Scale (Brooker & Waugh 2007, with permission)

Box 7.2 The main features of delirium

- Rapid onset, e.g. hours, days, weeks.
- Fluctuating behaviour – comes and goes or increases/decreases in severity.
- Disturbed level of consciousness, e.g. drowsy or hyperalert.
- Reduced ability to focus or concentrate, easily distracted.
- Rambling, incoherent, switching from one subject to another.
- Hallucinations.
- Suspicious or paranoid thinking.
- Agitated movements.
- Hypoactive – withdrawn, lacking motivation or energy.

It is important to be able to determine the difference between a chronic cognitive impairment such as dementia and an acute problem like delirium. Box 7.2 shows the main features of delirium.

The confusion assessment method (CAM) is a useful screening tool to use to help identify delirium (Inouye et al 1990) (see Box 7.3).

Reflection point

Think of a confused patient who you have cared for during your medical placement. Did you recognise any of the four features of the CAM tool? Were you aware that this patient had delirium? Consider what you might do differently in the future when caring for a confused patient.

With experience, you will be able to identify delirium quite quickly, especially if you are aware of the kinds of patients who are more likely to develop it and are actively looking out for it.

As delirium is a sign that your patient is acutely unwell, it is vitally important that

 Activity

Talk to your mentor and begin to identify those patients most at risk and then start to look out for the features described in the CAM assessment.

you act on it quickly. As a student nurse, your main priority should be making the nurse and doctor looking after the patient aware of your assessment. Be prepared to explain how you feel your patient's mental state has changed and refer to the CAM criteria.

Treating and managing delirium

The most important aspect of managing delirium is to identify and treat the underlying cause, for example infection, dehydration, polypharmacy (a person who is prescribed multiple medications). While the cause is being sought and treated, the management of the patient's confused state and the prevention of complications are largely the role of the nursing staff. Consider the following case history 7.1.

The following should be the main themes of the nursing care and management of a patient with delirium such as Mohammed:

Box 7.3 Confusion assessment method (CAM)

If features 1 and 2 and either 3 or 4 are present, your patient is likely to be suffering from delirium:

Feature 1 – acute onset and fluctuating course

This information would usually be obtained from a family member or carer and is shown by positive responses to the questions: Is there evidence of an acute change in mental status from the patient's baseline? Does the (abnormal) behaviour fluctuate during the day, that is tend to come and go, or increase and decrease in severity?

Feature 2 – inattention

This feature is shown by a positive response to the following question: Did the patient have difficulty focusing attention, for example being easily distracted or having difficulty keeping track of what was being said?

Feature 3 – disorganised thinking

This feature is shown by a positive response to the following question: Was the patient's thinking disorganised or incoherent, such as rambling or irrelevant conversation, unclear or illogical flow of ideas or unpredictable switching from subject to subject

Feature 4 – altered level of consciousness

This feature is shown by any answer other than 'alert' to the following question: Overall how would you rate this patient's level of consciousness? Alert (normal), vigilant (hyperalert), lethargic (drowsy, easily aroused), stupor (difficult to arouse) or coma (unarousable).

- Provide frequent orientation and explanations – patients may not remember where they are or why they are in hospital. Regular gentle reminders may help to relieve some anxieties. Always introduce yourself and tell the patient what you are there to do.
- Avoid any unnecessary moves within the ward or between wards. Sometimes it is necessary to move a patient to another ward, for example to receive specialist care or to another bed within a ward (to be barrier nursed or to be seen more closely from the nurses' station). This should be avoided if at all possible in a patient with delirium, as a move will disorientate them more. As a student, you will not have any control over if or where patients move, but as you progress and begin learning to manage a ward or group of patients, this will be something you need to take into consideration. Good forward planning as to which bed to place a delirious patient in before they get to the ward is ideal.
- Involve relatives – patients with delirium often respond better to people they know. Involving relatives as much as they would like in the care of the person with delirium will often help to keep the person calm during drug administration, at mealtimes, etc. Be careful not to place too much pressure on relatives to be involved, but welcome any involvement they wish to have.

Case history 7.1

Mohammed is a 55-year-old male who has presented at accident and emergency with a 5-day history of worsening shortness of breath and a productive cough. He has a history of COPD. He is transferred to the medical ward accompanied by his wife. On arrival to the ward he is agitated and is trying to pull out his intravenous cannula and IV fluids. He doesn't want to stay in hospital and his wife has to persuade him to stay.

When you speak to his wife she says that he is not normally confused, but has become increasingly confused over the last 3 days, especially at night. Mohammed speaks English and when you speak to Mohammed he says he is fine and doesn't need to be in hospital. He keeps interrupting you, saying that he is being kept here against his will. He is not able to answer any questions about his usual state of wellbeing or activities of daily living and is unable to focus on what you are trying to explain to him, constantly asking to go home.

Later in the evening when his wife has left the ward, he pulls out his intravenous cannula and falls over trying to get out of bed to get to the toilet. When the nursing staff get to him, he has been incontinent of urine on the floor.

The likely underlying cause for Mohammed's delirium is a chest infection. This would be confirmed by doctors through a physical assessment, chest X-ray and blood tests.

Activity

Use the CAM tool to identify the signs that suggest this patient has delirium.

- Provide reassurance and explanations – this needs to be for the family as well as the patient. The patient will be anxious as they may not remember where they are or why things are happening to them. The relatives will be anxious as they are seeing their loved one in a distressed state. Explaining why the person has delirium, what it is and how long it is likely to last will help to reassure the patient and their family.
- Reduce environmental stimulation and ensure good lighting – unfamiliar noises such as equipment beeping, call bells and telephones ringing, televisions or radios in other rooms or by other beds can confuse the person with delirium more. Therefore, keeping noise to a minimum will help to promote calm. The dark can be very disorientating and frightening for someone with delirium so, where possible, leave a night light on.

- Encourage independence and mobility – early mobilisation and return to a usual routine (e.g. toileting, washing and dressing) will prevent the person with delirium becoming too dependent and prevent functional decline. The more frail and dependent a person is, the more susceptible they are to developing delirium.
- Ensure hearing aids are working and glasses are clean – if the person with delirium has a hearing or visual impairment and this is not corrected, it will make them more confused and disorientated.
- Control pain – pain in itself can cause delirium, so managing pain appropriately is an important aspect of managing delirium.
- Ensure adequate food and fluid intake – patients with delirium often don't eat and

drink as much as they should do. It is important that they are encouraged and assisted to eat and drink regularly. By employing some of the techniques above to manage agitation and allowing enough time at mealtimes and easy access to food and drink throughout the day, it should be possible to ensure an adequate food and fluid intake. But remember, depending on the underlying cause of the delirium, their fluid intake requirements may have increased so intravenous or subcutaneous fluids may be necessary too. As a patient with delirium may be agitated and likely to pull out any intravenous or subcutaneous lines, you should aim to use these as a means of hydration for as short a time as possible, encouraging oral fluids as often as you can. It may be necessary to give intravenous or subcutaneous fluids overnight if the patient is restful, as they may be less likely to pull them out.

- One-to-one nursing – sometimes it is necessary to provide one-to-one nursing for a patient with delirium, particularly if they are at high risk of falling or are not concordant with essential therapy, for example oxygen. This should only be necessary for a short period of time while the treatment for the underlying cause gets underway. If you are asked to provide one-to-one care then following the actions mentioned above should be the aim of the care you give.

 Activity

You now have the knowledge to care for someone with delirium. Using this information, write a care plan for the management of Mohammed's delirium.

By adhering to the above principles of care it is also possible to prevent delirium occurring, especially in those patients that are at more risk of developing it than others.

In most patients, delirium resolves as the underlying cause is treated. You may find that some patients will remember different aspects of their delirium which they may find distressing. If they do mention this to you, don't be afraid of explaining what happened when they were delirious as this may help to reassure them that they are not imagining things that did not happen. It may help them to speak to a counsellor who specialises in this or a member of the mental health team. Speak to your mentor about the services available in your organisation and how referrals are made. In some cases, delirium doesn't resolve completely – it may take longer in some patients than others. If there is a concern that delirium is not resolving, the patient should be referred to a specialist mental health team. Again, ask your mentor if you can be involved in making the referral and, if possible, be with the patient when they are assessed by the specialist team. This will give you a good insight into how they are assessed and an opportunity to ask more questions about delirium.

Within the NMC Domain, Communication and Interpersonal Skills (NMC 2010), there are adult field-specific competencies that require nurses to demonstrate that they 'interact with people who find it hard to communicate for any reason' and 'to people who are anxious or in distress'.

There are also NMC Domains for nursing practice and decision making which incorporate adult field-specific competencies that will require you to 'recognise and interpret signs of normal and changing health, distress or capability' and 'recognise the early signs of acute illness in young people, adults and older people, accurately assess and start appropriate and timely management of those at risk of clinical deterioration who are acutely ill or need emergency care'.

Caring for a patient with delirium can be anxiety provoking when you are unfamiliar with it so seek support from your mentor

Activity

Now look carefully at the learning outcomes for your medical placement and try to identify how caring for a patient with delirium could help you to achieve some of them. Discuss them with your mentor.

and other staff on the ward. Ask them how they approach such patients, what sort of things they find work well and what don't work so well. Watch the way they communicate with the person and seek out role models with good communication skills. As a more experienced student, use the opportunity to reassure your junior student colleagues and role model your own developing communication skills.

How to detect and recognise the deteriorating patient in your medical placement

Most hospitals will have an early warning scoring system for observations of vital signs to detect patients who are deteriorating. If a patient observation of vital signs scores a certain number, you will be expected to take action. In acute hospitals, there is usually a team of nurses and doctors who will be contactable by bleep and these teams are often called outreach teams.

Who is in the outreach team?

The outreach team usually belongs to a high-dependency or intensive care unit and are contacted by any member of the hospital staff if a patient's observations score indicates deterioration. They normally carry bleeps, hospital aircalls or mobile phones and will come and assess a patient when contacted. The team is normally made up of anaesthetists, physicians and nurses and is a 24-hour service. In some areas there may be another system for out of hours which involves contacting the site nurse practitioners or senior nurses/matrons.

The purposes of these outreach teams are to (Intensive Care Society 2002):
- Avert admission to critical care.
- Facilitate timely admission to critical care and discharge back to the ward.
- Share critical care skills and expertise through an educational partnership.
- Promote continuity of care.
- Ensure thorough audit and evaluation of outreach services.

 Activity

Find out if your placement uses an early warning score. Discuss with your mentor how to use it and how it works. Find out if there is an outreach service in your placement area? How do you contact them? Who is in the team? Is it possible for you to spend a day with them during your placement?

The purpose of this score is to improve patient outcome by detecting and acting upon early signs of deterioration in hospitalised patients. This score was developed because we do not have the facilities to monitor all patients in high-dependency or intensive care beds. It allows us to identify the deteriorating patient before the situation becomes too profound and to treat the patient in a timely fashion.

In November 2007, NICE guidelines were published stating a need for track and trigger systems. They recommended the use of a scoring system that incorporates the monitoring of oxygen saturations (NICE 2007).

The Modified Early Warning Score (MEWS) is a simple scoring system suitable for use at the bed side; it is now based on seven physiological parameters:

1. Systolic BP.
2. Pulse rate.
3. Respiratory rate.
4. Oxygen saturations.
5. Temperature.
6. AVPU score (neurological status).
7. Urine output.

This system works on a structured scoring system and simple algorithm leading to timely recognition of the deteriorating patient (Table 7.1).

The following articles will give you further insight into assessing an acutely unwell patient and the use of an early warning score:

Steen C (2010). Prevention of deterioration in acutely ill patients in hospital. Nursing Standard 24(49):49–57.

Higgins Y, Maries-Tillott C, Quinton S et al., (2008) Promoting patient safety using an early warning system. Nursing Standard 22(44):35–40.

As a student you will be undertaking the observations of vital signs and it will be important that you understand about this score and how to report and document it. Your mentor should inform you about this during your orientation to the ward and you may even get the opportunity to go round with the team or receive some teaching directly from the team.

Consider the medical placement scenarios on pages 124 and 125, involving Mr X and Mr R, where the outreach team was involved. These are not real life scenarios but are compiled by an outreach nurse, Claire Mcmullen, who has vast experience of working as an outreach sister. They are aimed at making you think about what your actions would be if you were the nurse undertaking these observations. Take time to think about what you would have done in the following scenarios.

Table 7.1 Example of Modified Early Warning Score

				Modified Early Warning Score			
	3	2	1	0	1	2	3
Heart rate (bpm)	≤40		41–50	51–100	101–110	111–129	≥130
Systolic BP (mmHg)	≤85		86–100	101–170	171–190	191–200	≥200
Respiratory rate (bpm)	≤8			9–20	21–25	26–29	≥30
Temperature (°C)	≤35.0	35.0–35.9		36.0–37.9	38.0–38.9		≥39.0
CNS		New confusion		Alert	Voice/ agitation		Pain/ unresponsive
SpO_2 (%)	≤85	85–90	91–93	≤94			
Urine output (mL/h)	≤30			31–199			≥200

⬥ Activity

Please use the MEWS provided and work out the score for each set of patient observations below:

1. Temperature 37 °C, BP 100/80, pulse 100, respirations 21, responds to voice and is passing 35 mL urine/hour.
2. Temperature 36.5 °C, BP 130/80, pulse 75, respirations 14, patient is alert and passing 40 mL urine/hour.
3. Temperature 36.5 °C, BP 90/60, pulse 120, respirations 26, patient is alert and hasn't passed urine for the last 5 hours.
4. Temperature 34 °C, BP 100/60, pulse 45, respirations 12, patient is responding to painful stimuli and hasn't passed urine for the last 2 hours.

⬥ Activity

Mr X is a 67-year-old man admitted via accident and emergency with a cough, shortness of breath and low O_2 saturations (77%). He was discharged home from hospital 3 weeks ago following a 1-week stay on the intensive care ward.

Observations in accident and emergency

- Self-ventilating on 60% oxygen via face mask.
- Oxygen saturation 81%.
- Respiratory rate 22.
- Pulse 119.
- BP 110/57.
- Temperature 37.7.
- MEWS 7.

Patient transferred to ward

- Outreach called at 16:00 by doctor as he was concerned about the patient's breathing.
- Nurses did not call about high MEWS.
- Patient assessed using ABCD.

Observations by outreach

- Oxygen saturation 71% on 4-L O_2 via nasal specs.
- Respiratory rate 25.
- Equal air entry, bilateral wheeze, bilateral crackles.
- Pulse 118.
- BP 113/48.
- Temp 37.9.
- Patient reports he has not passed any urine all day (no fluid balance chart).
- MEWS 9.

Mr X was started on high-flow 15-L O_2 via a reservoir bag (60%). A medical specialist registrar was called to see him, a full plan was written, nebulisers were given and IV fluid was started. He was reviewed regularly overnight and went home the next day.

Activity

Mr R is a 66-year-old man admitted to hospital with shortness of breath and treated for exacerbation of COPD. He was transferred to the medical ward.

Past medical history

- Lung fibrosis.
- COPD.
- Discharged from intensive care 1 month ago after intubation and ventilation, following pulseless electrical activity arrest secondary to tension pneumothorax.

Outreach involvement

- Critical care outreach called by nursing staff as MEWS 4.
- Nurse reported that she had called the doctor and he had seen Mr R. The doctor informed the nurse that Mr R was fine and just needed a bit more oxygen.
- The staff nurse was not convinced that the patient was fine and decided to seek further help.

Observations

- ABCD.
- Patient sitting on the side of the bed.
- Very short of breath.
- Unable to complete full sentences.
- On O_2 face mask 40%.
- Saturation 92%.
- Respirations 30.
- Very poor air entry on the right side.
- Pulse 120.
- BP 110/47.
- Temp 37.
- MEWS 6.

Outcome

- Urgent chest X-ray ordered.
- Senior member of the team called.
- Chest X-ray showed right-sided pneumothorax.
- Chest drain inserted.
- Patient improved.

Summary

During this chapter you have been focusing on how to assess vital signs and recognise the changes within a patient's physical and mental health status. The activities and reflection points should help you to recognise and respond to the deteriorating patient on a medical placement whatever field of nursing you are in.

This chapter has also touched on the importance of communication when you are nursing your patients and this will be explored in more detail in Chapter 8.

References

Brooker, C., Waugh, A., 2007. Foundations of nursing practice: fundamentals of holistic care. Mosby, Edinburgh.

Holland, K., Jenkins, J., Solomon, J., et al., 2008. Applying the Roper–Logan–Tierney model in practice, 2nd ed Churchill Livingstone, Edinburgh.

Inouye, S., Van Dyck, C., Alessi, C., et al., 1990. Clarifiying confusion: the confusion assessment method. Annals of Internal Medicine 113 (12), 941–948.

Intensive Care Society, 2002. Guidelines for the introduction of outreach services: standards and guidelines. Intensive Care Society, London.

Jamieson, E.M., Whyte, L.A., McCall, J.M., 2007. Clinical nursing practices, 5th ed. Churchill Livingstone, Edinburgh.

Kelsey, J., McEwing, G., 2008. Clinical skills in child health practice. Churchill Livingstone, Edinburgh.

National Institute for Health and Clinical Excellence, 2007. Acutely ill patients in hospital: recognition of and response to acute illness in adults in hospital. NICE, London.

National Institute for Health and Clinical Excellence, 2010. Delirium: diagnosis, prevention and management. NICE, London.

Nunn, A.J., Gregg, I., 1989. New regression equations for predicting peak expiratory flow in adults. British Medical Journal 298, 1068–1070.

Nursing and Midwifery Council, 2010. Standards for pre-registration nursing education. NMC, London.

Further reading

Bellomo, R., Goldsmith, D., Uchino, S., et al., 2004. Prospective controlled trial of effect of medical emergency team on postoperative morbidity and mortality rates. Critical Care Medicine 32 (4), 916–921.

Buist, M., Bernard, S., Nguyen, T.V., et al., 2004. Association between clinical abnormal observations and subsequent in-hospital mortality: a prospective study. Resuscitation 62, 137–141.

Cuthbertson, B.H., Boroujerdi, M., McKie, L., et al., 2007. Can physiological variables and early warning scoring systems allow early recognition of the deteriorating surgical patient? Critical Care Medicine 35 (2), 402–409.

Department of Health, 2000. Comprehensive critical care. DH, London.

Fuhrmann, L., Lippert, A., Perner, A., et al., 2008. Incidence, staff awareness and mortality of patients at risk on general wards. Resuscitation 77 (3), 325–330.

Goldhill, D.R., White, S.A., Sumner, A., 1999. Physiological values and procedures in the 24 h before ICU admission from the ward. Anaesthesia 54, 529–534.

Hillman, K., Bristow, P.J., Chey, T., et al., 2001. Antecedents to hospital deaths. Internal Medicine Journal 31, 343–348.

Jacques, T., Harrison, G.A., McLaws, M.L., et al., 2006. Signs of critical health problems and emergency responses (SOCCER): a model for predicting adverse events in the inpatient setting. Resuscitation 69 (2), 175–183.

Kause, J., Smith, G., Prytherch, D., et al., 2004. A comparison of antecedents to cardiac arrests, deaths and emergency intensive care admissions in Australia and New Zealand and the United Kingdom – the ACADEMIA study. Resuscitation 62, 275–282.

MERIT Study Investigators, 2005. Introduction of the medical emergency team (MET) system: a cluster-randomised controlled trial. Lancet 365, 2091–2097.

Richardson, R., 2008. Clinical skills for student nurses: theory, practice and reflection. Reflect Press, Devon.

Websites

British Geriatric Society guidelines on delirium: http://www.bgs.org.uk (accessed July 2011).

Centre for Excellence in Teaching and Learning – a clinical skills resource: http://www.cetl.org.uk (accessed July 2011).

Let's Respect resources: http://www.nmhdu.org.uk/our-work/mhep/later-life/lets-respect/ (accessed July 2011).

Answers

Temperature

7.1 Our body temperature represents the balance between heat gain and heat loss.

7.2 The body requires its temperature to remain stable for optimum cellular function. A body temperature above or below the normal range will affect total body function. It should be measured on admission and at regular intervals thereafter.

7.3 Common methods of checking temperature include tympanic thermometers and tempadots. When using any piece of equipment to check temperature, it is important to follow the manufacturer's instructions to ensure an accurate reading. When using tympanic thermometers, it is important to check the following:
- The probe must be placed snugly in the ear canal to prevent air entering the ear around the probe and giving a false low reading.
- The probe cover must be installed correctly.
- The lens must be clean and free from cracks.
- Avoid using the thermometer within 2–3 minutes of the last reading as this does not give the machine long enough to recalibrate.
- Always use the same ear and record on the chart.
- When checking the temperature of a patient who has been lying down, don't use the ear on the side they were lying on as this may give a false high reading.

Tempadot thermometers must be stored correctly in order to give accurate readings (check manufacturer's instructions).

7.4 A normal body temperature is between 36 °C and 37.5 °C.

7.5
- A low-grade pyrexia (raised temperature), up to 38 °C, could be the result of mild infection, allergy or a disturbance of body tissue, e.g. trauma, surgery, malignancy, thrombosis.
- A moderate- to high-grade pyrexia, 38–40 °C, could be the result of wound infection, chest infection or urinary tract infection.
- A hyperpyrexia, 40 °C and above, could be the result of bacteraemia or damage to the hypothalamus, e.g. stroke, hyperthyroidism. An incompatible blood transfusion can also cause a raise in temperature.
- A low temperature, below 36 °C, could be the result of environmental temperature or a decline in metabolic rate resulting in a decrease in all bodily functions.

7.6 You may have considered the following:
- Positioning.
- Remove excess clothing.
- Offer pain relief/antipyretic, e.g paracetamol.
- Offer a fan if it makes her more comfortable.
- Undertake vital signs for temperature, pulse, BP, respiration and oxygen saturation.
- Offer psychological support.

Pulse

7.7   The pulse is a wave-like sensation that can be felt in any of the arteries lying close to the surface of the body. It reflects the heart rate.

7.8   As the pulse reflects the heart rate, any change in the pulse will indicate a change in the functioning of the heart. It is important to measure the pulse on admission and at regular intervals after that to monitor differences, detect trends or other defects.

7.9   Although dinamaps are commonly used to measure pulse rate, it is much more accurate to measure the pulse manually. The pulse most often used is the radial pulse as this is the most readily accessible. A pulse is measured by placing your second or third fingers along the appropriate artery and applying gentle pressure. The thumb and forefinger have pulses of their own that may be mistaken for the patient's pulse, so should not be used. The pulse should be counted for a full 60 seconds to give sufficient time to detect any irregularities. As well as counting the pulse rate, you should also note whether the rate is regular or irregular and whether the pulse is strong or weak. Any changes should be reported to the trained nurse looking after that patient. There is a temptation to just take the reading from the Dinamap but this will not tell you whether the pulse is regular or strong or weak.

7.10 In adults, a normal pulse rate would be 60–100 beats per minute.

7.11 A fast heart rate, over 100 beats per minute, could be the result of pain, raised temperature, stress, dehydration, bleeding, drugs and heart disease. A slow heart rate, under 60 beats per minute, could be the result of drugs or low temperature.

Blood pressure

7.12 Blood pressure is the force exerted by the blood against the walls of the blood vessels.

7.13 Blood pressure is an important indicator of cardiac function and blood volume. Consequently, changes in BP can indicate a serious deterioration of a patient's health problem. It should be monitored on admission and at regular intervals afterwards to detect any changes quickly.

7.14 Most nurses now rely on dinamaps to check a patient's BP but, where possible, you should also learn how to take BP manually. When using a dinamap, there are certain things you must do to ensure the reading is accurate:

- Where possible, ensure the dinamap is fully charged before you use it so that you don't have to turn it on and off between each patient. Sometimes the first reading taken after switching on is inaccurate.
- Ensure that it is clean.
- Ensure the BP cuff is the right size for your patient. Cuffs that are too small could lead to an abnormally high result. With dinamaps, cuffs that are too large may not sit snugly enough on the patient's arm to provide an accurate reading.
- Ensure the cuff is placed level with the heart and the centre of the bladder of the cuff covers the brachial artery.
- Ensure the dinamap has been checked regularly by service engineers.
- If you are unable to get a reading from a dinamap or are unconfident about the result, check it manually.

Any changes should be reported immediately to the nurse in charge of the patient.

7.15 Blood pressure will vary between individuals and will depend on whether they are sitting, standing, have just stood up, etc. An average BP for an adult can range from 100/60 mmHg to 140/90 mmHg.

7.16 A low BP, with a systolic (top number) of less than 100, could be the result of dehydration, drugs, bleeding, hypovolaemic shock, septic shock, incompatible blood transfusion or postural drop. A high BP, with a systolic of above 170, could be the result of exercise, stress, raised temperature, pain, circulatory overload, early compensatory sign of shock or heart disease.

7.17 You may have considered the following:

- Hypovolaemia – may be due to Mustafa being nil-by-mouth and dehydrated or bleeding.
- Ask Mustafa how he is feeling. Is he feeling thirsty?
- Has he recently vomited or had melaena?
- Repeat the observations of vital signs for temperature, pulse, BP, respiration and oxygen saturations.
- Check the capillary refill – is it delayed?
- Inform the nurse in charge who will inform the doctor.
- If Mustafa is allowed to drink, encourage oral fluids.

Respiration

7.18 The mechanism for supplying the body with oxygen and removing carbon dioxide.

7.19   You will sometimes hear the diagnosis type 1 and type 2 respiratory failure. Respiratory failure occurs when pulmonary gas exchange is sufficiently impaired to cause hypoxaemia with or without hypercarbia.

Type 1	PO_2	↓	hypoxia
	PCO_2	↓	hypocarbia
Type 2	PO_2	↓	hypoxia
	PCO_2	↑	hypercarbia

7.20   As oxygen is a necessary requirement for all bodily functions, a change in respiratory rate is often the first indication that something is wrong with a patient's health. It will often change up to 24 hours before a change in pulse, BP or temperature. It should be checked on admission and at regular intervals thereafter.

7.21   Respiratory rate is checked by counting the total number of breaths taken in 1 minute. Inspiration and expiration count as one breath. It is important to count for a full minute to detect any irregularities, and the depth and pattern of breathing can be noted at the same time. Often patients will alter their breathing rate when they know someone is watching it, so it is easier to count the respirations after taking the pulse so the patient is not aware of what you are doing. This is one of the observations that students often find difficult to measure accurately.

7.22   A normal adult respiratory rate is 12–20 breaths per minute.

7.23
- Is the patient short of breath at rest? If yes, can the patient talk in sentences? Is the patient using all his accessory muscles to breath?
- Is the patient short of breath on exertion? If yes, how much can the patient do before getting short of breath?
- Does the patient sound wheezy?
- Is the patient snoring? This is a sign of obstruction.
- Is the patient rousable? Can they maintain their airway? What position should they be in?
- What is the patient's respiratory rate?
- What are the patient's oxygen saturations?
- Is the patient on oxygen? If so, how much? Is this prescribed?
- Is the patient sitting upright? If lying flat, sitting up may help breathing.

7.24   A raised respiratory rate could be the result of respiratory distress, chest infection, heart failure, sepsis, deterioration in metabolic or cardiovascular function, trauma, embolus or haemorrhage, anaemia, obstruction of the airway, chronic respiratory health problems, bronchospasm (wheeze), injury, fluid overload or cardiac failure. A low respiratory rate could be the result of respiratory depression, drugs (e.g. morphine can cause respiratory depression), central nervous system damage.

7.25 You may have considered the following:
- Positioning to enhance lung surface area and therefore gaseous exchange.
- Does Henry have home oxygen?
- Nebulisers – is Henry prescribed these?
- Check oxygen saturation.
- What is normal for Henry?
- How is Henry feeling?
- Discuss the above with the registered nurse.
- Provide psychological support.
- The multidisciplinary team may need to be contacted by the registered nurse – community matron, doctor, physiotherapist.

Pulse oximetry

7.26 It is a non-invasive way of measuring the level of oxygen saturation in arterial blood.

7.27 As oxygen is essential for all bodily functions, a decrease in oxygen level can have serious consequences for the patient. It should be measured on admission and at regular intervals thereafter.

7.28 Oxygen saturation is measured using an electronic device called a pulse oximeter. This transmits light from one side of the probe to the other through the finger (toes and earlobes can also be used). To ensure an accurate reading, you must do the following:
- Check that the probe is clean.
- Check that the machine is within its service date.
- Do not use a finger on the same arm you are checking the BP.
- The site must be clean, warm and well circulated – you may need to warm or rub the skin first.
- Remove any nail polish from finger or toe nails.
- Movement of the patient can affect readings – if you need to secure the probe with tape, don't do it too tightly.
- Look for a good waveform on the monitor to ensure a good reading.
- Always rely on clinical judgement rather than the value displayed on the machine.

7.29
- For post-operative monitoring as patients recover from anaesthesia.
- On medical wards for patients with respiratory illness, especially those requiring oxygen therapy, patients with COPD or asthma or for those on sedatives.
- When patients undergo procedures such as endoscopy which may require respiratory depressant sedatives.
- During transport of patients who are at risk of cardiorespiratory instability.
- To assess tissue viability following vascular grafting or when intra-arterial catheters are used – this will indicate decline in pulsatile flow.
- To reduce the need for arterial blood gas sampling.

7.30 The normal range for an adult would be 95–100%, BUT this may vary depending on any underlying problems the patient may have.

7.31 A low saturation could be the result of chest infection, chronic lung disease, a decrease in peripheral circulation or deterioration of any bodily function.

Peak expiratory flow rate

7.32
- This is one of the most common lung function recordings taken on a medical ward by the nurse and is a measure of the maximum flow rate (in litres per minute) an individual can generate on a short sharp blow, starting at full inspiration.
- It is essential that the patient understands that it is not the volume of air that is expired that is crucial but the greatest force/rate with which he/she can expire it.
- Peak expiratory flow is a good indicator of severity of obstruction and is often used for patients who suffer from asthma.
- The mini-peak flow meter is most commonly used on wards as it is cheap and light. It measures from 60 to 800 litres per minute.

7.33 To detect worsening asthma, to help diagnose asthma, to show how a client is responding to treatment.
When to use:
- At home, in the morning and evening.
- Before taking a bronchodilator and 10 minutes after treatment to assess effect. This is known as pre- and post-peak flow readings.
- When the chest is tight or breathing is difficult.
- As a baseline prior to a patient having a procedure.
How to use:
- Set the indicator to zero.
- Take a full breath in through the nose or mouth.
- Hold the breath, with the mouth open – do not relax.
- Put the meter into the mouth. Close the lips around the mouthpiece and ensure a tight seal.
- Blow out as hard and as quickly as you can.
- Read the value and record.
- Repeat this twice more and take the best of three.

7.34 Depends on age, height and sex:
- Boy, 4'10' = 350 L/min.
- Woman, 30 years, 5'3' = 475 L/min.
- Man, 50 years, 5'9' = 600 L/min.
Readings should be 20% either side.
Your organisation should have a chart with predictive readings, usually based on or adapted from Nunn and Gregg (1989).

7.35 You may have considered the following:
- Keeping Imran informed about what is happening to reduce his anxiety.
- Assisting him to change position to maximise gaseous exchange.

- Look at the prescription chart with a registered nurse. Are the following prescribed – oxygen, bronchodilators, steroids?
- Inform the doctor of his vital signs to ensure he is reviewed and assessed.
- Increase the regularity of your vital signs monitoring to detect a change in his condition.
- Take peak flow measurements before and after his bronchodilators to assess their effectiveness.

8 Communication within medical placements

- To explore communication within multidisciplinary teams within medical placements
- To explore why communication is so important for the medical patient's wellbeing
- To determine the importance of accurate record keeping
- To identify learning opportunities to develop communication skills within placements

Introduction

Wherever you are in your medical placements and regardless of your field of nursing, you will have learning outcomes that require you to demonstrate competence in communication and interpersonal skills (Nursing and Midwifery Council (NMC) 2010,). Your NMC-approved programme based on the 2010 Standards and Competencies has a generic competence for communication and interpersonal skills alongside the NMC Essential Skills Clusters for 'care, compassion and communication' (NMC 2010). The NMC states that 'all nurses must use excellent communication and interpersonal skills. Their communication must always be safe, effective, compassionate and respectful' (NMC 2010, p. 15).

Some of you will be achieving competencies with the NMC (2008) Standards, which also have a significant number of competencies related to effective communication skills. As well as engaging with different sets of competencies, your curriculum documentation will be different for each university, but all of your programmes will incorporate the NMC Domains and Essential Skills Clusters. Some of you may have skills-based outcomes, activities and reflections in addition to these, and it is important that you are aware of what you need to achieve in relation to communication and interpersonal skills within your placements. You will need to adapt your communication strategies depending on who you are speaking to and where you are placed.

There are four key areas for you to focus on during your medical placement:

1. The relationship with the patient and their significant others.
2. Professional relationships with colleagues and the multidisciplinary team.

3. What information to give at handover or patient reporting period.
4. Record keeping.

This book may help you to meet some of these essential communication skills:

Sully P, Dallas J (2010) Essential communication skills for nursing and midwifery. Essential skills for nurses' series, 2nd ed. Mosby, Edinburgh

 Activity

During the theoretical component of your course, you will have been taught about the NMC Code (NMC 2008). Now that you are in your placement, think about how this is put into practice. You could consider the following:

1. Think about why it is important to maintain and regulate professional standards.

2. Are you able to think about examples from practice? How is confidentiality maintained? What records are left by patients' beds? How are patient records accessed and who can access them?

3. How do you answer the phone and what information are you allowed to give? Observe and listen to how other members of the nursing team deal with telephone queries.

4. Are patients asking you difficult questions? How can you answer them in a professional manner? How do other members of staff answer these questions?

Thinking back to my own practice, I can remember times when I have been providing personal care for a patient and they have asked me what is wrong with the patient in the next bed. I learnt to politely explain that I would never discuss their health problem with another patient as that would be unprofessional and, therefore, I am unable to discuss another patient's diagnosis with them.

When answering the phone it is really important to state the name/number of the ward, who you are and your title and to ask the person at the end of the phone how you can help them.

With regards to record keeping, the NMC (2009) produced very comprehensive guidelines, but it is important to remember that records at the end of a bed could be looked at by anyone visiting and should contain nothing that provides demographic data or diagnosis.

Reflective practice is now part of nursing and many of your learning outcomes will require you to reflect about your practice. There are many models of reflection that you will have been introduced to at your university (Johns 1996, Gibbs 1988). Nursing involves situations that are complex and we need to make sense of these situations in order to build on the relationship between practice and theory. Whatever model or framework you use for reflection, they normally contain the following considerations (Gibbs 1988):

- Description of the experience/event – what happened?
- Feelings – what were you thinking and feeling?
- Evaluation – what was good and bad about the experience?
- Analysis – what sense can you make of the situation?
- Conclusion – what else could you have done?
- Action plans – if it occurs again, what would you do?

It is important to keep a reflective journal. This may be an essential part of your professional development portfolio (PDP) recording where not only will you wish to keep a reflective diary/journal, but also those specific to your attainment of goals agreed with a personal tutor or mentor. Many students carry a small notebook with them to enable them to jot down interesting thoughts and actions. The journal can act as a prompt when you are meeting with your mentor, promote deeper learning and also be useful as evidence for future academic assignments.

 Activity

Speak with your mentor and allocate some time to discuss your reflections on action during your placement.

It may help you to read the following articles about reflection and the student nurse:

O'Donovan M (2007) Implementing reflection: insights from pre-registration mental health students. Nurse Education Today 27(6):610–616

de Sales T, Beddoes L (2007) Using reflective models to enhance learning: experiences of staff and students. Nurse Education in Practice 7(3): 135–140

The relationship between nurse, patient and carers

The therapeutic relationship between nurse, patient, family and next of kin starts from the moment the patient walks through the door – how we greet, non-verbal cues, treating with respect, being polite, not overreacting or taking offence to patient comments which are often made in times of stress. Sometimes it is important to explain

to the patient why some things cannot be taken care of immediately and keeping them informed about their condition. This has the overall aim of making patients feel safe and cared for and developing a relationship of trust whereby the nurse acts as the patient's advocate. We live in a diverse society and need to treat every person as an individual and seek to understand their philosophy of health and their spiritual needs while they are in hospital. This therapeutic relationship lays the foundations for future emotional support and possibly dealing with difficult questions. The following tips can help.

 Tip

- Introduce yourself as a patient's named nurse for the day.
- Admit lack of knowledge but willingness to find out.
- Undertake a quality admission.
- Spend time listening and answering questions.
- Think about how you would want to be treated.

 Reflection point

If you were a patient in your medical environment, how would you wish the nurse to communicate with you?
The communication skill that I have learnt through placement is how to use the therapeutic relationship in practice where a patient will confide in you their fears and emotions in certain situations and to listen.
(Emma Hankin, first-year student)

Professional relationship with colleagues and the multidisciplinary team

Each medical ward/placement will have its own culture and philosophy of care. You will gain far more from the placement if you seek to integrate and build relationships with the team and immerse yourself in the ward culture. You need to appreciate that your learning needs are important but patient needs will always come first for the staff on the ward, given their accountability for care delivery.

You need to take ownership of your own learning and make positive proactive contributions to the team which, in turn, will help you meet your learning outcomes. This will result in a good working relationship between mentor and student. If you can demonstrate that you are able to actively participate within the ward setting, greater opportunities will arise. Here are some examples of the learning opportunities that you could access:

- Multidisciplinary team forums – care planning meetings.
- Participating in ward rounds – usually a consultant will have set days and times for ward rounds. Ward rounds take place by the patients' beds and a registered nurse, consultant and a team of doctors with other healthcare professionals discuss with the patient how they are progressing. A clinical assessment and examination are often made by the consultant and actions to be taken are discussed with the patient and documented.
- Making referrals under supervision of your mentor on behalf of patients to clinical nurse specialists, district nurses, discharge coordinators and others.
- Spending time with the clinical nurse specialists who link with the medical placement.
- Liaising with social workers, physiotherapists, occupational therapists, bed managers and site nurse practitioners.

 Activity

In Chapter 4, patient journeys and examples of learning pathways were explored. This is an ideal opportunity for you to speak with your mentor to ensure that you are accessing all the learning opportunities possible with regard to understanding about the work of other health and social care colleagues.

You will see that you will have some learning outcomes that require you to communicate with other disciplines and to have some understanding of their role. This was one of the actions from several high-profile healthcare investigations in the UK which criticised staff for not being able to communicate effectively, such as the Bristol Royal Infirmary Inquiry (2001), the Climbie case (Department of Health 2003) and the case of Baby P (Laming 2009).

Try to think of your placement as the centre of your learning environment but also speak to your mentor and co-mentor to try to understand the opportunities that you could be accessing. Remember

Activity

Ask your mentor if you can attend a multidisciplinary forum such as a multidisciplinary meeting, care planning meeting or goal setting meeting. How did the registered nurse communicate with the team? What roles did people take within the team? What contribution did each discipline make? What was the purpose of the meeting? How were the outcomes of the meeting captured?

that your mentor is not a mind reader and it is up to you to be open about what your learning needs are and, most importantly, those you have to achieve as part of your practice assessment expectations.

The kinds of information you may gain during one of these meetings might be the following:

- A member of the medical team might have spoken about the current health status of a patient.
- The physiotherapist may have discussed the mobility needs of the patient.
- The occupational therapist may have provided information regarding their ability to self-care, the assistance they require and the condition of their home environment.
- The social worker may have discussed the resources available to support the person at home.
- The nurses will have discussed how the patient is managing their activities of daily living on the ward.
- The views and wishes of the patient and their family/significant others will have been provided either by the patient and family themselves, if present, or by any member of the team who has discussed this with them.
- A member of the team will have taken the role of record keeper to ensure that all decisions are documented.
- The outcome of the meeting will usually be plans for discharge, goals that need to be met prior to discharge and referrals to any other members of the team not present.

If you are a first-year student, your medical placement may be your first encounter with patients and you may worry about how to approach them and what to say. It can be difficult for you to determine what it is you are actually supposed to be learning, however, do not worry as this is a normal reaction. Try not to compare yourself to other students who may have a background in health care and appear confident already.

Some pre-registration nursing programmes will give you a skills schedule or booklet with various nursing competencies for you to achieve. Examples of competencies could be: 'the student introduces himself/herself to patients' or 'the student introduces himself/herself to patients, staff and others in a professional manner' which you will automatically do when you meet a patient or take over their care from someone else. You may be asked to undertake a patient's vital signs, and before you do that you will introduce yourself and explain what you would like to do and gain their agreement. This simple interaction is very important and will demonstrate that you are communicating with your patient. It also indicates that you understand about gaining a patient's consent (informed consent).

This article may help you understand what is meant by informed consent:

Chaloner C (2007). An introduction to ethics in nursing. Nursing Standard 21 (32):42–46. Online. Available at: http://nursingstandard.rcnpublishing.co.uk/archive/article-an-introduction-to-ethics-in-nursing (accessed July 2011).

Activity

> Observe your mentor when she/he communicates with patients. How does your mentor promote a professional yet caring image to the patient?

We live in a very diverse world where English may not be a patient's first language and within your daily communication with patients and staff you will be required to demonstrate that you are able to respect diversity and respond to differences while maintaining a person-centred approach.

You may also come across patients who live a very different life from you and you may never have come across some of the relationships or lifestyles that your patient has. Medical patients will often be admitted to the ward with a diverse range of conditions, which will affect them physically and psychosocially. Patients will come from a diverse cultural background and have different beliefs about health and living. You may find that your personal and professional values and beliefs are challenged and you may find that providing non-judgemental care is more difficult in some circumstances. It is important for you to think about the values and prejudices that you have and reflect on how this impacts on your nursing care and your ability to provide non-judgemental care.

 Activity

> Discuss with your mentor how you could adapt your communication skills if you were caring for a patient who did not speak very much English.

You may find this a useful book to read:

Holland K, Christine Hogg (2010). Cultural awareness in nursing and healthcare, 2nd ed. Edward Arnold, London.

Chapter 5 of this book examines culture care: knowledge and skills for implementation in practice.

An RCN publication that may also be of interest is:

Mootoo J (2005). A guide to cultural and spiritual awareness. RCN, London.

This Website provides Department of Health guidance for the NHS:

Department of Health (2009) Religion or belief: a practical guide for the NHS: http://www.dh.gov.uk/prod_consum_dh/groups/dh_digitalassets/documents/digitalasset/dh_093132.pdf (accessed July 2011).

The nursing handover

It is important for you to identify and inform your mentor about what you need to know, and sometimes to remind them of what you already know and the level you are at in your training. Medical wards can be unpredictable and fast paced with patients with a variety of health problems, and you may be overwhelmed with information and have difficulty identifying and extracting relevant information that needs to be passed on to other colleagues. You need to ensure that you communicate with the trained staff throughout the shift (see Ch. 1). The registered nurse may appear busy but is still there to support and supervise you. It is important that you recognise the resources available to you on the ward, for example other students, assistant practitioners, healthcare assistants, nurse consultants, clinical nurse specialists and therapists.

Sometimes it is difficult to know what you should be letting staff know about, but this comes with experience. You will learn to undertake risk assessments, for example risk assessments that will tell you if someone is at risk of malnutrition, falls or pressure ulcers (see Ch. 6). You will learn to inform the registered nurse and other healthcare professionals during your shift and in handover. You will begin to understand the normal values for observations for vital signs and to inform someone when they are abnormal or have returned to normal. You will learn to identify when a patient's condition changes and how soon you need to inform someone.

Much of the information is now found electronically and you will need to ask your mentor for your own log-on code to ensure that you adhere to the Data Protection Act (1998).

Between shifts, staff will have a handover period. This is done differently in different organisations and there is usually a policy to support this process. In the majority of your placements, the following will be communicated (handed over) away from the patient area to maintain confidentiality (see Table 8.1):

- The patient's name, age and diagnosis.
- Past medical history.
- Resuscitation status.
- Infections.

An article that will help to inform you more about handover:

Chaboyer W, McMurray A, Wallis M (2010). Bedside nursing handover: a case study. International Journal of Nursing Practice 16:27–34.

Generally nurses are then allocated to a group of patients who are under the care of a team of nurses led by a team leader/named nurse. They then move to the bedside to handover more specific aspects of care using the documentation at the end of the bed or the electronic patient records. This handover usually includes patients' reactions as well. For example, a nurse may say to a patient: 'Did you have your chest X-ray?' or 'Did the physiotherapist see you this morning? How did it go?'

The shift handover period is an ideal arena for you to develop your skills and confidence when communicating about the care that has been delivered to the patients in your care while providing an opportunity for clarification of issues you may not fully understand and teaching by others. As a senior student, you are expected to contribute to handover. As a less experienced student, you should be encouraged to do this. You can make notes during handover but there should never be anything in your notes that would identify who a patient is – notes should be shredded/destroyed after your shift (NMC 2008). Many nurses carry a small pocket-sized note book.

Nursing handover can be difficult for the less experienced students to understand. Make sure that you question anything you do not understand, although maybe that would have to wait until the end of the

Table 8.1 Handover period	
Office handover	**Bedside**
Name	Allocated nurses for group of patients will receive handover
Age	from the nurses on the previous shift
Allergies	The patient should be included in the handover
Consultant	The allocated nurses must introduce themselves to the
Diagnosis	patient if they have not met that patient before
Planned treatment	Handover must include:
Investigations carried	
out/scheduled	• care plans
Resuscitation status	• medication charts
	• fluid balance chart
	• observation charts

handover itself. Take a note of various patient diagnoses reported. Some of the conditions you will come across are listed in Box 8.1.

Activity

On your medical placement, think about any handover you received from the registered nurses regarding your allocated patients. Think about what you would say if you were handing over information about the patients that you cared for that day. Ask your mentor if you can practise handing over your patients to them. Get them to ask questions about the care, why it was delivered and what evidence underpins that care. Reading about the way in which patients with certain health problems may experience the signs and symptoms of their illness and the medications they might be taking will help you with care delivery and also ensure that you are giving safe and effective care to a group of people who are in a vulnerable situation.

It will be helpful for you to look after one to three patients in an early-stage placement and try to provide person-centred care under direct supervision for these patients. This is one of the competencies expected of you at progression point 1 (NMC 2010).

As a third-year student, you should start to look after a caseload of patients and you should be contributing to multidisciplinary forums rather than just observing. You should be handing over your caseload of patients verbally and in writing under the supervision of a registered nurse. At progression point 3, you are expected to 'inspire confidence and provide clear direction to others ... manage time effectively ... negotiating with others in relation to balancing competing and conflicting priorities.'

Box 8.1 Conditions that might be referred to at handover

- Congestive cardiac failure.
- Left ventricular failure.
- Atrial fibrillation (arrythmias).
- Confusional states.
- Diabetes.
- Cerebral vascular accidents.
- Dehydration.
- Sickle cell.
- HIV/AIDS and related disorders.
- Myocardial infarction.
- Unstable angina.
- Liver failure.
- Pancreatitis.
- Chronic obstructive pulmonary disease.
- Asthma.
- Tuberculosis.
- Pneumonia.
- Leg ulcers.
- Anaemia.
- Gastrointestinal (GI) bleed.
- Enteral feeding.
- Pulmonary embolus.
- Deep vein thrombosis.

It allows me to care for a wide range of acutely ill patients with a whole variety of conditions; enables me to develop myself as a nurse who is able to work under pressure and in demanding situations, and also gives me the opportunity to work alongside various other healthcare professionals, e.g. physiotherapists, social workers, clinical nurse specialists.

(Nicola Cooper, first destination staff nurse)

Situation, background, assessment, recommendation and response

The NHS is often criticised for poor communication, however there are few tools that actively focus on how to improve communication, in particular verbal communication. Effective handover between shifts is vital to protect patient safety and assist with delivering high standards of care. The transfer of a patient's care to another person/team is the point at which the patient is most vulnerable on their journey through the hospital. Gaps in communication can lead to breakdowns in continuity of care, inappropriate treatment and potential harm to the patient.

Originally used in the military and aviation industries, 'situation, background, assessment, recommendation and response' (SBARR) was developed for health care by Dr M Leonard and colleagues (2004) from Kaiser Permanente in Colorado, USA. In one healthcare setting, the incidence of harm to patients fell by 50% after implementing SBARR. SBARR is an easy to remember mechanism that can be used to frame conversations, especially critical ones. It enables you to clarify what information should be communicated between members of the team and how. It can also help develop teamwork and foster a culture of patient safety. The tool can be used to shape communication at any stage of the patients' journey.

The tool consists of standardised prompt questions within four sections, to ensure that staff are sharing concise and focused information. It allows staff to communicate assertively and effectively:

- Situation: state what is happening at the present time.
- Background: explain the circumstances leading up to the situation.
- Assessment: state pertinent assessment findings.
- Recommendation: state what needs to be done and in what time frame.
- Response: how long?

Case history 8.1

You are looking after Mrs Hamer, a 64-year-old, who you have been caring for on medical day care. She returned to the unit a couple of hours ago having had a colonoscopy. You respond to a call from another patient and when you go back to Mrs Hamer you find her on the floor. She is alert and says she has fallen but has terrible pain in her hip. You call the registered nurse who instructs you not to move Mrs Hamer but to carry out a full assessment and then use the SBARR tool to inform the doctor.

Activity

Use the SBARR tool in Figure 8.1 to collate the information that you would need to inform the doctor of the situation.

The above situation would require documentation in the nursing notes and completion of an incident form. Record keeping is another way in which nurses are required to communicate.

Reflection point

Consider why and where we document (refer to Boxes 8.2 and 8.3).

Record keeping

The NMC (2009) outlines what is expected of nurses and midwives in relation to record keeping which is seen as an integral part of

Fig 8.1 SBARR tool

Your name:	Date:	Time:

Situation

I am calling about (patient name): ....

Under the care of (consultant name): ....

The patient is **for Resus** ☐ or **DNAR** ☐

• I am afraid that the patient is going to arrest ☐

I am concerned because:

I have just assessed the patient personally. I am concerned because the observations show (tick all that apply):

• The blood pressure is >200mmHg ☐ or <100mmHg ☐ or >30mmHg below usual ☐

• The pulse is >130bpm ☐ or <50bpm ☐

• The respiratory rate is <10 ☐ or >28 ☐

• The temperature is <35.5 °C ☐ or >38°C ☐

• The conscious level is deteriorating ☐

• The patient's general condition is deteriorating ☐

• The urine output in the last two hours is:

Background

The patient was admitted on: ....

The admitting diagnosis was: ....

Their past medical history includes: ....

The patient's mental status is:

• Alert & orientated to person, place & time ☐

• Confused ☐

• Agitated ☐

• Lethargic but conversant ☐

• Drowsy & not talking clearly ☐

• Comatose – eyes closed, not responding to stimulation ☐

The skin is:

• Warm & dry ☐

• Pale and/or clammy ☐

• Sweaty ☐

• The extremities are warm ☐ or cold ☐

Continued

Fig 8.1—cont'd

Background (continued)

The patient is ☐ or is not ☐ on oxygen

• The patient has been on ____ (l/min) or (%) oxygen for ____ minutes/hours

• The pulse oximeter reading is ____ %

• The oximeter does not detect a good pulse and is giving erratic readings ☐

Assessment

I think that the problem is:

The problem seems to be cardiovascular ☐ respiratory ☐ sepsis ☐ neurological ☐

• I don't know what the problem is but the patient is deteriorating ☐

• The patient is very unstable and we need to act quickly ☐

Recommendation

I would like you to (say what you think should be done):

• I think the patient should be transferred to a critical care area ☐

• Please talk to the patient or family about resuscitation status ☐

• Please ask for a consultant to review the patient ☐

Are any tests needed?

CXR ☐   ABG ☐   ECG ☐   Bloods ☐   Septic screen ☐

Response

• How often should I do vital signs?

• Is there any treatment I should start?

• If the patient does not improve when should I call you again?

• Please come and see the patient right away ☐

nursing and midwifery practice. It is no surprise then that record keeping is part of the NMC Domain, Communication and Interpersonal Skills, and is included within the NMC Essential Skill Clusters (2010). By the end of your first year, there is an expectation that you 'communicate effectively both orally and in writing so that the meaning is always clear' and, for entry to the register, you will be expected to provide 'accurate and comprehensive written and verbal reports based on best available evidence' (NMC 2010, p. 8). See Table 8.2 for examples of using appropriate language.

> I ensured everything I do helped me to
> adhere to the Nursing and Midwifery
> Council code of conduct and to the trust

policies. The NMC states that every care we give to patients should be documented and that before giving care consent should be sought.

(Patricia Moyo, third-year student nurse)

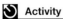 **Activity**

Read the NMC (2009) *Record Keeping: Guidance for Nurses and Midwives* and find out how this is applied by registered nurses within your medical placement. Are there any local policies that support this NMC guidance?

Rules of good documentation

Documents should:

– be written in black ink, clearly, in a manner that cannot be erased
– be accurate, factual and consecutive
– be written as soon after the event has occurred as possible
– be written with patient and/or carer involvement
– be timed, signed, dated and have name printed alongside and countersigned by a registered nurse
– have any alterations crossed through with a single line, signed and dated.

Box 8.2 Why do we document?

■ To ensure quality patient care.
■ To ensure continuity of care.
■ For good communication between staff.
■ For better communication and dissemination of information between members of the interprofessional healthcare team.
■ To detect changes in patients' clinical condition early.
■ For accurate account of treatment.
■ For legal requirements.

Box 8.3 Where do we document?

■ Fluid charts.
■ Food charts.
■ Observations of vital signs and scoring systems to detect deterioration.
■ Risk assessments, e.g. pressure sores, falls, malnutrition.
■ Blood sugar readings.
■ Continence charts.
■ Care plans/patient records.
■ Electronic patient records.
■ Incident reports.

Table 8.2 Using objective language instead of subjective language

Subjective	Objective
Diet taken fair	Half of diet consumed
Appears restless	Thrashing about in bed
IV running well	Dextrose 5% infusing at 125 mL per hour Site clear
Usual night	Requested pain medication for headache
Medication × 1 for pain	Oral analgesia given at 00:30
Catheter minimal drainage	Catheter drained 200 mL in 6 hours
Sacrum red	Grade 2 pressure ulcer on sacrum measured and wound care plan implemented
Fair morning or no complaints	Patient has rested on bed all morning and says she feels a bit better today
Good night	Patient says she slept quite well last night
All due care given	There is no objective statement for all due care given, you must document the care you have given according to the patient's care plan

You will find the following article helpful: McGreehan R (2007). Best practice in record keeping. Nursing Standard 21(17):51–55.

Legal requirements

Patients' records may be used as evidence in a court of law to answer a complaint or negligence claim. There are a number of policies which set out patients' rights in accessing their healthcare records:
• Health records are defined as 'information about the physical or mental health or condition of an identifiable individual made by or on behalf of a health professional in connection with the care of the individual' (NMC 2009).
• Data Protection Act 1998: regulates the storage and protection of patient

information. Data can only be used for the specific purpose for which it was collected. Data cannot be disclosed without patient consent. Individuals have the right of access to information held about them (subject to exemption, i.e. crime).

Data Protection Act 1998 – eight principles
1. Fairly and lawfully processed.
2. Processed for limited purposes.
3. Adequate, relevant and not excessive.
4. Accurate and up to date.
5. Not kept for longer than necessary.
6. Processed in line with rights.
7. Secure.
8. Not transferred to other countries without adequate protection.

Consider this: you are on placement and you do not have a computer log-on code for the electronic records. You have just undertaken the vital signs for six patients and they need to be put into the computer. The registered nurse says that you can use his/her user name and password to access the information. What would your answer be?

You would have to say no and explain that you would be happy to do this if you were given your own log-on code. To input data using someone else's log-on code contravenes the Data Protection Act because the information would indicate that the registered nurse had documented these data and not you.

Freedom of Information Act 2000
This Act grants a general right of access to all types of information held by public health authorities that is not covered by the Data Protection Act. Certain information that is deemed sensitive can be withheld with a reason given.

 Activity

> Ask your mentor what they would do if a patient asked to see their medical notes.

Patients are allowed to see their medical notes and organisations will have policies in place to support this. Patients will be required to book an appointment with a consultant through his/her secretary to ensure that they have someone there who can answer any queries while they are reading their notes.

Accurate and timely record keeping is an integral part of nursing and nursing notes must be clear and complete. The patients that you are looking after will all have a plan of care and, as a student, you will be contributing to this care plan under the

Activity

> Find out where patients' care plans are kept and look at how they are written and individualised. Now look at the nursing notes to understand how they relate to the care plan.

supervision of a registered nurse. Documentation varies depending on where you are placed and it is important that you are familiar with this.

Care planning

- What is written in the nursing notes must relate to the patient's care plan.
- If care plans are numbered, the corresponding number can be used in the nursing notes to evaluate that problem.
- Once something is no longer a problem, discontinue the care plan – you will have less to write.

Activity

> Now practise writing a care plan for one of the patients you have looked after and show it to your mentor. An example of a care plan can be found in Holland et al (2008). You can use this to practise using a framework for the assessment and planning of care process.

Activity

> Look at the example of nursing notes in Figure 8.2. Would you consider this to be good record keeping?

Date and timed	Nursing Report	Signature
1/3/06	Admitted with UTI. Appears confused. Prescribed antibiotics.	
4/3/06	S/B Drs. Condition improving. Rash probably due antibiotic. Drug stopped. Aim home soon.	NBL
5/3/06	Self caring. No complaints. Aim for discharge in next few days.	PS
6/3/06	Confused this am. Assistance given with hygiene Intake poor.	
night	Slept well. No complaints.	LP
7/3/06	Self caring this am. No complaints.	GT
night	Slept well. No complaints.	
8/3/06 1800	Daughter stated that her mother seemed more confused than usual. Reassured that it was due to infection. Dr. to review.	SOPER
0130	Pt found collapsed. Cardiac arrest call put out and CPR commenced. Given Adrenaline x4 and CPR for 20 mins. RIP. Daughter informed by telephone.	NR

NHA 828

Surname	Other names	Consultant	Ward	Religion
Talarcyk	Greta		3	

Fig 8.2 Nursing report

Complete the wordsearch to evaluate what you have learnt.
(Answers on page 152.)

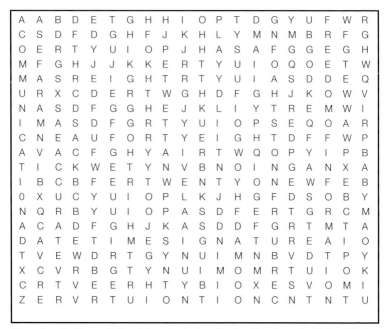

A	A	B	D	E	T	G	H	H	I	O	P	T	D	G	Y	U	F	W	R
C	S	D	F	D	G	H	F	J	K	H	L	Y	M	N	M	B	R	F	G
O	E	R	T	Y	U	I	O	P	J	H	A	S	A	F	G	G	E	G	H
M	F	G	H	J	J	K	K	E	R	T	Y	U	I	O	Q	O	E	T	W
M	A	S	R	E	I	G	H	T	R	T	Y	U	I	A	S	D	D	E	Q
U	R	X	C	D	E	R	T	W	G	H	D	F	G	H	J	K	O	W	V
N	A	S	D	F	G	G	H	E	J	K	L	I	Y	T	R	E	M	W	I
I	M	A	S	D	F	G	R	T	Y	U	I	O	P	S	E	Q	O	A	R
C	N	E	A	U	F	O	R	T	Y	E	I	G	H	T	D	F	F	W	P
A	V	A	C	F	G	H	Y	A	I	R	T	W	Q	O	P	Y	I	P	B
T	I	C	K	W	E	T	Y	N	V	B	N	O	I	N	G	A	N	X	A
I	B	C	B	F	E	R	T	W	E	N	T	Y	O	N	E	W	F	E	B
O	X	U	C	Y	U	I	O	P	L	K	J	H	G	F	D	S	O	B	Y
N	Q	R	B	Y	U	I	O	P	A	S	D	F	E	R	T	G	R	C	M
A	C	A	D	F	G	H	J	K	A	S	D	D	F	G	R	T	M	T	A
D	A	T	E	T	I	M	E	S	I	G	N	A	T	U	R	E	A	I	O
T	V	E	W	D	R	T	G	Y	N	U	I	M	N	B	V	D	T	P	Y
X	C	V	R	B	G	T	Y	N	U	I	M	O	M	R	T	U	I	O	K
C	R	T	V	E	E	R	H	T	Y	B	I	O	X	E	S	V	O	M	I
Z	E	R	V	R	T	U	I	O	N	T	I	O	N	C	N	T	N	T	U

(Reproduced with permission of Anne Levington, Practice Experience Facilitator at Barts and the London NHS Trust)

8.1. How many years does the NHS need to keep adult records? [5]
8.2. How many years does the NHS need to keep child records? [9]
8.3. What 'C' assists in the dissemination of information? [13]
8.4. What 'A' ensures that documentation is precise and concise? [8]
8.5. What is the 'D', 'T' and 'S' that must be documented on all patient records? [4, 4, 9]
8.6. What is the parliamentary Act the grants patients the right to request to view their records? [7, 2, 11]
8.7. Within how many hours must a patient's record be written? [10]

Summary

This chapter has explored communication within multidisciplinary teams in medical placements and why it is important for medical patients' wellbeing. The importance of accurate record keeping has been outlined and how it is integral to the role of the nurse. Learning opportunities have been identified to help you to develop your communication skills within your placements.

References

Department of Health, 2003. Lord Laming: the Victoria Climbie inquiry. Department of Health, London.

Gibbs, G., 1988. Learning by doing: a guide to teaching and learning methods. Further Education Unit, Oxford Polytechnic, Oxford.

Holland, K., Jenkins, J., Solomon, J., et al., 2008. Applying the Roper–Logan–Tierney model in practice, 2nd ed. Churchill Livingstone, Edinburgh.

Johns, 1996. Using the reflective model of nursing and guided reflection. Nursing Standard 11 (2), 34–38.

Laming, The Lord, 2009. The protection of children in England: a progress report. The Stationary Office, London. Online. Available at: http://news.bbc.co.uk/1/shared/bsp/hi/pdfs/12_03_09_children.pdf (accessed July 2011).

Leonard, M., Graham, S., Bonacum, D., 2004. The human factor: the critical importance of effective teamwork and communication in providing safe care. Quality and Safety in Healthcare 13, i85–i90.

Nursing and Midwifery Council, 2008. The code: standards of conduct, performance and ethics for nurses and midwives. NMC, London.

Nursing and Midwifery Council, 2009. Record keeping: guidance for nurses and midwives. NMC, London.

Nursing and Midwifery Council, 2010. Standards for pre-registration nursing education. NMC, London.

The Bristol Royal Infirmary Inquiry, 2001. The inquiry into the management of care of children receiving complex heart surgery at the Bristol Royal Infirmary. Online. Available at: http://www.bristol-inquiry.org.uk/ (accessed July 2011).

Further reading

Arnold, E.C., Boggs, K.U., 2007. Interpersonal relationships: professional communication skills for nurses, 5th ed. Saunders, Edinburgh.

Burnard, P., Gill, P., 2008. Culture, communication, and nursing. Pearson Education, Harlow.

Caldwell, P., Horwood, J., 2007. From isolation to intimacy: making friends without words. J Kingsley, London.

Dunn, K., 2005. Effective communication in palliative care. Nursing Standard 20 (13), 57–64.

Edwards, K., 2011. What prevents one to care. Nursing Times 107, 25–27.

Godsell, M., Scarborough, K., 2006. Improving communication for people with learning disibilities. Nursing Standard 20 (30), 58–65.

Griffith, R., 2004. Putting the record straight: the importance of documentation. British journal of Community Nursing 9 (3), 122–125.

Kraszewski, S., McEwen, A., 2010. Communication skills for adult nurses. Open University Press, Maidenhead.

Mccabe, C., Timmins, F., 2006. Communication skills for nursing practice. Palgrave Macmillan, Basingstoke.

Moloney, R., Maggs, C., 1999. A systematic review of the relationship between written manual nursing care planning, record keeping and patient outcomes. Journal of Advanced Nursing 30 (1), 51–57.

O'Leary, K., Thompson, J., Landler, M., 2010. Patterns of nurse–physician communication and agreement on the plan of care. Quality and Safety in Health Care 1 (3), 195–199.

Taylor, H., 2003. An exploration of the factors that affect nurses' record keeping. British Journal of Nursing 12 (12), 751–758.

Turner, D., Beddoes, L., 2007. Using reflective models to enhance learning: experiences of staff and students. Nurse Education in Practice 7 (3), 135–140.

Whittington, K., Hodgson, L., 2010. The complexities of caring for a patient with an ICD in end-stage heart failure. Cardiac Nursing 5 (12), 568–575.

Answers to wordsearch

8.1. EIGHT.

8.2. TWENTY ONE.

8.3. COMMUNICATION.

8.4. ACCURATE.

8.5. DATE, TIME, SIGNATURE.

8.6. FREEDOM OF INFORMATION.

8.7. FORTY EIGHT.

9 Nutrition and effective elimination

Introduction

Much has been written, particularly in the media, about malnutrition in hospitals and the lack of assistance some patients get to eat and drink (Age Concern 2006, O'Regan, 2009). Malnutrition is defined by the Malnutrition Advisory Group (2003) as:

> *a state in which a deficiency, excess or imbalance of energy, protein and other nutrients causes measurable adverse effects on tissue/body form (body shape, size and composition), function or clinical outcome.*

According to a report by Age Concern in Age Concern, 2006, 6 in 10 older patients in hospital were either malnourished or at risk of becoming malnourished. Malnourished patients are more likely to succumb to infection, stay longer in hospital and require more intensive nursing care.

Read the original *Hungry to be Heard* (Age Concern 2006) and the more recent update *Still Hungry to be Heard* (Age UK 2010) reports to understand more about the nutritional issues facing patients when admitted to hospital and the steps that nurses and hospitals can take to prevent it.

Ensuring adequate food and fluid intake is an essential role of the nurse and it plays a significant part in the recovery of patients on acute medical wards. Even as a very junior student nurse, you will be expected to start helping patients to eat and drink and assess their nutritional status, and planning care to meet nutritional needs will become an important skill for you to learn. Nutrition and fluid management is a significant part of the Essential Skills Clusters (Nursing and Midwifery Council (NMC) 2010a). At entry level to the register, it will be expected you can do the following:

- Assist patients to choose a diet that provides an adequate nutritional and fluid intake.
- Assess and monitor the nutritional status of a patient and, in partnership, formulate an effective plan of care.
- Assess and monitor the fluid status of a patient and, in partnership with them, formulate an effective plan of care.

- Assist patients in creating an environment that is conducive to eating and drinking.
- Ensure that those unable to take food by mouth receive adequate fluid and nutrition to meet their needs.
- Safely administer fluids when fluids cannot be taken independently.

This chapter aims to help you identify the knowledge and skills required in meeting the nutritional needs and elimination needs of a patient and to identify how you could meet your learning outcomes while in a medical placement.

Why is it such an important part of recovery?

Often when someone is unwell, eating a large meal will be the last thing they feel like doing, and those recovering from an acute illness in hospital may have little or no appetite at all. A good balanced diet is an essential part of recovery from illness.

Immune system

A number of nutrients are required to maintain a healthy immune system. This will be particularly important for the patients you are nursing on a medical ward. Some may already have a compromised immune system due to long-term medical conditions, for example HIV and tuberculosis, or as a result of treatment they have received recently or past surgical procedures such as chemotherapy/radiotherapy, transplant surgery and splenectomy. Their immune system may be compromised due to their current medical condition such as anaemia, infection and malnutrition (see Montague et al 2005).

Certain patients with a compromised immune system will need to be nursed in a specific way (reverse barrier nursing) in a single room to prevent them from contracting infections from others.

Tissue growth and wound healing

The repair of tissues and production of new cells are essential for the body to heal itself. Protein is the essential nutrient required for this. When weight is lost quickly, muscle mass is usually lost rather than fat. A patient on bed rest due to an acute illness can lose up to 12% of their muscle strength every week. Consequently, a high-protein diet is often necessary for patients recovering from an acute illness. In order for the body to use protein efficiently, it needs to get its energy from alternative sources, so carbohydrate and fat are important sources of energy (see Table 9.1).

 Activity

> Take some time to find out which foods contain the essential nutrients you need. Do you eat a balanced diet? Think about the patients on your placement – are they getting all the nutrients they need?

Nutritional assessment

An assessment of a patient's nutritional status is an important part of the initial assessments carried out when a patient is admitted to a medical ward. Each organisation will have their own policy about which assessment/screening tool is used and the timescale within which it must be completed. The National Institute for Health and Clinical

 Activity

> Ask your mentor about the tools used and the procedures/guidelines for nutritional assessment in your placement area. Learn how to use these in your assessment of patients' needs.

Table 9.1 Importance of nutrition for good health

Nutrient	Why we need it
Protein	Cell growth, wound healing, production of antibodies
Fats and carbohydrates	Energy sources
Vitamin A	Essential for healthy immune system, eyesight and skin
Vitamin B complex	Formation of antibodies
Vitamin B_{12}	Helps maintain a healthy nervous system, important in formation of red blood cells
Vitamin C	Important in the formation of collagen, aids the absorption of iron and maintains capillaries, bones and teeth
Vitamin D	Promotes absorption of calcium, important in maintaining healthy bones
Calcium	Helps build and maintain strong bones, vital for nerve function, muscle contraction and blood clotting
Potassium	Assists in regulation of acid-base balance, protein synthesis, metabolism of carbohydrates, normal body growth and normal electrical activity of the heart
Sodium	Regulates fluid balance and blood pressure
Iron	Prevents anaemia
Niacin	Helps the body to process sugars and fatty acids and maintain enzyme function, important for development of nervous system
Zinc	Helps with cell formation
Fibre	Stimulates digestive tract, prevents constipation, encourages growth of good bacteria in large intestine, slows down carbohydrate absorption

Excellence (NICE; 2006a) guideline recommends that all hospital in-patients are screened for risk of malnutrition on admission and weekly thereafter.

Assessment of nutritional status will be an ongoing process while the patient is in hospital. You may be required to repeat an assessment with a screening tool at various intervals but observation and communicating with the patient about their nutritional needs will be just as important. If you are unsure what your role is in monitoring the nutritional status of your patients, talk to your mentor about it. This will be something you could

include in your learning outcomes as there are competencies in assessing nutritional status at both the second progression point and entry to the register within the Essential Skills Clusters (NMC 2010a).

Competencies at the second progression point
- Takes and records accurate measurements of weight, height, length, body mass index and other appropriate measures of nutritional status.

- Assesses baseline nutritional requirements for healthy people related to factors such as age and mobility.

Competency at entry level to the register

- Makes a comprehensive assessment of people's needs in relation to nutrition, identifying, documenting and communicating level of risk.

Screening tools

There are many nutritional screening tools available for use. One widely used validated tool is the Malnutrition Universal Screening Tool or MUST (British Association for Parenteral and Enteral Nutrition (BAPEN) 2008). There are five steps to the MUST tool which give you an overall score between 0 and 6. The tool then provides some management guidance to inform your care plan.

Step 1: Measure height and weight to get a body mass index (BMI) score using the chart provided.

Step 2: Note percentage unplanned weight loss and score using tables provided.

Step 3: Establish acute disease effect and score.

Step 4: Add scores from steps 1, 2 and 3 together to obtain overall risk of malnutrition.

Step 5: Use management guidelines and/or local policy to develop care plan.

Step 1 – calculating body mass index

To calculate a patient's BMI, you need to know their height and their weight. Body mass index is an assessment of body composition and gives you an indication as to whether a patient is underweight, normal weight, overweight or obese. It should not replace your clinical judgement, but should be used to guide your assessment. The BMI chart (see http://www.bapen.org.uk/pdfs/must/must_page2.pdf (accessed July 2011)) also gives you a score of 0 to 2 which is the first step of the MUST assessment.

When a patient is acutely unwell, it is not always easy to obtain their weight and height. The patient may know what their weight is or it may have been recorded recently at an out-patient appointment and be in their medical records. If so, this may give you a guide to work from until you are able to gain an accurate weight. However, most placement areas will have weighing scales that allow patients to sit down while being weighed or, alternatively, there may be a hoist that can weigh a patient who is bed bound. Measuring height can be more difficult if the patient is unable to stand. BAPEN (2008) recommends using ulnar length to estimate height as an alternative (see http://www.bapen.org.uk/pdfs/must/must_page6.pdf (accessed July 2011)).

Step 2 – percentage of unplanned weight loss

To determine the percentage of your patient's unplanned weight loss in the last 3–6 months, you will need to know what their weight was before they lost weight. The patient may be able to tell you or give you an idea of what this was. Or they may be able to tell you how much weight they think they have lost. Once you have determined whether they have lost less than 5%, between 5% and 10% or more than 10% of their body weight, you can then compare to this using the weight loss score table provided by BAPEN (see http://www.bapen.org.uk/pdfs/must/must_page4.pdf (accessed July 2011)) which will attribute a score of 0–2 to add to the score from step 1.

Step 3 – establish acute disease effect

If your patient is acutely unwell and is likely to be unable to eat for more than 5 days, an additional score of 2 is added at this step.

Step 4 – add scores together

By adding the scores from the first 3 steps together you will get an overall score telling you the patient's risk of malnutrition. The flow chart from BAPEN (http://www.bapen.

org.uk/pdfs/must/must_page3.pdf (accessed July 2011)) includes recommended management guidelines. The ward/ department you are working in may have locally adapted guidelines so make sure that you are aware of these. Remember, as with all assessments, your clinical judgement is equally important and you may feel that although your patient doesn't have a score indicating a high risk of malnutrition, they still require input from a dietician or close monitoring (see Aston et al (2010) for more information about decision making in practice).

Monitoring food intake

The mealtime routine in hospitals has changed considerably over the last two decades or so with the role of the registered nurse in mealtimes decreasing and care assistants and kitchen personnel playing a greater role in serving meals and removing meal trays at the end of mealtimes (Xia & McCutcheon 2006). This has resulted in the production of best practice statements, such as the *Essence of Care* (Department of Health 2010) food and drink benchmark (see Box 9.1), to reinforce that it is the registered nurse's overall accountability and responsibility to ensure patients receive adequate nutrition and hydration while in hospital.

Many other members of the multidisciplinary team will be interested in a patient's food intake as it will influence the decisions they make when treating the patient. You may find that doctors, dieticians and speech and language therapists, among others, will ask you about a patient's intake, therefore it is important that you are familiar with the food monitoring charts used in your placement area and how to complete and interpret them. Accuracy is vital when completing a food monitoring chart.

Box 9.1 *Essence of Care* food and drink benchmark

- People are encouraged to eat and drink in a way that promotes their health.
- People and carers have sufficient information to enable them to obtain their food and drink.
- People can access food and drink at any time according to their needs and preferences.
- People are provided with food and drink that meet their individual needs and preferences.
- People's food and drink are presented in a way that is appealing to them.
- People feel the environment is conducive to eating and drinking.
- People who are screened on initial contact and identified at risk receive a full nutritional assessment.
- People's care is planned, implemented, continuously evaluated and revised to meet individual needs and preferences for food and drink.
- People receive the care and assistance they require with eating and drinking.
- People's food and drink intake is monitored and recorded.

Activity

Look at the two charts in Figure 9.1. Which one tells you more about the patient's intake?

Fig 9.1 Examples of completed food charts

Breakfast	Toast and marmalade
Lunch	Cheese and onion sandwich Refused dessert
Supper	Chicken, mashed potatoes, carrots Sponge pudding and custard
Snacks	Food brought in by relatives

Breakfast	1 slice of toast and marmalade Offered cereal or porridge but declined
Lunch	½ cheese and onion sandwich Offered dessert but delined
Supper	5 forkfuls of chicken, 2 forkfuls of mashed potato 4 small slices of carrot ½ bowl of sponge and custard
Snacks	2 small cakes and packet of crisps from relatives

Both of these charts could be for the same patient but chart **B** clearly shows that the patient's intake is not so good. This is not clear from chart **A** which merely documents what the patient was given and not the exact amount they ate. Food monitoring charts should be completed as soon as the meal is finished, before the tray has been removed, so that you can look at what is left on the patient's plate.

This also gives you the opportunity to ask the patient about their meal. Is there a reason they haven't eaten much? Maybe they feel nauseous or they didn't like the food, they may be worrying about a forthcoming test or investigation, they may be in pain or have found the food difficult to manage without assistance, adapted cutlery, etc. Once you know the reason your patient isn't eating, you can act upon it – tell the registered nurse looking after them or report it to their doctor.

Not all patients will be able to tell you why they aren't eating so it is important that you investigate all possible causes (see next section) – this could end up as a process of elimination, but knowing about your patient's medical and social history will certainly help.

If the food monitoring chart is being completed by someone else, such as a care assistant working with you, make sure you check the chart regularly and speak to the patient if their intake is poor. It is the registered nurse's responsibility to ensure that patients receive adequate nutrition while they are in hospital and, as a student nurse, you can begin to develop your skills in monitoring and acting upon the risk of malnutrition among your patients. Speak to your mentor about your role in this and include it in your learning outcomes. Nutritional monitoring is a skill that is required in all areas of nursing, so the skills you develop in your medical placement will benefit you in future placements.

Encouraging your patients to eat and drink

If you have identified a patient who is not eating and drinking well, it is essential to determine why and then plan their care accordingly. There could be many reasons why a patient who is able to eat and drink isn't eating or drinking well. The following are just some of the possible reasons:

- Not liking the food.
- Too much food on the plate – being overfaced.
- Food not presented nicely and does not look appetising.
- Food not culturally appropriate.
- Food too hot/cold.
- Texture of food difficult to chew/swallow.
- Knife and fork difficult to hold.
- Not being able to sit up properly in chair/bed to eat.
- Positioning of bedside table/tray.
- Noise.
- Environmental temperature – too hot, too cold.
- Poorly fitting dentures.
- Loose or painful teeth.
- Sore gums, tongue, lips.
- Pain.
- Anxiety.
- Confusion.
- Nausea, constipation.
- Lack of energy or motivation.
- Depression.
- Pain on swallowing.
- Indigestion or epigastric pain.
- Fear of diarrhoea, wind or abdominal pain.
- Food allergies or intolerances.
- Fasting for a religious reason.

⊙ Reflection point

Think of a patient in your placement who is not eating and drinking well. What factors may be contributing to their poor appetite? What could you do about it?

The following articles may be interesting to read as you reflect on the factors affecting your patient:

Chappiti U, Jean-Marie S, Chan W (2000). Cultural and religious influences on adult nutrition in the UK. Nursing Standard 14 (29):47–51.

O'Regan P (2009). Nutrition for patients in hospital. Nursing Standard 23(23):35–41.

There will be many more reasons and you must consider all of these when determining why your patient has a reduced food intake. Talking to the patient and their carers or relatives will help you to understand if this is a new problem or something which has been an issue prior to their acute illness. This will influence your plan of care.

There are a number of strategies that can help encourage and monitor patients' food intake. Some of these are nationally recognised in the UK, such as the use of red trays and protected meal times (Age UK 2010), as being best practice and you will be likely to find them happening in your medical placement area.

As you progress through your training, you are likely to have a number of competencies related to supporting patients who are having problems eating and drinking. For example, in the Essential Skills Clusters (NMC 2010a), at your second progression point it will be expected that you can do the following:

- Identify people who are unable to, or have difficulty in, eating or drinking and report this to others to ensure adequate nutrition and fluid intake is provided.
- Follow local procedures in relation to meal times, for example protected mealtimes, indicators of people who need additional support.
- Ensure that people are ready for the meal; that is, in an appropriate location, position, offered an opportunity to wash hands, offered appropriate assistance.
- Recognise and respond appropriately and report when people have difficulty eating or swallowing.
- Adhere to an agreed plan of care that provides for individual differences, for example cultural considerations and psychosocial aspects, and provide adequate nutrition and hydration when eating or swallowing is difficult.

In 2007, the Council of Europe Alliance, which included the Department of Health, RCN, BAPEN, National Patient Safety Agency (NPSA) and others, produced 10 key characteristics of good nutritional care in hospitals (see Box 9.2).

 Activity

How well are these and the other initiatives detailed below being implemented in your placement area? Talk to ward staff and your mentor about the importance placed on meal times and nutritional care and any of the challenges they may face.

Red trays

In some hospitals, red trays are often used to serve food to patients who require assistance with eating or require prompting to eat and close monitoring. The red tray provides a visible signal to all care and catering staff that this patient needs assistance and that the tray should not be removed until a member of nursing staff is happy that the patient has received the assistance they require.

Protected meal times

Protected mealtimes are designed to reduce the number of interruptions patients receive during the hour or hour and a half that meals are served. This ensures that patients are able to eat their meal in quieter surroundings without being interrupted by doctors, therapists, etc., wanting to assess them or carry out treatment and investigations.

Essence of care benchmarking

The Essence of Care (DH 2010) food and nutrition benchmark sets out standards of best practice to assist healthcare practitioners in auditing their current standard of nutritional care and implementing improvements in nutritional care.

Box 9.2 Ten key characteristics of good nutritional care in hospitals (Council of Europe Alliance 2007)

- All patients are screened on admission to identify the patients who are malnourished or at risk of becoming malnourished. All patients are rescreened weekly.
- All patients have a care plan which identifies their nutritional care needs and how they are to be met.
- The hospital includes specific guidance on food services and nutritional care in its clinical governance arrangements
- Patients are involved in the planning and monitoring arrangements for food service provision.
- The ward implements protected meal times to provide an environment conducive to patients enjoying and being able to eat their food.
- All staff have the appropriate skills and competencies needed to ensure that patients' nutritional needs are met. All staff receive regular training on nutritional care and management.
- Hospital facilities are designed to be flexible and patient-centred with the aim of providing and delivering an excellent experience of food service and nutritional care 24 hours a day, every day.
- The hospital has a policy for food service and nutritional care which is patient-centred and performance managed in line with home country governance frameworks.
- Food service and nutritional care are delivered to the patient safely.
- The hospital supports a multidisciplinary approach to nutritional care and values the contribution of all staff groups working in partnership with patients and users.

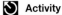 **Activity**

If any of these are in place in your placement area, ask your mentor if you can be involved in carrying out an audit as part of the essence of care benchmarking or another local audit of nutritional care and practice. The essence of care benchmarks can be found at: http://www.dh.gov.uk/en/Publicationsandstatistics/Publications/PublicationsPolicyAndGuidance/DH_119969 (accessed July 2011).

The role of the dietician

The role of the hospital dietician is to assess and advise on the nutritional care of patients with special dietary needs. These may be needs that are associated with a chronic medical condition, such as diabetes, or may be patients whose nutritional intake is compromised because of their acute medical condition such that they require a special or modified diet or supplementary or artificial feeding. Find out who the dietician is in your placement area. Speak to your mentor about possibly spending some time with the dietician to understand their role and the variety of supplementary and artificial feeding options available in your organisation. Box 9.3 gives some examples of departments or staff associated with nutrition in hospital that you could meet or spend time with during your placement.

Fortified/modified diets

For those patients who are able to eat normally, but have a reduced appetite or increased protein needs such as during wound healing, a diet fortified with protein can be prescribed by the dietician. This could be in the form of protein powder added to their usual meals or by drinking fortified drinks or eating fortified puddings between meals. There are also high-fat supplements that can be given as a liquid medicine to increase calorie intake of those who are malnourished. Patients with swallowing problems may also require a diet modified to meet their needs, for example soft or pureed, and the dietician can ensure that such a diet meets their nutritional requirements. The following Website

provides information on swallowing problems (dysphagia) which may be useful: http://www.dysphagiaonline.com/en/pages/home.aspx (accessed July, 2011).

Nasogastric feeding

Nasogastric (NG) feeding is commonly used as a temporary measure to maintain nutritional intake when a patient is unable to maintain their nutrition orally. On a medical ward this is likely to be because of a swallowing problem (dysphagia) or because they have a reduced level of consciousness. It involves passing a fine-bore (feeding) tube through the nasal cavity, through the pharynx and down the oesophagus into the stomach. Caution must be taken to ensure that the tube is placed correctly before feeding commences, and subsequently, each time the tube is used for medication administration or feeding, by aspirating 2 mL of fluid and testing using pH paper (NPSA 2005). See Dougherty and Lister (2011) for more detailed information about this.

The placing of an NG tube is an important skill and one that you may encounter frequently on a medical ward,

---

Box 9.3 Examples of learning opportunities around nutrition

Dietician

Understand their role, how they assess patients' nutritional status and decide on treatment options.

Nutrition nurse

If the organisation you are placed in has a specialist nurse for nutrition, find out their role within the multidisciplinary team.

Catering

Find out where patients' food comes from, how it is distributed throughout the organisation and what range of meals are available.

Pharmacy

Find out how total parenteral nutrition is prepared and distributed from the pharmacy.

especially if the ward you are on accepts patients who have had a stroke. Consult your placement documentation and talk to your mentor about whether this skill is appropriate for you to learn now. Even if it is too early for you to begin to learn to pass an NG tube, the care of the patient with an NG tube is something you can learn now. Your mentor will be able to guide you through best practice, but also consider referring to a clinical procedures reference text such as Dougherty and Lister (2011) for a detailed description and evidence-based rationale.

Gastrostomy feeding

If artificial feeding is required over a longer period of time, a gastrostomy, often referred to as a percutaneous endoscopic gastrostomy (PEG) or radiologically inserted gastrostomy (RIG), is the preferred option. This places a feeding tube directly into the stomach through an incision in the stomach wall. This procedure occurs while the patient is sedated. Caring for a patient with a PEG/RIG tube requires good infection control practice to keep the gastrostomy site clean and healthy, especially during the initial healing process. Talk to your mentor about how to care for a patient with a gastrostomy and include this in your learning outcomes.

Total parenteral nutrition

Total parenteral nutrition (TPN) is the administration of a feeding solution intravenously, usually through a central venous catheter. You may not see it very often on a medical ward but it is used when a patient's gut needs complete rest or is obstructed and feeding enterally is not possible.

The following article describes the various alternative feeding methods described above in more detail along with important nursing care considerations:

Whiteing N, Hunter J (2008). Nursing management of patients who are nil by mouth. Nursing Standard 22 (26):40–45.

Read the following case history and answer the questions below.

You may have considered a number of reasons why Mary is reluctant to eat. There may be a medical cause for her loss of appetite and recent weight loss, for example a malignant tumour in her gastrointestinal tract, and this is being investigated. This

---

■ Case history

Mary Smith is 69 years old and has been admitted to hospital with anaemia. She is waiting to have a gastroscopy and a colonoscopy to help identify the cause of her anaemia. She has lost weight recently and you notice that she is refusing most of the meals offered to her on the ward. When you talk to Mary about her appetite, she says that she doesn't feel very hungry and the amount of food served on the plates puts her off wanting to eat any of it. She also finds some foods difficult to swallow. At home, she would usually eat small meals of plain food, as spicy or rich foods tend to upset her stomach and she often gets indigestion if she is not sitting at a table when eating. Mary also has arthritis in her hands and sometimes drops the knife and fork, which she finds embarrassing when there are other patients nearby.

◆ Activity

■ What factors may be influencing Mary's reluctance to eat?
■ What could you do to encourage Mary to eat more while in hospital?

could also be causing nausea and pain which should be assessed and controlled appropriately with analgesia and antiemetics. As she does not feel hungry, she is being overfaced with her meals. Giving her smaller portions and encouraging her to eat small amounts or snacks throughout the day may result in her intake being greater than if she is only offered three large meals a day. Her swallowing difficulties need to be investigated; she should be referred to a speech and language therapist for assessment. They will be able to advise on the right consistency of food for Mary to manage. You should try to assist Mary to choose foods from the menu that she would usually eat at home. If there are no options that she likes, speak to the catering manager and dietician about alternatives available. Pain from indigestion will prevent Mary from eating so it is important that she is assisted to sit in a position that is comfortable to her when eating, for example at a table and not in bed. An occupational therapist may be able to provide adapted cutlery that would be easier for Mary to use due to her arthritis, and she may prefer to eat in private (you could draw the screens around her bed) if she does not want other people to see her eating.

Encouraging fluid intake

If your patients are not eating very well then it is also likely that they are not drinking enough fluid either. Monitoring fluid intake and output is an important skill to develop and you need to become proficient in interpreting fluid balance and reporting any imbalances promptly to the team looking after the patient. A fluid imbalance is an early indication that your patient's condition is deteriorating.

As with patients who are not eating well, the first step is to determine why your patient is not drinking enough fluid. The following are some reasons you may want to consider:

- Drinks not within reach, e.g. table or locker too far away.
- Difficulty holding cup/beaker.
- Fresh water not available, e.g. water in the jug has been sitting on the table all day.
- Drinks not cold enough or not hot enough (if tea, coffee, etc.).
- Sore mouth, gums, tongue, lips.
- Person doesn't like plain water or drinks that are available.
- Unable to sit up in a comfortable position to drink.
- Lack of energy or motivation.
- Depression.
- Confusion.
- Fear of incontinence.

These are just some possible explanations. It is important that you speak to your patients to ask them why they are not drinking. They may not be aware of how important drinking fluid is for their general health and recovery.

In some organisations, a red beaker or jug is used, like the red tray, to clearly identify to staff which patients need assistance or encouragement to drink. In most cases you will need to regularly prompt patients to drink. It is better for them to take small amounts of water regularly than to just drink large glasses of water at specific times. The hot drinks served in hospitals are often not served by nursing staff and it easy therefore to assume that by providing patients with a jug of water, their fluid needs will have been met. Consider some ways in which you could encourage a patient to drink more fluids:

- Ensure chilled, fresh water is available (not just stale water in a jug).
- Encourage fluids from early in the morning as many patients may not want to drink in the evening for fear of needing the toilet in the night.
- Find out which drinks your patients like and ask relatives to bring in juice, herbal or fruit teas, etc.
- Offer water alongside tea and coffee.
- Every time you have contact with a patient, fill their glass and encourage them to have a drink.

- Involve them in completing their fluid balance chart so they can see how much they are drinking.
- Ask friends and relatives to prompt the patient to drink while they are visiting.
- Encourage intake of foods which have a high fluid content, e.g. cereal with milk, soup, jelly.

Oral care

Good oral hygiene is essential if patients are to feel able to eat and drink well. Many patients won't be able to maintain their own oral hygiene while in hospital or they won't have the resources to do it effectively. Where possible, encourage your patients to clean their teeth with a normal toothbrush and toothpaste twice a day, as they would at home. You may need to provide them with a toothbrush, toothpaste and clean water to be able to do this.

Speak to your mentor about the resources available for patients who don't have a supply of their own. For those who are unable to manage their own oral hygiene, assisting them to clean their teeth, gums and oral mucosa gently with a toothbrush and toothpaste is generally the best option. See the article by Huskinson and Lloyd (2009) for more information about the importance of good oral care for patients in hospital.

 Activity

> Speak to your mentor about any local guidelines/protocols for mouth care. What resources are available to provide mouth care in your placement area?
>
> You are likely to find that a number of your learning outcomes concern helping those who have eating, drinking and swallowing difficulties. These form a large part of the nutrition and fluid management Essential Skills Clusters (NMC 2010a).

(!) Reflection point

> Reflect on what you have read so far in this chapter and identify how you could meet the following competencies from the second progression point in the Essential Skills Clusters (NMC 2010a) in your current placement area:
>
> ■ Under supervision, help people to choose healthy food and fluid in keeping with their personal preferences and cultural needs.
>
> ■ Maintain independence and dignity wherever possible and provide assistance as required.
>
> ■ Identify people who are unable to, or have difficulty, eating or drinking and report this to others to ensure adequate nutrition and fluid intake is provided.
>
> ■ Follow local procedures in relation to meal times, e.g. protected meal times, indicators of people who need additional support.
>
> ■ Ensure that people are ready for the meal, i.e. in an appropriate location, position, offered an opportunity to wash hands, offered appropriate assistance.
>
> ■ Recognise and respond appropriately and report when people have difficulty eating or swallowing.

Monitoring fluid balance

On your medical ward you will find many patients who require fluid balance monitoring. You may think to yourself, why is this important? You may not always understand why someone requires fluid balance monitoring.

There will be a multitude of reasons for this including cardiac failure, renal failure and cerebral vascular accident, and it is important for you to understand why your patient's fluid balance requires such careful monitoring. It can become just a habit to fill out the forms but it is important for you to understand why your patient requires this close monitoring. Your mentor/co-mentor can help you with this.

There are multiple reasons for monitoring fluid balance and some of the reasons that patients on a medical ward may require this are outlined in Box 9.4.

It is important that you discuss the fluid balance requirements of your patient with your mentor and understand the rationale for this.

One means of assisting with assessing a patient's fluid balance is measuring and recording his or her fluid intake and output to observe for trends over given time periods. If the patient is critically ill, these trends may occur over short time periods and will therefore be assessed more frequently – hourly or 4-hourly. If the patient is not critically ill, observation would be over longer periods of time. Again you can check with your mentor or co-mentor whether you are assessing the fluid balance on an hourly basis or over a longer period of time.

Box 9.4 Reasons for monitoring fluid balance

- Fluid restriction – for electrolyte balance.
- Renal failure.
- Diuretic therapy.
- The patient has cardiac failure.
- Intravenous infusions are in progress.
- A urinary catheter is present and drainage needs to be recorded.
- The patient is nil by mouth.
- The patient requires close monitoring to ensure adequate hydration.
- The patient is losing fluid from drains, nasogastric tube.
- The patient has diarrhoea and vomiting.
- Enteral feeding is in progress.
- The patient is on opiates and may be drowsy and needs prompting to drink.
- Post-procedure/operation.

Quiz: fluid balance

Try the following quiz to test your knowledge about fluid balance.
(Answers on p. 181.)

9.1. Approximately what percentage of the human body is made up of water?
   a. 45%
   b. 60%
   c. 50%
   d. 75%

9.2. Which of the following patients require fluid balance monitoring?
   a. Patient with diarrhoea
   b. Patient with cardiac failure
   c. Dyspnoeic patient on continuous oxygen
   d. All of the above

9.3. What is the minimum acceptable urine output for a patient with normal renal function?
   a. 0.5 mL/kg/h
   b. 1 mL/kg/h
   c. 2 mL/kg/h
   d. 10 mL/kg/h

9.4. What does body water contain?
  a. Sodium and potassium
  b. Magnesium and bicarbonate
  c. Sodium, potassium, chloride, bicarbonate, calcium and magnesium
  d. Water only
9.5. Which of the following are important interventions for a patient with dehydration?
  a. Administration of IV fluids
  b. Regular skin and mouth care
  c. Accurate fluid balance monitoring
  d. Physiotherapy
  e. Close monitoring of vital signs
  f. High-fibre diet

The following case history will help you to identify the fluid requirements of a patient and the subsequent care he requires.

Most hospitals will have policies for cannula care supported by care plans to prevent infection and to ensure patency. Make sure that you are able to access these. The phlebitis score is widely used and considered best practice for identifying cannula-related problems (see Fig. 9.3).

The fact that George has a cannula does not mean that he should stop drinking. George will be able to stop IV fluids if he can drink enough and he needs to be informed of this.

■ **Case history**

George is 67 years old and was admitted to your medical ward 2 days ago with an exacerbation of his chronic obstructive pulmonary disease. He has been diagnosed with pneumonia and is pyrexial at 38°C. George's hyperpyrexia is causing him to sweat profusely and he does not feel like eating or drinking very much. He has oxygen 2 L administered via nasal specs, requires 4-hourly salbutamol nebulisers via air, oral steroids and IV antibiotics. He weighs 12 stone.

To calculate his fluid requirements, convert his weight into kg and multiply your answer by the number of mL/kg identified in his age group (see Table 9.2).

You will also need to consider the insensible loss when calculating fluid balance. This includes :

  – sweating
  – faeces
  – breathing.

Normal insensible fluid loss would be approximately 500 mL a day, however if a patient has pyrexia, diarrhoea or is tachypnoeic, the insensible loss will increase. Therefore, it is important to consider your observations of vital signs when you are calculating fluid balance. There are also other ways to assess fluid balance.

Figure 9.2 shows George's fluid balance chart for the last 24 hours:

Previous balance = −980 mL
Total input   = 1030 mL
Total output   = 1510 mL

Now try and answer the following questions (answers on p. 181):

9.6. What is the balance for this last 24 hours?

9.7. When you take into account the balance for the previous 24 hours, what is the balance?

9.8. Do you need to factor any insensible loss into this balance? Explain your answer.

9.9. Is this balance adequate for George (consider weight and age)? Explain your answer.

9.10. Would it be important for you to look at George's electrolyte balance?

9.11. What nursing actions could you suggest?

9.12. How much fluid intake does George need to ensure that he is adequately hydrated?

During the ward round, the medical team decides to start George on some IV fluids. The doctor prescribes 1000 mL normal saline over 8 hours. Your IV giving set administers drops at 20 drops/minute. Using the formula in Box 9.5, calculate the drops/minute for this prescription.

This improves George's fluid intake, however George now has an intravenous cannula and, as his nurse, you also need to be aware of the requirements for cannula care (see Ch. 19 in Brooker & Waugh 2007).

Table 9.2 Fluid requirements by age/weight

Adult patient age group (age range years)	Fluid requirements (mL/kg)
Young adult 16–30	40
Average adult 25–55	35
Older patient 56–65	30
Older patient 66–75	25–30
Elderly patient >75	25

(Source: Finestone & Greene-Finestone 2003)

When you are a junior student, you will observe the registered nurse admitting the patient and discussing their activities of daily living with them including eating, drinking and elimination. As you progress during your training, you will start to become more involved in this process. The mentor will continuously assess you, and gradually you will start to take the lead during admissions and to make your own assessment of the activities of daily living. During this assessment you will be considering whether they need to have close monitoring of their fluid balance and you will need to explain your rationale for this to your mentor. This includes explaining why a patient might not need close fluid balance monitoring. Practice makes perfect and you need to expect to get it wrong sometimes, but that is how you will learn. Fluid balance is only one of the ways in which we monitor our patients' conditions and it can never be taken in isolation. As a registered nurse, you will be expected to 'use a range of diagnostic and clinical skills, complemented by existing and developing technology, to assess the nursing care of

Time	Oral	Input other	Input other	Urine output	Other output
06:00		IV antibiotic 100 mls		350 mls	
07:00					
08:00	Tea 100 mls				
09:00					
10:00					
11:00	H_2O 100 mls			200 mls	
12:00		IV antibiotic 100 mls			
13:00	Tea 150 mls				
14:00					
15:00					
16:00	H_2O 30 mls				
17:00				350 mls	
18:00		IV antibiotic 100 mls			
19:00					
20:00	Tea 150 mls				
21:00					
22:00		IV antibiotic 100 mls			
23:00	H_2O 100 mls			250 mls	
24:00					
01:00					
02:00					
03:00					
04:00				360 mls	
05:00					
Total	630 mls			1510 mls	

Fig 9.2 George's fluid balance chart

Box 9.5 Formula to calculate drops/minute

Calculation of intravenous infusion rates

Standard giving sets deliver 20 drops per mL.
Blood giving sets deliver 15 drops per mL.

Formula for calculating drops per minute

$$\text{drip rate per minute} = \frac{\text{volume of infusion (mL)} \times \text{no. of drops per mL of giving set}}{\text{infusion time in minutes}}$$

individuals undergoing therapeutic or
clinical interventions' (NMC 2010b).

Elimination

This section will address the various aspects
of elimination and the role you will play in
assisting patients to manage their
elimination needs. Some patients admitted
to a medical ward will not have any problems
managing their elimination and toileting
needs, but others may be significantly
affected. This will depend on their illness, the
treatment they are receiving and the extent to
which they are incapacitated by these.

Urinary incontinence

Urinary incontinence can be defined as 'the
complaint of any involuntary leakage of
urine' (NICE 2006). It can be caused by any
number of illnesses or treatments or an
abnormality in the lower urinary tract.

A common cause of urinary incontinence
in medical patients is a urinary tract
infection (UTI). Symptoms of a lower UTI
include pain (dysuria), a burning sensation
on passing urine and increased frequency.
The diagnosis of a UTI will be made
following the collection of a urine
specimen.

You will be asked to collect a mid-stream
specimen of urine (MSU) for many of your
patients as it is an important diagnostic tool.
Often a ward-based 'dipstick' test will suffice

in detecting any problems, but sometimes
a specimen will need to be sent to the
laboratory for further tests and to
determine antibiotic sensitivity (see
Tables 9.3 and 9.4).

Also see this resource for a demonstration of
specimen collection:

http://www.cetl.org.uk/learning/specimen-swab-collection/player.html (accessed July
2011).

(●) Reflection point

Think about how you would explain to a
patient that you need a urine sample
from them: include why you need it,
what it involves and what you need the
patient to do. Consider how a patient's
culture and/or religious beliefs may
affect how they feel about this. For
example, a male patient may not feel
comfortable being assisted by a female
nurse to do this and vice versa.

Assessment and causes of urinary incontinence

If your patient does not have a UTI or they
are still having problems with urinary
continence once their UTI has been treated,
it is important that their continence is
assessed. Incontinence is not a part of
normal ageing and should always be

Phlebitis score

All patients with an intravenous access device should have the IV site checked every shift for signs of infusion phlebitis. The subsequent score and action(s) taken (if any) must be documented on the cannula record form.

The cannula site must also be observed:
- When bolus injections are administered
- IV flow rates are checked or altered
- When solution containers are changed

IV site appears healthy	**0**	**No signs of phlebitis** • Observe cannula
One of the following is evident: • Slight pain near IV site • Slight redness near IV site	**1**	**Possible first signs of phlebitis** • Observe cannula
Two of the following are evident: • Pain at IV site • Swelling • Redness	**2**	**Early stages of phlebitis** • Resite cannula
All of the following are evident: • Pain along path of cannula • Redness • Swelling	**3**	**Medium stages of phlebitis** • Resite cannula • Seek medical advice • Consider treatment
All of the following are evident and extensive: • Pain along path of cannula • Redness • Swelling • Palpable cord	**4**	**Advanced stage of phlebitis/ start of thrombophlebitis** • Resite cannula • Seek medical advice • Consider treatment
All of the following are evident and extensive: • Pain along path of cannula • Redness • Swelling • Palpable venous cord • Pyrexia	**5**	**Advanced stage of thrombophlebitis** • Resite cannula • Seek medical advice • Initiate treatment

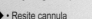

Fig 9.3 Phlebitis score (Reproduced with permission of Andrew Jackson, Consultant Nurse, Intravenous Therapy and Care, The Rotherham NHS Foundation Trust)

Table 9.3 Collecting a mid-stream sample of urine

Action	Rationale
Explain the procedure to your patient, what it will involve and why you need a urine specimen Gain their consent	Informed consent is required for all procedures and your patient will be able to assist you if they understand what they need to do
Collect your equipment You will need a sterile pot to collect the specimen in, gloves, a specimen pot to send the sample to the laboratory, gauze and clean water	In preparation for collecting the sample
Assist your patient to the toilet and ensure they have privacy	To maintain the privacy and dignity of your patient
Ask the patient, or assist them, to clean their urethral meatus In women, this should be done by cleaning from front to back	To prevent contamination of the sample from any bacteria around the urethral meatus
Explain to the patient that you do not want the first few mLs of urine passed It is helpful if the patient is able to stop mid-flow of urine	The first few mLs will contain any bacteria from the urethra
Collect the required amount of urine in the sterile pot	To prevent contamination of the sample from non-sterile products, e.g. bed pan
Transfer the sample to the specimen pot for the lab and label the specimen with patient details straight away	Label immediately to prevent a mistake in identifying the sample
Document in the patient's notes that a sample has been sent	To communicate to the rest of the team
Arrange for the sample to be sent to the lab according to ward policy and procedure	To ensure prompt collection and analysis

assessed and investigated. Sometimes patients may have been experiencing problems for a number of months or years and felt too embarrassed to approach their GP for help. In these cases especially, this may be the only opportunity to help our patients so we must encourage them to discuss their problem by approaching the subject sensitively. This may mean reflecting on your own feelings about incontinence; if you feel embarrassed about the subject then this will make it difficult to discuss this with your patient.

◐ Reflection point

Consider how you might feel if you were experiencing continence problems and how you would want your nurse to discuss the subject with you. Talk to your mentor about the best ways to broach the subject with a patient.

Table 9.4 Performing a urine dipstick

Action	Rationale
Explain the procedure to your patient, what it will involve and why you need a urine specimen Gain their consent	Informed consent is required for all procedures and your patient will be able to assist you if they understand what they need to do
Assist your patient to the toilet and ensure they have privacy	To maintain the privacy and dignity of your patient
Ensure your patient has a bed pan or similar clean vessel to pass urine into	To allow you to remove the sample from the toilet to perform the dip stick test
Wearing gloves, remove the reagent strip from its container and dip the stick in the urine sample, ensuring all the coloured areas are covered in urine	To ensure all of the reagents come into contact with the urine sample
Remove the stick from the sample at an angle to prevent reagents from running into each other	To ensure the accuracy of the testing
Following the manufacturer's instructions, wait and compare the changes on the reagent strip with those accompanying the strips	To allow the reagent to mix with the sample
Dispose of the strip and urine sample appropriately	To prevent cross-infection
Document the test results in the patient's notes and inform the medical team	To ensure test results are acted upon promptly
Ensure the container of reagent strips remains closed at all times	Moisture can reduce the effectiveness and accuracy of the strips

You may find some useful information on the Bladder and Bowel Foundation and NHS Choices Websites:

http://www.bladderandbowelfoundation.org (accessed July 2011).

http://www.nhs.uk/livewell/incontinence/pages/incontinencehome.aspx (accessed July 2011).

There may be a continence specialist nurse in your placement area that you could talk to or spend time with.

Before talking to a patient about incontinence, it is a good idea to ensure that

 Activity

Find out if there is a continence specialist nurse in your placement area. How do you contact them for advice or to refer a patient to them? See if there is a possibility of you spending some time with them during your placement.

your own knowledge about incontinence and what can be done about it is up to date. This will help when reassuring your patient that it is something they should talk about and have investigated.

Read the following article to enhance your knowledge of this problem:

Hanzaree Z, Steggall MJ (2010). Treatment of patients with urge and stress urinary incontinence. Nursing Standard 25 (23):41–46.

A thorough assessment is important to determine the cause of incontinence and this should begin with a detailed history of signs and symptoms. Examples of some of the questions you may want to ask can be found in Box 9.6.

The answers to these questions will help a specialist nurse or doctor decide what further investigations are required to diagnose the cause of the incontinence and the possible treatments available. This process may take some time and will not necessarily happen while your patient is in hospital, but it is important that the appropriate referrals are made and that nursing staff do all they can to manage the patient's incontinence while they are in hospital.

The completion of a bladder diary is another simple way we can assist a specialist in assessing incontinence. The frequency and volume of incontinence should be documented in the bladder diary for a minimum of 3 days. This will help to establish the pattern of incontinence and can assist with management on the ward. Getting your patient involved in completing the diary, if they are well enough and are able to, while they are in hospital can help them to feel in control of their situation.

There are four main types of urinary incontinence: stress, urge, overflow and functional.

Stress incontinence

Stress incontinence is a leaking of urine when laughing, coughing, sneezing or any other movements that put pressure on the bladder. It is the most common form of incontinence in women, particularly after pregnancy, childbirth and menopause. It is caused by the bladder neck sagging and descending abnormally as a result of a lack of oestrogen, poor muscle support, nerve damage, a decrease in collagen or fractures and surgery to the hip or pelvis.

Box 9.6 Assessment of urinary incontinence

How long have you had the problem?
Do you leak urine when you laugh, cough, sneeze or jump?
How much urine do you leak?
Does it only happen during the day or at night as well?
Do you always know when you have leaked urine?
Do you feel the need to empty your bladder before leaking urine?
Do you feel a sudden strong urge to pass urine and have to go quickly?
Do you leak urine before you reach the toilet?
How often do you pass/leak urine?
Do you find it hard to start to pass urine?
Has your flow of urine changed, e.g. weaker, stops and starts, takes longer than before?
Does your bladder feel empty after passing urine?
Do you have any problems physically getting to the toilet?
Have you had any abdominal or gynaecological surgery (women only) in the past?
Have you had children and was it a traumatic birth (women only)?

Urge incontinence

Urge incontinence or overactive bladder syndrome is when the person feels the need to pass urine, but is unable to inhibit bladder contraction, thus resulting in leaking of urine suddenly when an urge is felt. Patients with urge incontinence may empty their bladder during sleep, after drinking small amounts of water or hearing running water or touching water. It is also common to have symptoms of both urge and stress incontinence and this is referred to as mixed urinary incontinence.

Overflow incontinence

Overflow incontinence occurs when the bladder fails to contract and empty adequately resulting in overflow leakage. It is often caused by nerve damage, spinal injury, neurological conditions, such as Parkinson's, or an obstruction in the urinary tract, for example an enlarged prostate gland in men.

Functional incontinence

In functional incontinence the bladder functions normally but the person is not able to interpret the bladder signals or cannot respond appropriately to the signals. This could be because they are cognitively impaired or have had a stroke or brain injury, or it could be because they cannot physically get to the toilet in time due to poor mobility, pain or drowsiness. This type of incontinence is common in hospital patients and is the type that, as nurses, we can do the most to prevent and manage well. Keeping a bladder diary can help to identify a pattern of incontinence, especially if the patient is cognitively impaired. From this, a timed or prompted voiding regime can be put into place. This involves assisting your patient or prompting them to use the toilet at set intervals or at certain times of the day.

Urinary catheterisation

You may find a number of patients in your placement area with a urinary catheter in place. The usual reason for this is to assist in close monitoring of fluid balance. Some patients may require their fluid balance to be monitored hourly and, consequently, catheterisation is the only way to ensure this is done accurately. Other patients may have a long-term catheter and will have been admitted with it. Incontinence is not an indication for catheterisation and you will find that the medical team try to avoid urinary catheterisation unless absolutely necessary. This is because of the increased risk of complications associated with catheters, namely infection. Urinary catheters should be removed at the earliest opportunity (Pratt & Pellowe 2010, Dailly 2011).

 Activity

Now that you are aware of the risks associated with urinary catheterisation, think of the patients on your ward who currently have a urinary catheter. You should be able to answer the following questions for each of them. If you are not sure, ask your mentor or the nurse looking after the patient:

1. Why does your patient have a catheter?
2. When was it put in?
3. What type of catheter is it – long/short term?
4. What is the plan for removing it?

 Activity

Think about the patients in your placement area. How many of them could benefit from prompting and assistance to use the toilet regularly? Discuss with your mentor how this could be implemented for your patients.

This information is important in reducing the risk of catheter-associated infection. The longer a catheter is in place, the greater the risk of infection, so knowing why it was put in initially and what the plan is for removing it should be questions that are routinely asked during nursing handover.

Catheterisation is a skill you will need to master and you should discuss with your mentor the opportunities that may become available during your placement to either observe or attempt catheterising a patient. Different placement areas will stock different types of catheter. Ask your mentor to show you where they are kept and familiarise yourself with the different types, particularly male and female catheters, different sizes, what they are made from, long term and short term. Also learn about the different types of catheter bags available and when it is appropriate to us them.

Read Chapter 20 by Martin Steggall in Brooker and Waugh (2007) for more detailed information on the care of a patient with a urinary catheter.

Faecal incontinence

As with urinary incontinence, faecal incontinence is a difficult and embarrassing subject for a patient to discuss. Therefore, it needs to be addressed sensitively. Some patients may not want to tell you they have a problem so it is important that we include questions about incontinence in our nursing assessments to allow patients an opportunity to talk about it. Certain groups of people are thought to be at high risk of faecal incontinence (see Box 9.7) so attention should be paid to ensuring a full assessment of patients within these groups. A good history of symptoms from your patient will help you and the team looking after them determine what might be the cause and possible treatments.

As with urinary incontinence, a good record of your patient's bowel habits will help the specialist team in investigating the cause of incontinence. A simple bowel chart which records the frequency and consistency of stool together with a complete food and fluid chart will be necessary. Again, encourage your patients to complete these themselves wherever

---

Box 9.7 Groups at high risk of faecal incontinence

- Frail older people.
- People with loose stools or diarrhoea from any cause.
- Women following childbirth (especially following third- and fourth-degree obstetric injury).
- People with neurological or spinal disease/injury (e.g. spina bifida, stroke, multiple sclerosis, spinal cord injury).
- People with severe cognitive impairment.
- People with urinary incontinence.
- People with pelvic organ prolapse and/or rectal prolapse.
- People who have had colonic resection or anal surgery.
- People who have undergone pelvic radiotherapy.
- People with perianal soreness, itching or pain.
- People with learning disabilities.

(NICE 2007)

---

possible. The Bristol Stool Chart in Figure 9.4 (Lewis & Heaton 1997) is a good example of a tool used to record bowel movements that all team members will understand (see Ch. 21 in Brooker & Waugh (2007) for more information about assessment of faecal elimination and management of faecal incontinence).

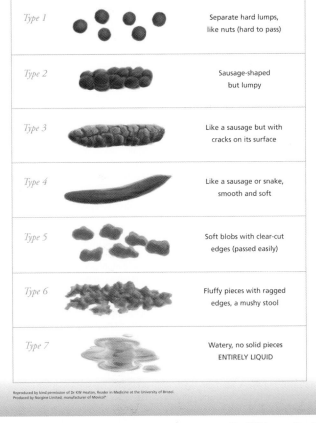

THE BRISTOL STOOL FORM SCALE

Type 1	Separate hard lumps, like nuts (hard to pass)
Type 2	Sausage-shaped but lumpy
Type 3	Like a sausage but with cracks on its surface
Type 4	Like a sausage or snake, smooth and soft
Type 5	Soft blobs with clear-cut edges (passed easily)
Type 6	Fluffy pieces with ragged edges, a mushy stool
Type 7	Watery, no solid pieces ENTIRELY LIQUID

Reproduced by kind permission of Dr KW Heaton, Reader in Medicine at the University of Bristol.
Produced by Norgine Limited, manufacturer of Movicol®

Fig 9.4 The Bristol Stool Chart (Reproduced by kind permission of Dr KW Heaton, Reader in Medicine at the University of Bristol. © 2000 Norgine Pharmaceuticals Ltd.)

You might find this article helpful: http://en.wikipedia.org/wiki/Bristol_Stool_ Scale (accessed July 2011).

Management of incontinence on the hospital ward

As investigation and treatment of urinary and faecal incontinence can take some time, it is an important role of the nurse to ensure the patient is able to manage their continence appropriately while in hospital. There are a number of ways you can ensure this happens:

Good communication Ensuring your patient feels able to talk to you about their continence problems and is reassured that any questions or issues they have will be dealt with sensitively and promptly is the crucial first step.

Toilet access Ensure your patient is in a bed close to the toilet or, if they are unable to get to the toilet on their own, ensure that they have a nurse call bell to hand at all times and that it is answered promptly. Good signs (ideally with pictures and words) directing people to the toilet will help, especially if your patient has memory problems or does not speak English as they may be too embarrassed to ask. If your patient has mobility problems, ensure they have been referred to the physiotherapist and any walking aids needed are close at hand.

Toilet facilities Ensure the toilet facilities are clean and offer privacy to your patients. Ensure there are sufficient products in the toilet to help your patients if they have been incontinent (e.g. fresh pads, pants, wipes etc.).

Continence aids Discuss with your patient which aids will suit them. Men may wish to wear a penile sheath attached to a catheter bag to help manage urinary incontinence. Patients will have different preferences with regards to the size of pad they wear and

how and when it is changed. Prompt attention to help your patients change or manage their continence aid is essential.

Prompting or timed voiding As described above, this can help some patients to remain continent and should always be tried while the patient remains in hospital.

Assessment of fluid and food intake Good documentation of intake and output is essential to assist assessment of incontinence. Speak to your mentor or the dietician about specific dietary advice you could give a patient with urinary or faecal incontinence.

Review medication Many medications can exacerbate incontinence. Try to familiarise yourself with some of the common drugs that may cause a problem with continence. Speak to your mentor about which drugs these may be and then look them up to find out more about them.

Dignity Maintaining your patients' dignity when talking about continence, helping to maintain personal hygiene and managing incontinence aids is the most important aspect of continence care.

Involve the multidisciplinary team If your organisation has a continence nurse specialist, they will be a key member of the team to be involved. Physiotherapists can help to manage incontinence, especially where mobilising to the toilet is a problem. Specialist physiotherapists are often trained to teach pelvic floor exercises, which strengthen the pelvic floor muscles and can help with stress and urge incontinence as well as faecal incontinence. If your patient struggles to manage their clothing when in the toilet, an occupational therapist can help. On discharge, it is important to make sure that your patient is properly followed up if they are still experiencing problems. They may need a referral to the district nurse or the continence nurse specialist.

Read the following case history and answer the questions.

Case history

Mrs Peters is 52 years old and has been admitted with a chest infection. She is very short of breath and is using oxygen continuously. While helping her to prepare to have a wash one morning, you notice that there is a pair of urine-soaked knickers in a bag in her locker.

1. How would you approach Mrs Peters about this?
2. Think about how you would start the conversation and the kind of questions you might want to ask her (look back to Box 9.6).

After talking to Mrs Peters, she tells you that she hasn't had a problem with incontinence before but, at the moment, every time she coughs she leaks urine and is very embarrassed as she cannot get to the toilet due to her breathlessness.

Activity

Write a care plan for managing Mrs Peters' incontinence while she is in hospital. Consider any further assessments/tests she may need, how you can help her to manage her incontinence and relieve her embarrassment, and any other members of the multidisciplinary team you would involve in her care.

Summary

Assessing and assisting patients to maintain their nutritional status will be a key part of your learning outcomes and competencies for your medical placement. The Essential Skills Clusters (NMC 2010a) have a section dedicated to nutrition and fluid management, so whatever stage you are at in your training, this will be an area that you need to continue to develop in. Aspects of the other skills clusters, such as care, compassion and communication, will also be relevant, particularly when caring for a patient with continence problems. This chapter should have given you plenty of ideas to identify learning opportunities within your placement to meet these learning outcomes, and all of the skills and knowledge you develop in these areas will be transferable to other placement settings.

References

Age Concern, 2006. Hungry to be heard. Age Concern, London. Online. Available at: http://www.scie.org.uk/publications/guides/guide15/files/hungrytobeheard.pdf (accessed July 2011).

Age UK, 2010. Older patients: still hungry to be heard. Age UK, London. Online. Available at: http://www.ageuk.org.uk/latest-news/archive/older-patients-still-hungry-to-be-heard/ (accessed July 2011).

Aston, L., Wakefield, J., McGown, R., 2010. The student nurse guide to decision making in practice. Open University Press, Maidenhead.

British Association for Parenteral and Enteral Nutrition, 2008. The MUST toolkit. BAPEN, Redditch. Online. Available at: http://www.bapen.org.uk/musttoolkit.html (accessed July 2011).

Brooker, C., Waugh, A., 2007. Foundations of nursing practice. Mosby, Edinburgh.

Chappiti, U., Jean-Marie, S., Chan, W., 2000. Cultural and religious influences on adult nutrition in the UK. Nursing Standard 14 (29), 47–51.

Council of Europe Alliance, 2007. 10 key characteristics of good nutritional care in hospitals. Online. Available at: http://www.nrls.npsa.nhs.uk/resources/?entryid45=59865 (accessed July 2011).

Dailly, S., 2011. Prevention of indwelling catheter associated urinary tract infections. Nursing Older People 23 (2), 14–19.

Department of Health, 2010. Essence of care 2010. The Stationery Office, London. Online. Available at: http://www.dh.gov.uk/en/Publicationsandstatistics/Publications/PublicationsPolicyAndGuidance/DH_119969 (accessed July 2011).

Dougherty, L., Lister, S., 2011. Royal Marsden Hospital manual of clinical nursing procedures, 8th ed. Wiley–Blackwell, Chichester.

Finestone, H.M., Greene-Finestone, L.S., 2003. Rehabilitation medicine: 2. Diagnosis of dysphagia and its nutritional management for stroke patients. Canadian Medical Association Journal 169 (10), 1041–1044.

Huskinson, W., Lloyd, H., 2009. Oral health in hospitalised patients: assessment and hygiene. Nursing Standard 23 (36), 43–47.

Lewis, S.J., Heaton, K.W., 1997. Stool form scale as a useful guide to intestinal transit time. Scandinavian Journal of Gastroenterology 32 (9), 920–924.

Malnutrition Advisory Group, 2003. Press release: malnutrition and the wider context. MAG, BAPEN, Redditch.

Online. Available at: http://www.bapen.org.uk/res_press_rel9.html (accessed July 2011).

Montague, S., Watson, R., Herbert, A., 2005. Physiology for nursing practice, 3rd ed. Elsevier, Edinburgh.

National Institute for Health and Clinical Excellence, 2006a. Nutrition support in adults: oral nutrition support, enterral feeding and parenteral nutrition. NICE, London. http://guidance.nice.org.uk/CG32/Guidance/pdf/English (accessed July 2011).

National Institute for Health and Clinical Excellence, 2006b. Urinary incontinence: the management of urinary incontinence in women. NICE, London.

National Institute for Health and Clinical Excellence, 2007. Faecal incontinence: the management of faecal incontinence in adults. NICE, London.

National Patient Safety Agency, 2005. Reducing the harm caused by misplaced nasogastric feeding tubes. NPSA, London. Online. Available at: http://www.nrls.npsa.nhs.uk/resources/?EntryId45=59794 (accessed July 2011).

Nursing and Midwifery Council, 2010a. Essential skills clusters. NMC, London.

Nursing and Midwifery Council, 2010b. Standards for pre-registration nursing education. NMC, London.

O'Regan, P., 2009. Nutrition for patients in hospital. Nursing Standard 23 (23), 35–41.

Pratt, R., Pellowe, C., 2010. Good practice in the management of patients with urethral catheters. Nursing Older People 22 (8), 25–29.

Whiteing, N., Hunter, J., 2008. Nursing management of patients who are nil by mouth. Nursing Standard 22 (26), 40–45.

Xia, C., McCutcheon, H., 2006. Mealtimes in hospital – who does what? Journal of Clinical Nursing 15, 1221–1227.

Further reading

Lawson, L., Peate, I., 2009. Essential nursing care: a workbook for clinical practice. Wiley–Blackwell, Chichester.

Richardson, R., 2008. Clinical skills for student nurses: theory, practice and reflection. Reflect Press, Devon.

Solomon, J., 2008a. Eating and drinking. In: Holland, K., Jenkins, J., Solomon, J., Whittam, S. (Eds.), Applying the Roper–Logan–Tierney model in practice. 2nd ed. Churchill Livingstone, Edinburgh (Chapter 6).

Solomon, J., 2008b. Eliminating. In: Holland, K., Jenkins, J., Solomon, J., Whittam, S. (Eds.), Applying the Roper–Logan–Tierney model in practice. 2nd ed. Churchill Livingstone, Edinburgh (Chapter 7).

Ward, D., 2002. The role of nutrition in the prevention of infection. Nursing Standard 16 (18), 47–52.

Websites

Department of Health's Nutrition Action Plan: http://www.dh.gov.uk/en/Publicationsandstatistics/Publications/PublicationsPolicyAndGuidance/DH_079931 (accessed July 2011).

NHS Institute for Innovation and Improvement, The Productive Series: http://www.institute.nhs.uk/quality_and_value/productivity_series/productive_ward.html (accessed July 2011).

Royal College of Nursing, Nutrition Now: http://www.rcn.org.uk/newsevents/campaigns/nutritionnow/tools_and_resources/workshop (accessed July 2011).

Answers

9.1. b

9.2. d

9.3. a

9.4. c

9.5. a, b, c and e

9.6. −ve 480 mL.

9.7. −ve 980 mL + −ve 480 mL = −ve 1460 mL.

9.8. Yes. Insensible loss will be more than 500 mL per day because he is tachypnoeic, pyrexial and sweating.

9.9. No. According to his age and weight, George needs between 1900 mL and 2280 mL fluid every 24 hours.

9.10. Yes. He is in a negative balance and could be losing vital electrolytes, which could cause complications.

9.11. Encourage George to drink, explain rationale, find out what George likes to drink, try to reduce pyrexia, discuss intravenous fluids with doctors.

9.12. Due to insensible loss and taking into account negative balance of around 1500 mL, the required fluid balance for his age and weight is at least 3 L over the next 24 hours.

10 Medicines management

CHAPTER AIMS

- To provide an overview of policy and procedure associated with medicines management
- To provide an Introduction to the commonest medicines used for patients in medical placements
- To consider how to assess the effect of the medicines administered
- To identify opportunities to develop knowledge and skills in medicines management throughout the patient journey

Introduction

Regardless of your field of nursing or year of training, you will have learning outcomes that focus on medicines management because it is one of the Nursing and Midwifery Council (NMC) Essential Skills Clusters (NMC 2010) from year 1 to entry to the register. Box 10.1 provides some examples of the Essential Skills Cluster – Medicines Management (NMC 2010).

In every ward you are placed on, all of your patients will have one thing in common – a prescription chart. Some patients will have very few medications prescribed while others may have more than one chart. Medications can be a daunting area for students and you may wonder when you should start to learn about medications.

You need to start being involved in administering medication to your individual patients as early as possible, or as appropriate to your individual course of study and practice requirements. Many medications you come across will belong to common groups of drugs, for example antibiotics, analgesics and cardiac drugs. You need to start learning some of the common medications used, side effects, cautions and routes. It can be quite nerve wracking at first and you may find that your hands shake as you try to dispense medications into the receptacle in front of a qualified nurse. You may also feel that you are very slow and that you are holding up your mentor and making patients wait.

You are not alone, but it is not something that should be rushed. It is essential that you know what you are doing and why you are doing it, and it must always be under supervision. If you have not yet covered this topic in theory at university, then please refer to the NMC, university and trust guidelines for the administration of medications.

Box 10.1 Examples of the Essential Skills Cluster – Medicines Management

At the end of the first year, a student nurse needs to be competent in medicines calculations for tablets, capsules, liquid medicines and injections and International System of Units (SI) conversion.

By the end of the third year, many skills are identified such as the following:

■ Drug pathways and how they act.
■ Related anatomy and physiology.
■ Observation and assessment.
■ Effects of medicines and other treatment options.
■ To meet standards for medicines management *(NMC 2010)*

 Activity

Read the NMC *Standards for Medicines Management* (2008a), your university and placement guidelines, and then discuss your role in medicines management with your mentor.

An example of the guidelines you might read about are:

■ Custody, prescribing and administration of medication.
■ Self-administration of medicines policy.
■ Medical devices policy.
■ Controlled drugs policy.
■ Injectable medicines policy.
■ Safe storage of medications.

 Activity

Find out where medicines are stored in your placement area and discuss the rationale for their storage with your mentor. An excellent insight learning day (spoke placement) is to spend a day with the pharmacist, who is very much the expert in both drug administration and the legal aspects of this.

Nurse prescribing and patient group directives

Within your medical placements you may be exposed to a range of nurses who have completed an advanced course in nurse prescribing. Only those who have undergone appropriate training and are registered with the NMC as an independent prescriber can prescribe (NMC 2006). It must also be judged that it is part of the nurse's role. Some clinical nurse specialists, advanced nurse practitioners, practice nurses, district nurses, health visitors and community matrons will have completed this course and will have undergone intensive supervision and academic assessment to meet the competencies required (Kaufman 2010).

 Activity

Ask your mentor if there are any practitioners within your area who are nurse prescribers and find out if you can spend some time with them to discuss their role and how it fits in with day-to-day medicine administration by nurses in placement.

Self-administration

In some of your medical placements, patients may be self-administering their medication and there should be a policy within the organisation that supports this practice. Nurses must assess that the patient is willing to do this, has the knowledge and is not forgetful or confused before self-administering their medication. It can work very effectively for patients as they do not need to wait for a nurse to administer their medication and they are able to have control over this aspect of their care. Within the essential skills clusters, there is an expectation that student nurses will 'involve people and carers in administration and self-administration of medicines' (NMC 2010) and from your second year this will be one of your learning outcomes under the supervision and guidance of your mentor.

There is also an assessment that can be undertaken when admitting or discharging a patient. Nurses can make arrangements for medication to be packaged in different ways to aid compliance. This can be arranged on discharge to allow health and social care practitioners within the community to help patients take their medicines. The NMC expects nurses to continually assess their patients regarding the appropriateness of the medication compliance aid. Patients who have been taking long-term medication are usually very knowledgeable about their medication. The following are examples of compliance aids:

- Blister packs: the medication is packaged with the days of the week highlighted.
- Dosette boxes: the medication will be placed in a box with separate compartments for days and times by a nurse to ensure that the patient does not get muddled about which medication to take and when. This is very helpful when a patient has multiple medications to take every day (Fig. 10.1).

 Activity

When a patient is being discharged from your placement (if in hospital), what arrangements can be made for a patient who needs help to administer their own medications? Who would you need to refer the patient to and what information would they require? What policies would support this?

Covert administration

Covert administration of medicines means administering medicines to your patient without their knowledge, for example disguising it in food or drink. This is not considered good practice (NMC 2008a). If your patient is refusing their medicines, it is important that you first establish why they do not want to take them. Often it will be because they don't know what they are or why they need to take them. Spending some time explaining the medicines and reassuring your patient may be all that is needed for your patient to agree to take their prescribed medicines.

Fig 10.1 Dosette box (Brooker C, Waugh A (2007) with permission)

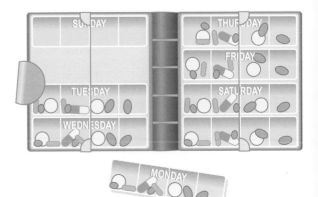

An interesting article for you to read: Griffith R, Griffiths H, Jordan S (2003). Administration of medicines part 1: the law and nursing. Nursing Standard 18 (2):47–51. Online. Available at: http://nursingstandard.rcnpublishing.co.uk/archive/article-administration-of-medicines-part-1-the-law-and-nursing (accessed July 2011).

If you are not sure about the medicines, use this as an opportunity to brush up on your own knowledge. Your patient may be having difficulty swallowing their tablets and it may be possible to order them in a different preparation, for example as a liquid. Crushing medication could also affect its metabolism/absorbance and may alter the affect of the drug. This could cause harm to the patient.

It may be that your patient does not understand the importance of the medicines and the potential side effects of not taking them. In this case, the team looking after the patient will need to determine if the patient has capacity to decide whether to take the medicines (see Ch. 6 for a discussion on capacity). Within the Essential Skills Clusters (NMC 2010) there is an expectation that 'people can trust the newly registered graduate nurse to work within the legal and ethical frameworks that underpin safe and effective medicines management'.

If it is decided that a patient does not have the capacity to make the decision, the multidisciplinary team, along with those who know the patient best (e.g. relatives/carers), must make a decision in the best interests of the patient and this may be to administer medicines covertly. If this is the case, how and when the medicines are given must be decided and documented clearly in the patient's notes. This decision must also be regularly reviewed.

As you progress in your nurse training, your learning outcomes will incorporate ethical issues in relation to medicines and consent. You will need to be able to demonstrate that you are aware of religious, cultural and ethical beliefs pertaining to medications and that you are sensitive to these issues.

This Website provides information to patients regarding Ramadan and there is a comprehensive section relating to medicines:

http://www.nhs.uk/Livewell/
healthyRamadan/Pages/
Healthyramadanhome.aspx (accessed July 2011).

 Activity

Have any patients been reluctant to take their medications within your placement areas? Discuss the actions that you have taken with your mentor.

The reasons patients give might include the following:

- Can't swallow tablets.
- Too many tablets.
- Feel sick or afraid of vomiting.
- Don't understand why they need them.
- Diuretics make them incontinent.
- Confusion.

Medicines management for controlled drugs

Since the fourth report of The Shipman Inquiry (2004) there has been tighter legislation in relation to controlled drugs, and nurses need to familiarise themselves with the latest NMC, Department of Health and local trust and university policies. As a student, you will be placed in a variety of placements – community, independent sector and acute sector trusts – and will need to make sure that you are aware of the placement policies regarding controlled drugs. The NMC (2008a) emphasises that student nurses must be involved in the administration of all medicines when they are deemed competent by a registrant and also feel confident and competent themselves. One of the essential skill outcomes states that 'people can trust the newly registered graduate nurse to safely order, receive, store and dispose of medicines (including controlled drugs) in any setting' (NMC 2010).

Controlled drugs are kept in a double-locked cupboard and the nurse in charge will hold a separate set of keys to this cupboard. These keys are not to be left on hooks in the office nor on the ward desk, but on the person of the key holder at all times.

The national guidance for drugs considered to be controlled drugs can be found here:

http://www.homeoffice.gov.uk/
publications/alcohol-drugs/drugs/drug-licences/controlled-drugs-list (accessed July 2011).

 Activity

Read the controlled drugs policy for the hospital you are placed in and note the role of the student nurse in the administration of controlled drugs. Compare this with your university administration of medicines policy, which you will have used in any clinical simulation activities concerning medicines management, and discuss this with your mentor.

❓ Quiz: management of controlled drugs

Here is a quiz to help you with the above activity.
(Answers on p. 197.)

10.1. Are student nurses allowed to give any medication without supervision?

10.2. Which of these policies do student nurses need to read and understand prior to taking part in drug administration?
   a. Medicines management (NMC 2008a)
   b. Administration of medicines (university guidelines)
   c. Policy for the custody and administration of medicines
   d. Fasting and medicines in Ramadan
   e. Policy for safe use of medical devices
   f. Injectables policy.

10.3. A staff nurse checks paracetamol with you in the clinical room and then asks you to take the medication to Mrs Smith in bed 8. Would you say yes or no? Explain your answer.

10.4. Mrs Patel is confused and refusing her antibiotic which she really needs. The staff nurse crushes the tablet and disguises it in a spoon of porridge and asks you to give this to the patient. Would you agree to this? Explain your answer.

10.5. Your patient requires a subcutaneous injection of insulin which the staff nurse allows you to draw up under his/her supervision. The staff nurse then takes you to the patient and allows you to administer the injection. Would you agree to do this? Explain your answer.

10.6. You have just undertaken a blood glucose measurement which is 10 mmol. The patient is on an insulin infusion which is currently running at 1 mL/hour. The prescription states that the infusion should run at 2 mL/hour if the blood glucose is 10 mmol. You inform the staff nurse and she tells you to increase the rate on the pump. Would you agree to do this? Explain your answer.

10.7. What is a controlled drug?

10.8. Who would need to be present when preparing and administering a controlled drug?
   a. Registered nurse and student nurse
   b. Registered nurse, healthcare assistant and student nurse
   c. Two registered nurses
   d. Two registered nurses and a student nurse
   e. Registered nurse and clinical assistant practitioner.

10.9. Where are controlled drugs kept?

10.10. Who has the keys for the controlled drugs?

10.11. When can a student nurse administer medications under supervision?
   a. First year
   b. Second year
   c. Third year.

10.12. A patient is prescribed 0.1 mg thyroxine. The registered nurse asks you to come along to observe. The nurse checks the medication against the prescription chart and then counts out $10 \times 100\ \mu g$ tablets. She asks you to come with her and administer them to the patient. What is your response?

As a student nurse, you will need to become involved with medications under the direct supervision of a registered nurse wherever you are placed. As a third year student nurse, you will be required to be assessed undertaking a medicines management assessment as part of your nursing programme. Details of medicines management assessments are given in Box 10.2.

This can seem daunting and you may feel that you already have enough to cope with,

---

Box 10.2 Medicines management assessments

- Prepare the medicines trolley or use patients' own dispensary appropriately.
- Check the prescription sheets and initially identify medication to be given at the prescribed time.
- Check that prescriptions are written in accordance with the medicines administration policy of the practice area.
- Check the medication for:
  - expiry date
  - correct time
  - dosage
  - route
  - signed
  - special instructions relating to its administration.
- Check for allergies:
  - check for allergies wristband
  - check prescription chart or notes for allergies.
- Explain details of side effects of medications to the assessor and explain how these side effects can be managed if they occur.
- Administer medication to patients with regard to the local medicines policies and NMC *Standards for Medicines Management* (2008).
- Ascertain the patient's understanding of the reasons for the administration of medications.
- Ensure that oral medicines have been ingested by the patient.
- Demonstrate/describe the actions to be taken in situations of non-compliance of patients with prescribed medication.
- Be able to give an account of the legislation governing the administration and storage of scheduled poisons and controlled drugs.
- Be able to discuss the role of the student nurse in the administration of controlled drugs.
- Be able to discuss and demonstrate the procedure to follow when administering blood and blood products.
- Be able to explain what the term 'patient group directive' means.

including exams, objective structured clinical examinations, assignments and practice-based assessments. It is important for you to consider what type of learner you are. There are many strategies for learning about medications. Some of the following may help:

- Make sure that you administer the medications for your group of patients according to trust, university and NMC guidelines. You will be doing this under the supervision of the registered nurse.
- Become involved with the administration of controlled drugs – make sure that you understand the policy for administering this medication. Who is able to sign the controlled drugs book? Who holds the keys to the controlled drug cupboard? Are the keys kept with the other medication keys or are they a separate bunch? How often do these medications need to be checked and by whom?
- Many patients will be given intravenous drugs. Make sure you look at and understand the policy for this and the training that is required for this procedure, as well as the rationale for the patient having to have these.
- When you administer medications to patients, do they have a right to be informed about each medication? Remember that they are partners in their care.
- Think about the dose, route, side effects and contraindications for the medications.
- Identify the different groups of drugs and three drugs that belong to each group. You will find that each group of drugs often has side effects in common.
- Maybe think of a mnemonic to help you learn the drug side effects.
- You could learn about three drugs a day and make notes about them.
- You may find it easier to link medications to patients' conditions.
- Try to find a book related to medicines that you find readable and easy to understand.

- Remember that everyone learns in a different way. Your mentor may also be able to give you advice.
- Ask your mentor to undertake a mock drug assessment with you. This could highlight your strengths and help you to understand where you need to develop.

 Activity

List the different routes of medication that can be administered and give examples of the routes and medication that you have been actively involved in administering within your practice area.

 Activity

Ask your mentor about administering drugs via a syringe driver. If possible, try to observe medication for a syringe driver being prepared by a staff nurse and see how the syringe driver is set up with the patient.

Determine what key skills are required to prepare and administer this kind of medication. If you are a third-year student, it may be appropriate for some of these to be included in your learning outcomes (see Further reading list for clinical skills texts that may be useful).

Drug calculations

It is really important to ensure that you are competent and accurate when undertaking calculations for medications. If you get the dose wrong, this could harm the patient – too low a dose could be ineffective and too high a dose could be toxic.

Drug calculations need practice and it is important that you let your mentor know if this is something you struggle with. Mentors can only help if they know what you need help with. Many nurses worry about calculations. They may not be natural mathematicians! However, calculations are something you can learn. If you know the formula, then you can work out the dose for the medication. You are never alone on a ward and there is always someone to check your calculation with.

You will find the following books helpful for drug calculations:

Downie G, Mackenzie J, Williams A (2011). Calculating drug doses safely. A handbook for nurses and midwives, 2nd ed. Churchill Livingstone, Edinburgh

Lapham R, Agar H (2009). Drug calculations for nurses: a step-by-step approach, 3rd ed. Hodder Arnold, London.

Acknowledging our limitations is part of the NMC Code (2008b), however there is a level of competence that needs to be achieved by a registered nurse before they can administer medications. Once you qualify, you will find that this competence is frequently tested by organisations to ensure patient safety.

Within all fields of nursing, the essential skills clusters expect student nurses to be competent in 'basic medicines calculations relating to: tablets and capsules, liquid medicines, injections including unit dose, sub-and multiple unit dose and SI unit conversion'.

Calculating drug dosages

Here are some common formulae used in calculations. (Refer to Table 10.1 for a list of common abbreviations and concentrations.)

Calculating amount of a solution needed to obtain a prescribed dose

Working out the amount of a solution you need to obtain the prescribed dose is achieved using the following formulae:

$$\frac{\text{dose prescribed}}{\text{dose in stock ampoule}} \times \text{volume of solution}$$

Table 10.1 Abbreviations and concentrations

Abbreviations	
g	gram
mg	milligrams
mcg/µg	micrograms
ng	nanograms
L	litre
mL	millilitre
mmol	millimole

Concentrations	
1 g	1000 mg
1 mg	1000 mcg
1 mcg	1000 ng

Calculating intravenous infusion rates
Giving sets
- Standard giving sets deliver 20 drops per mL.
- Blood giving sets deliver 15 drops per mL.
- Burettes/paediatric giving sets deliver 60 drops per mL.

Formula for calculating drops per minute:

$$\frac{\text{drip rate}}{\text{per minute}} = \frac{\begin{array}{c}\text{volume of} \\ \text{infusion (mL)}\end{array} \times \begin{array}{c}\text{no. of drops per} \\ \text{mL of giving set}\end{array}}{\text{infusion time in minutes}}$$

Calculating concentrations of drugs in solution

To work out the concentration of a solution (i.e. how many mg there are per mL), we use the following formula:

$$\frac{\text{quantity of drug in solution}}{\text{volume of solution}} = \text{mg/mL}$$

Working out the amount of drug in a solution

Some drugs that are presented in a 'percentage' solution will have the amount of drug per mL stated, either on the ampoule or in the accompanying literature. However, the following formula can be used to work out the amount of drug present in a given volume of fluid when it is presented in a percentage form:

(% of solution × 1000) ÷ 100 = mg/mL

Drug dosages in ratios

Some concentrations of drugs are presented as ratios (e.g. adrenaline (epinephrine) is available in concentrations of 1:1000 and 1:10 000):

- A 1:1000 solution means that 1 g is dissolved in 1000 mL.
- Therefore, 1000 mg are dissolved in 1000 mL.
- Therefore, 1 mg is dissolved in 1 mL.

The following formula can also be used:

(1 ÷ the ratio) × 1000 = mg/mL

What knowledge of medications is required?

Apart from the calculations, you need to consider the medications that are commonly used on your medical placements. For entry to the register, you will need to apply 'knowledge of basic pharmacology, how medicines act and interact in the systems of the body and their therapeutic action' (NMC 2010). It is easier to start with groups of medications, and the list in Box 10.3 is by no means exhaustive.

Once you have sorted out the groups of medications, specify the actual medications that are used on your ward. You need to know the general doses, routes and side effects of the drugs.

Box 10.3 Groups of medications

Cardiac drugs	Antiemetics
Diuretics	Vitamins
Antibiotics	Sedatives
Analgesics	Antituberculosis
Laxatives	Anticoagulants
Respiratory drugs	Steroids
Hypoglycaemics	Antidepressants
Bronchodilators	

Quiz

Ask yourself the following questions about the bronchodilator salbutamol.
(Answers on p. 197.)

10.13. What is the action of bronchodilators?

10.14. What routes can you use to administer salbutamol?

10.15. What is the usual dose for a salbutamol nebuliser?

10.16. What are the side effects of salbutamol?

10.17. What health problem is salbutamol commonly used for?

 ### Activity

Consider the action of antibiotics: what are they commonly used for?

Common antibiotics include amoxicillin, cefuroxime, ciprofloxacin, metronidazole, vancomycin and gentamicin. It is important to check blood levels prior to administration and to reduce the dose in renal failure.

Side effects include diarrhoea, allergy, rash, nausea, vomiting and anaphylaxis. It is imperative to know how to treat anaphylaxis as this is a medical emergency.

Quiz: medications

(Answers on p. 197.)

10.18. What are the side effects of opiates?

10.19. What two observations should you look at before administering cardiac drugs?

10.20. What are the side effects of antibiotics?

10.21. Name four groups of laxatives.

10.22. What groups do the following drugs belong to?
   a. metoclopramide
   b. furosemide
   c. prednisone
   d. salbutamol
   e. gliclazide
   f. flucloxacillin
   g. diclofenac
   h. morphine
   i. cyclizine.

10.23. What do you need to consider if a patient is on long-term steroids? What impact might this have on your nursing care?

10.24. What information might a patient who is taking salbutamol require?

10.25. Are there any special requirements for patients who are taking vancomycin or gentamicin?

10.26. What blood test do patients who are taking warfarin require and what is the antidote?

10.27. When, in relation to food, do you give a patient flucloxacillin?

Medicines management is an essential skill or nurses, and wherever you are in your placement you will be involved in the administration of medications under the supervision of a registered nurse. Despite all of the policies, guidance and knowledge for the administration of medications, errors still occur.

 Activity

> Discuss with your mentor what actions a nurse would need to take if they made an error in administering a medication.

The following article may be of help:

Jones SW (2009). Reducing medication administration errors in nursing practice. Nursing Standard 23(50):40–46.

Assessing the effect of medication you have given

When you are undertaking the administration of medicines during your medical placement, you will more than likely be administering analgesia to your patients. If a patient is prescribed analgesia, should you, as the nurse, administer it just because it is prescribed or should you assess the patient prior to administering the medication? This will provide your patient with an opportunity to tell you about any pain they are experiencing and will empower them to take an active role in their management. It is important that you understand how the patient is feeling prior to administering analgesia so that you can understand how effective the analgesia has been and document this. It can be difficult to assess pain in those who cannot respond verbally, however there can be physiological changes in respiration, blood pressure and pulse rate, nausea and sweating. Visually, the patient's body language, emotions or facial expression could also indicate that they are in pain. There are various pain assessment tools available including verbal descriptors, numerical rating scales and visual analogue scales that can help you to assess and evaluate pain.

When administering analgesia, it is important to think about the following:

- How much pain is the patient experiencing? Measure and record it in the nursing notes.
- Does the analgesia you are administering take the pain away?
- Could you offer anything else – repositioning, heat?
- Is the patient requesting analgesia before the next dose is due?
- Is the patient experiencing any side effects that you can help to reduce, e.g. offering aperients for constipation?

Refer to the example of visual analogue used at Newham University Hospital NHS Trust (Fig. 10.2).

Case history 10.1

You are looking after a 74-year-old man who is rehabilitating on an intermediate care ward recovering from pneumonia, which has left him very weak. You are about to administer his medicines under the supervision of a registered nurse. He is prescribed digoxin 125 μg once a day and bisoprolol 10 mg once a day. Before you administer the digoxin, you take his pulse and find that it is 52 bpm. What should you do?

(Answer on p. 198.)

Case history 10.2

Mrs Wells is a 73-year-old lady who is rehabilitating on a stroke unit. She has diabetes and usually takes three short-acting insulin injections a day and a longer acting insulin at night. At handover, the night staff inform you and your mentor that they have not been able to give the night dose of insulin because her blood sugar has been very low, requiring the patient to have sugary drinks and snacks. The doctor was informed overnight. The blood sugar prior to breakfast is within normal limits. Your mentor asks you about the actions that need to be taken by a registered nurse.

(Answers on p. 198.)

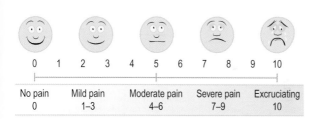

Fig 10.2 Example of visual analogue to help assess and evaluate pain used at Newham University Hospital NHS Trust

| No pain 0 | Mild pain 1–3 | Moderate pain 4–6 | Severe pain 7–9 | Excruciating 10 |

Summary

In this chapter you have explored the policies and procedures in relation to medicines management and considered the commonest medicines that your medical patients may have been prescribed. The role of the nurse in the administration of medicines is an important one and keeping up to date during your career is a must. Medication policies change and it is important that you always read and check the medicines policies in each placement area. You will become more confident and knowledgeable throughout your training but you will never know everything there is to know about medicines, as medical research continues to develop new medicines.

References

Brooker, C., Waugh, A., 2007. Foundations of nursing practice: fundamentals of holistic care. Mosby, Edinburgh.

Kaufman, G., 2010. Developing patient group directions for medicines management. Nursing Standard 24 (48), 50–56.

Nursing and Midwifery Council, 2006. Standards of proficiency for nurse and midwife prescribers. NMC, London.

Nursing and Midwifery Council, 2008a. Standards for medicines management. NMC, London.

Nursing and Midwifery Council, 2008b. The code: standards of conduct, performance and ethics for nurses and midwives. NMC, London.

Nursing and Midwifery Council, 2010. Essential skills clusters. NMC, London.

The Shipman Inquiry, 2004. Fourth report. The regulation of controlled drugs in the community. Department of Health, London. Online. Available at: http://www.shipman-inquiry.org.uk/reports.asp.

Further reading

Bennett, J., Dawoud, D., Maben, J., 2010. Effects of interruptions to nurses during medication administration. Nursing Manage 16 (9), 22–23.

Crocker, C., 2009. Following the patient journey to improve medicines management and reduce errors. Nursing Times 105 (46), 12–15.

Dougherty, L., 2002. Delivery of intravenous therapy. Nursing Standard 16 (16), 45–52.

Elliot, M., Liu, Y., 2010. The nine rights of medication administration. British Journal of Nursing 19 (5), 300–305.

Hyde, L., 2002. Legal and professional aspects of intravenous therapy. Nursing Standard 16 (26), 39–42.

Jenkins, K., Kirk, M., 2010. Heart failure and chronic kidney disease: an integrated approach. Renal Care 36, 127–135.

Jordan, S., Griffiths, H., Griffith, R.A., 2003. Administration of medicines part 2: pharmacology. Nursing Standard 18 (3), 45–54.

Kirby, M., 2008. A spoonful of sugar: helping older patients to take their medicines. British Journal of Primary Care Nursing: Cardiovascular Disease and Diabetes 5 (1), 21–23.

McIntosh, K., 2008. Medicines management. Nursing Times 104 (44), 18–20.

Tingle, J., 2010. Patient safety and health quality: recent reports from the CQC. British Journal of Nursing 19 (7), 45–55.

Nursing and Midwifery Council, 2010. Standards for pre-registration nursing education. NMC, London.

Answers

10.1. No.

10.2. All of them.

10.3. No, because you need the staff nurse to witness and supervise you to ensure that the medication is given to the correct patient.

10.4. No, for two reasons: i) disguising medication is not considered good practice by the NMC (2008a); ii) crushing the medication may alter the therapeutic properties of the medication.

10.5. Yes, if you are competent and the patient consents.

10.6. No, because as a student nurse you are not allowed to administer medications unsupervised.

10.7. Some prescription medicines contain drugs that are controlled under the Misuse of Drugs legislation. These are called controlled drugs.

10.8. Depending on the organisation this can vary, but if there are two registered nurses available, they should check the controlled drug with the student nurse as witness. Always check your university and organisational policy in relation to controlled drugs.

10.9. Controlled drugs are kept in a double-locked cupboard

10.10. The nurse in charge

10.11. a

10.12. No, because this would be a drug error – 0.1 mg thyroxine = 100 μg thyroxine, therefore only one tablet is required.

10.13. Bronchodilators cause the bronchi to dilate.

10.14. Oral, inhaler, IV.

10.15. 2.5–5 mg via a nebuliser, repeated up to 4 times a day.

10.16. Tachycardia, arrhythmia, headache, nausea, gastric irritation.

10.17. Asthma.

10.18. Commonly respiratory depression, constipation, itchiness, nausea, vomiting.

10.19. Blood pressure and pulse.

10.20. Anaphylactic shock, rash, diarrhoea, nausea and vomiting at toxic levels.

10.21. Osmotic, bulk forming, enemas, suppositories and stimulating.

10.22.

       a. metoclopramide: antiemetic.
       b. furosemide: loop diuretic.
       c. prednisone: steroid.
       d. salbutamol: bronchodilator.
       e. gliclazide: oral hypoglycaemic.
       f. flucloxacillin: antibiotic.
       g. diclofenac: non-steroidal anti-inflammatory.

      h. morphine: opiate.

      i. cyclizine: antihistamine.

10.23. Cushings syndrome, diabetes, gastric ulceration, thinning of the skin, hypertension, Addison's crisis.

- You would assess the patient for any history of gastric ulceration/irritation prior to administering steroids. If this is a problem for the patient, a proton pump inhibitor could then be prescribed by the doctor to prevent this side effect and maybe enteric-coated steroids prescribed.

- Check urinalysis for glucose.

- Weigh the patient to assess if the patient has gained weight and ask if they have noticed any changes in their appearance.

- Check blood pressure.

- Patient information and health education: the patient should be informed about the need to reduce steroids gradually under the supervision of a doctor to prevent Addison's crisis.

10.24.

- The action of the medication.

- Help with their inhaler technique or what to do with their nebuliser mask once the medication has finished.

- Side effects that they might experience: palpitations, tremors, headaches, anxiety.

- Peak flow: technique, information, peak flow diary.

10.25. Blood levels need to be taken to prevent toxic levels building up. Doctors usually need to gain microbiology consent prior to prescribing these.

10.26. The International normalised ratio test (INR). The antidote to warfarin is vitamin K, given in tablet or injectable form.

10.27. 30 minutes before food.

Case history 10.1 After discussion and under the supervision of a registered nurse, you could do the following. Omit both medicines for the time being, as both will reduce the heart rate, and contact the doctor to determine what she would like you to do. Ensure that the patient is kept fully informed and that every action you take is documented accurately in the nursing notes. The doctor may prescribe a lower dose of digoxin and ask you to omit the beta blocker, or she may ask you to omit both for today and say that they will review the patient on the ward round. Your role is to understand how the medications could affect your patient and inform the doctor if you feel that administering them might be contraindicated.

Case history 10.2 Ensure the patient has her breakfast, administer insulin for the morning and contact the diabetic nurse specialist and doctor to review the blood sugar. Ask the patient how she is feeling. Document any actions you take in the nursing notes and keep the patient informed of what is going on with her medication.

11 Medical investigations and medical day care

CHAPTER AIMS

- To understand the role of medical investigations and day care in the care of the medical patient
- To follow the journey through admission, procedure, recovery and home
- To understand the role of the nurse and other professionals within medical investigations
- To identify learning opportunities within medical day care/investigation units

Introduction

For your medical nursing learning experience you may find yourself placed in a medical day care unit or investigations unit. This may be for the whole of your placement or for a short period of time as an insight learning day or a longer 'spoke' placement. However long you will spending in the day care/investigation unit, it will be a great opportunity to care for a wide variety of patients with differing medical problems and experience the many roles of the nurse within the unit.

This chapter will start by explaining what medical investigations and medical day care are and will then take you through the journey of two patients attending a medical day unit – one to undergo a medical investigation and the other to receive medical treatment – and how you can meet your learning outcomes and identify learning opportunities with such patients.

What are medical investigations?

Many patients will be attending the unit to undergo investigations. The aim of these investigations will be to diagnose patients' problems so that they can receive appropriate treatment and care. In some ways, a medical investigation is similar to day surgery in that the patient will be admitted on the day of the procedure, usually be sedated or anaesthetised to undergo the procedure and then, after a period of recovery, discharged, again usually on the same day. The difference between medical investigations and day surgery is that medical investigations are usually diagnostic procedures compared to day surgery which is usually a treatment or a surgical intervention for an already diagnosed problem.

What is medical day care?

Patients attending medical day care will be receiving medical treatment for an ongoing medical problem. They may just attend on one occasion for treatment or may attend on a number of occasions over the course of a few days, weeks or months.

Where does medical day care take place?

Medical day care/investigation units are usually based within a hospital as they require access to theatres, radiology and pharmacy, among other departments that are generally hospital based. They can be found within both NHS and independent health services. The units usually operate on a 5-day, Monday to Friday basis and their hours will usually be from 7 or 8 a.m. to 8 or 9 p.m. Patients attending the unit can be out-patients or in-patients from other areas of the hospital. The out-patients will be admitted from their place of residence, for example home, intermediate care or nursing home, on the day of their investigation or treatment and then be discharged back to their place of residence from the unit on the same day once everything is completed. Some of the investigations carried out in the unit will be necessary investigations for in-patients on the wards as well. So patients will be brought from the ward at a specific time to have their investigation in the unit. Their preparation and recovery will take place on the ward they are staying on. If your placement is on a medical ward, intermediate care or a nursing home, then see if it is possible to arrange to accompany a patient who is going to the day care unit for an investigation.

 Activity

> Find the operational policy for the unit you are placed in. This will give you information on the types of patients seen, how they are referred to the unit and how the unit operates on a day-to-day basis. From this, you will be able to begin to plan some of your learning outcomes for your placement. The text by Howatson-Jones and Ellis (2008) provides good information on the range of settings medical day care may take place in along with the role of the nurse in these settings.

The journey through the medical day care and investigation unit

This section will take you through the journey of a patient attending a medical investigation unit using a case history approach. You will be encouraged to consider what the patient's needs may be and the role of the nurse in meeting these needs at each stage of their journey.

Medical investigations

Mr Murray is a 42-year-old bank manager who has been suffering from severe heartburn for the last month. He has tried over-the-counter indigestion remedies and they have had no effect. He recently had a shoulder injury from playing tennis and has been taking anti-inflammatory medication for pain relief. Over the last couple of days he has noticed that his stools have been black.

Before admission

Mr Murray makes an appointment to see his GP regarding the severe heartburn (epigastric pain) he has been experiencing.

After taking a full history, his GP is concerned that Mr Murray may be suffering from a peptic ulcer which may be bleeding, resulting in the black-coloured stool. To ensure Mr Murray receives the appropriate treatment, he will require a diagnostic gastroscopy. His GP writes to the gastroenterologist at his local hospital explaining the history of Mr Murray's problems and requesting a gastroscopy as an out-patient. He also arranges for Mr Murray to have a series of blood tests and commences him on a medicine called a proton pump inhibitor to begin treatment for a suspected peptic ulcer.

A few days later Mr Murray receives an appointment to attend the medical investigations unit at his local hospital for a gastroscopy in 3 weeks' time. He is required to be at the unit for 8 a.m. and he has been instructed not to eat or drink anything for 6 hours prior to this. He will also need to stop taking the medication prescribed to him by the GP 2 weeks before his appointment. He has a leaflet explaining more about a diagnostic gastroscopy to read. He is also asked to attend a pre-admission assessment appointment in 1 week's time. He has never been admitted to hospital or needed to attend hospital as an out-patient before.

Pre-admission assessment

Two weeks prior to his procedure, Mr Murray attends for his pre-admission assessment appointment. This is held at the out-patient department of his local hospital. A nurse conducts the pre-admission interview. The nurse talks through the history of Mr Murray's current health problem and asks about any previous medical history or other health problems that he currently has. The nurse also checks his blood pressure, pulse, temperature and respiratory rate. This is to help determine Mr Murray's suitability to undergo the procedure. The nurse then explains to Mr Murray what will happen on the day of the procedure, including what time he needs to be there and where to report to. She advises him about stopping eating and drinking 6 hours prior to admission and reminds him that he should now stop taking his proton pump inhibitor tablets. There is then an opportunity for Mr Murray to ask any questions he has about the procedure and coming into hospital.

The purpose of the pre-admission appointment is to help determine that the patient is medically stable to undergo the procedure and also to provide information to the patient, which will lessen the chance of them not attending on the day due to anxiety or fear. It also enables the nurses to plan for any particular needs the patient may have on the day of the procedure, such as hospital transport or special dietary requirements. These consultations can be carried out by doctors but are often done by nurses and can also be done over the telephone.

 Activity

What do you know about diagnostic gastroscopy? If you were Mr Murray, what questions might you have about the procedure?

Look at the following Website regarding diagnostic gastroscopy to learn more about what it is and why it is carried out:

http://www.nhs.uk/Conditions/ Diagnosticendoscopyofthestomach/ Pages/Introduction.aspx (accessed July 2011).

The following link contains a short video of a nurse explaining a pre-operative assessment, which would be similar to the one Mr Murray attended:

http://www.nhs.uk/nhsengland/ aboutnhsservices/nhshospitals/pages/ going-into-hospital.aspx (accessed July 2011).

On the day of admission

Mr Murray arrives at the medical investigation unit at 8 a.m. on the day of his gastroscopy. He has had nothing to eat or drink since the following evening. On arrival, he is greeted by a nurse and shown to a cubicle area with a trolley and a chair, and the nurse explains that she will return shortly to admit Mr Murray.

 Activity

Think back to the admission of a patient discussed in Chapter 5. What aspects of the admission process do you think are likely to apply to an admission to a medical investigation unit?

When the nurse returns, she begins by checking Mr Murray's personal details, name, address, date of birth and the contact details for his next of kin. She then takes a set of observations – blood pressure, pulse, temperature, respirations and oxygen saturations – to establish a baseline and to ensure that Mr Murray is in a fit condition for the investigation. Once these are recorded, she explains what will happen during the day. She explains the procedure to Mr Murray and asks if he has any concerns or questions. The nurse also checks that someone will be able to collect Mr Murray after his procedure as he will not be able to drive following his sedation and should not be alone overnight following the

 Reflection point

How might a person who has never been in hospital before feel when attending a day unit for a procedure? What anxieties and concerns may they have and how could you, as the nurse caring for them, alleviate some of these anxieties and concerns?

sedation. Mr Murray's admission may also include him being weighed, as the dose of some sedatives is calculated based on the weight of the patient.

Good communication skills are essential when caring for patients attending for an investigative procedure. Patients need to feel reassured and confident in the skills and knowledge of the health professionals caring for them. You will have learning outcomes or competencies regarding communication as it is one of the Nursing and Midwifery Council (NMC) Domains and an integral part of the NMC (2010a) Essential Skills Clusters – care, compassion and communication. For example, it is expected that you will do the following:

- Respect patients as individuals and strive to help them preserve their dignity at all times.
- Engage with patients in a warm, sensitive and compassionate way.
- Engage therapeutically and actively listen to patients' needs and concerns, responding using skills that are helpful, providing information that is clear, accurate, meaningful and free from jargon.
- Gain patients' consent based on sound understanding and informed choice prior to any intervention and that their rights in decision making and consent will be respected and upheld.

The following two articles, although written about day surgery, illustrate the need to develop a therapeutic relationship with your patient even though they are with you for a short length of time:

Rogan Foy C, Timmins F (2004). Improving communication in day surgery settings. Nursing Standard 19(7):37–42.

Mitchell M (2010). A patient-centred approach to day surgery. Nursing Standard 24(44):40–46.

The next person to see Mr Murray is the consultant gastroenterologist who will carry out the gastroscopy. He has come to complete Mr Murray's consent form with him.

Consent

For all medical or surgical procedures, from a blood test to major surgery, a person must first give consent. Consent must be both voluntary and informed. To be voluntary means that the person must make the decision whether or not to consent by themselves and not do so under pressure from anyone else; their doctor, family or friends. To be informed, the person must be given full information about what they are consenting to and involves the risks, the benefits, possible alternatives and what might happen if the procedure is not done. The person must also be capable or have the capacity to make the decision to consent or not (Department of Health 2009).

The following guidance for health professionals and patients on consent for treatment will be useful for you to read:
Department of Health (2001). Consent – what you have a right to expect. A guide for adults. DH, London.
Department of Health (2009). Reference guide to consent for examination or treatment, 2nd edn. DH London.

 Activity

Refresh your knowledge of the Mental Capacity Act (2005) as discussed in Chapter 6. It is important that you understand how capacity is assessed, to know that your patient has the capacity to consent to a procedure. The Department of Health reference guide cited above contains information about consent and capacity (see also Further reading list).

The doctor also discusses with Mr Murray how he will be sedated for the procedure. In gastroscopy, the level of sedation given is usually dependent on the patient, how anxious they are and how medically stable they are to receive sedation. Unlike a surgical procedure, there is rarely an anaesthetist present during a medical investigation unless the patent requires a full anaesthetic. For information about anaesthetics, refer to a specialist textbook.

Mr Murray is given the option of having a local anaesthetic spray to the back of his throat or an intravenous sedative to make him drowsy so that he will have little or no recollection of the procedure. As he has never been in hospital before, he is very anxious about the procedure so he opts for the sedative. A common sedative used in short procedures such as a gastroscopy is midazolam (see Skelly & Palmer, 2003 for information about conscious sedation).

 Activity

Using the online *British National Formulary* (BNF), look up midazolam and other similar sedatives that could be used. Take note of their side effects. What implications will this have for the care Mr Murray will receive once the procedure is completed?
http://www.bnf.org (accessed July 2011). (This site requires you to register once and then log in on subsequent visits, but registration is free and open to anyone.)

Once Mr Murray has signed his consent form, he now has to wait until it is his turn to go into the endoscopy suite for the procedure. As he waits, the nurse inserts an intravenous cannula into the back of his left hand using an aseptic technique. This is essential to reduce the risk of infection, both locally to the cannula site (phlebitis) but also systemically (septicaemia) (Brooker 2007). The cannula will be used to administer the sedative medication. (See Ch. 9 for more information on the care of a peripheral intravenous cannula).

 Reflection point

> Think how it feels to sit and wait for a procedure you are anxious about. What might make it easier for the patient who is anxiously waiting?

During the procedure

While you are on placement in a medical investigations unit or if you have the opportunity to accompany a patient to the unit to undergo a procedure, make sure you get the chance to be in the room while the procedure takes place. Speak to your mentor about the most appropriate place to stand to observe the procedure or, if you feel able, what role you could play in caring for the patient during the procedure. It is important that you gain the patient's consent to be present during their procedure.

There are likely to be a number of people in the room with the patient:

- The doctor or nurse endoscopist (a registered nurse who has undergone specialist training to perform gastroscopies) performing the procedure.
- A registered nurse who will be monitoring the patient's condition throughout the procedure.
- Another person who could be a registered nurse but could also be a healthcare assistant, clinical assistant practitioner or a technician who will be assisting with the preparation and cleaning of the equipment.
- A member of the team will also be documenting what is done during the procedure and the equipment used, and also receiving and preparing any specimens, e.g. tissue biopsies, to be sent to the laboratory.

Throughout the procedure, Mr Murray's pulse and oxygen saturations are monitored continuously to detect any possible complications. The nurse monitoring him will also check his respiratory rate and speak to him to reassure him and explain what is happening. Although he is sedated and is unlikely to remember the procedure, he may to some extent be aware of what is happening at the time and, as the procedure can be uncomfortable, he will require reassurance.

 Activity

> Speak to, and try to spend some time with, each member of the team during a gastroscopy or similar procedure to understand their role more fully.

Mr Murray's gastroscopy was completed successfully and confirmed that Mr Murray did have a peptic ulcer.

Post-procedure

Once the procedure is complete, Mr Murray is transferred back to the day unit to recover.

 Activity

> What do you think would be the role of the nurse in Mr Murray's recovery?

It will take a little while for Mr Murray to recover from the sedation he has had and he may sleep for a time after returning to the unit. The role of the nurse is important in monitoring his status and ensuring he recovers safely from the sedation and procedure, and to detect any complications early on.

Table 11.1 shows the nursing actions that are likely to form part of Mr Murray's post-procedure care plan and some placement areas may have specific documentation to record post-procedure care.

Table 11.1 Nursing actions likely to form part of Mr Murray's post-procedure care plan

Nursing action	Rationale
Mr Murray to be nursed on his side with oxygen if required	To maintain a patent airway while recovering from sedation
Record temperature, respiration rate, pulse, blood pressure and oxygen saturations at regular intervals and complete early warning score	To identify early signs of deterioration
Assess skin pallor and capillary refill	
Speak calmly to Mr Murray and reassure and orientate him as he begins to wake up from the sedation	To orientate him to his surroundings and relieve anxiety
Assess his level of comfort and pain	To identify possible complications and ensure he is comfortable and pain free
When Mr Murray is fully awake, encourage him to drink NB: if a patient has had a local anaesthetic spray to the back of their throat, they may need to wait a certain length of time before they can drink and need to be aware not to take hot fluids This should be documented in their notes by the endoscopist	To ensure he is able to drink comfortably and without problems

Mr Murray recovers from the procedure without complications and is able to have a drink before he leaves the unit. His intravenous cannula is removed. The nurse inspects his cannula site for signs of phlebitis such as redness or inflammation, infiltration (where fluid has infused into the surrounding tissue rather than the vein) and extravasation (where infiltration has occurred resulting in severe tissue damage such as necrosis). As none of these signs are present, the nurse applies a dry dressing and records this in his notes. (For more information on the complications of IV therapy, see Brooker 2007.)

The doctor who performed the procedure comes to speak to him before he is discharged to explain the results and to tell Mr Murray that he should continue on the proton pump inhibitor medication prescribed by his GP. The nurse who has been caring for him gives him an information leaflet about peptic ulcer disease and a leaflet about aftercare from a gastroscopy, explaining what to expect and who to contact if he has any concerns. His wife arrives to collect him and he is discharged from the unit.

A letter explaining the procedure results and ongoing care required will be sent to Mr Murray's GP to ensure his aftercare is appropriate. He will not need to see the consultant at the hospital again.

Medical day care

This section follows the journey of a patient attending the medical day care unit for a blood transfusion.

Mrs Singh is a 69-year-old widow who lives with her son and daughter-in-law. She has chronic kidney disease, diabetes and microcytic anaemia and her long-term conditions are monitored at home by a community matron who sees her once a week. Following a routine set of blood tests, her community matron informs her that her haemoglobin is 7 and she needs to attend the day care unit to receive a blood transfusion. The community matron has liaised with her GP and the consultant haematologist at the hospital who manages Mrs Singh's condition to arrange for Mrs Singh to be booked into the day unit in a few days' time.

Mrs Singh has attended the day unit for blood transfusions in the past so is familiar with where the unit is and what happens when she gets there. As her family are out at work during the day, the community matron arranges for the hospital transport service to collect Mrs Singh from home to take her to the unit.

On admission

On arrival at the hospital, the ambulance driver takes Mrs Singh to the medical day care unit where she is greeted by a nurse and taken to a recliner chair where she will sit while she receives her transfusion.

 Activity

> What is the nurse likely to ask Mrs Singh as part of her admission process?

The nurse checks Mrs Singh's personal details, name, date of birth and address and her next of kin details. She has Mrs Singh's medical notes so is aware of her previous medical history but checks and records what medications Mrs Singh is currently taking. Mrs Singh has brought her medicines with her and she tells the nurse which medicines

she is due to take while she is at the day unit. Mrs Singh's admission may also include her being weighed and providing a urine specimen for the nurse to perform a urine dipstick test on, to detect any possible problems such as a urine infection.

A doctor from the haematology team comes to see Mrs Singh, takes a history and performs a physical examination to ensure she is fit to receive the transfusion and there are no other problems that need to be addressed.

The nurse takes a set of observations to act as a baseline before she commences her blood transfusion and then inserts an intravenous cannula. She explains to Mrs Singh the process of the transfusion and answers any questions she may have. As Mrs Singh is familiar with the process of having a blood transfusion, she does not have any concerns about it.

 Activity

> If a patient has not received a blood transfusion before, what concerns or questions do you think they may have? Revise your own knowledge about what a blood transfusion is and how it works by looking at this Website: http://www.nhs.uk/conditions/Blood-transfusion/Pages/Introduction.aspx (accessed July 2011).

Not all people are happy to receive blood transfusions due to personal feelings and beliefs and also religious beliefs. It is well known that many Jehovah's witnesses do not believe in receiving blood transfusions. As nurses, it is important that we respect and try to understand what our patients' concerns about blood transfusion may be. In the NMC (2010b) Domain, Professional Values, it states that:

> *All nurses must practise in a holistic, non-judgmental, caring and sensitive manner*

that supports social inclusion and recognises and respects diversity and the beliefs, rights and wishes of individuals of all ages, groups and communities. Where necessary, they must challenge inequality, discrimination or exclusion from access to care.

 Activity

Spend some time finding out how culture and religion may influence a person's beliefs about their health and wellbeing. 'Cultural awareness in nursing and healthcare' (Holland and Hogg, 2010) is a good introductory text to read. The following Website may also have useful resources for you to look at: http://ethnomed.org/ (accessed July 2011).

Patients may have many different beliefs about their health and illness that are connected to their cultural and religious beliefs.

Mrs Singh's transfusion

Table 11.2 outlines the plan of care for Mrs Singh during her blood transfusion.

Being able to identify a deteriorating patient is an essential skill that you will need to develop. As you progress through your training, you are likely to have learning outcomes and competencies about monitoring a patient's condition and detecting a change in a patient's condition. The NMC (2010a) Essential Skills Cluster, Medicines Management, will also be relevant as blood is classed as a drug and should be administered and monitored as such.

Table 11.2 Plan of care for Mrs Singh during her blood transfusion

Nursing action	Rationale
Check that the blood has been prescribed correctly	To avoid error in identification and administration of blood
Explain the rationale for the transfusion to Mrs Singh and gain her consent to receive the transfusion	To reassure her and give an opportunity to ask any questions. Verbal consent must be gained before any blood transfusion
Ask Mrs Singh to state her name and date of birth – check this against the blood and the prescription	Pre-transfusion checks should take place at the patient's bedside/chair. Use of open-ended questions to check identity prevents the patient saying 'yes' to a question they may not have heard or understood
Check the blood group, unit number and expiry date on the blood unit. Check the quality of the unit	To ensure that the blood is the correct type, has not expired and has not been damaged
Check the name, date of birth and hospital number on the patient's ID band against the demographics on the blood unit	To ensure the right unit of blood is being given to the right patient

Continued

Table 11.2 Plan of care for Mrs Singh during her blood transfusion—cont'd

Nursing action	Rationale
A second staff member checks the name, date of birth and hospital number on the patient's ID band against the demographics on the blood unit, independently of the first checker	Two members of staff must check to avoid error Checks must be made independently to avoid staff relying on each other to check the details
Carry out a baseline set of vital signs	
Wash hands using six-stage technique and dry thoroughly Wearing gloves, prime the giving set and start the transfusion according to the prescription	To reduce the incidence of infection when manipulating the cannula
Explain to Mrs Singh the importance of alerting staff if she begins to feel unwell	To aid the early identification of a transfusion reaction
Observe Mrs Singh throughout the transfusion for signs of a reaction – fever, chills, tachycardia, hyper- or hypotension, collapse, rigors, flushing, urticaria, bone, muscle, chest and/or abdominal pain, shortness of breath, nausea, generally feeling unwell, respiratory distress Stop transfusion immediately if she has a transfusion reaction and contact medical team	To aid the early identification of a transfusion reaction
Monitor and record vital signs as per hospital policy	Blood pressure, temperature, pulse and respirations should be measured pre-transfusion, 15 minutes into the transfusion and at the end of each unit as a minimum The observations should be done more frequently in certain situations (e.g. if the patient cannot communicate/has significant cardiovascular disease/patient is in a side room/transfusion is happening at night)
Ensure the transfusion is completed in the correct time frame	Maximum time for a red cell transfusion is 4 hours
Ensure traceability documentation is completed as per hospital policy	It is the law that hospitals are able to trace all blood components administered A record of all transfusions must be kept in the hospital lab for 30 years

Read the Royal College of Nursing (2004) guidance on good practice in blood transfusions:
http://www.rcn.org.uk/__data/assets/pdf_file/0009/78615/002306.pdf (accessed July 2011).

Mrs Singh was monitored by the nursing staff throughout her transfusion and was given drinks and her lunch while at the day care unit. She also had her lunchtime medication as usual, which she self-administered.

Post-transfusion

Once the transfusion was complete, Mrs Singh was seen again by the doctor from the haematology team and discharged. The nurse removed her intravenous cannula and inspected the cannula site for redness, inflammation and pain. The site was fine so a dry dressing was applied. The nurse then contacted the hospital transport service to let them know that Mrs Singh was ready to be taken home.

 Activity

> Consider what the role of the nurse would be once Mrs Singh's blood transfusion is complete.

The doctor and the nurse completed a discharge summary which will be sent to Mrs Singh's GP explaining the care and treatment she received and requesting that her full blood count be checked again in a few days' time.

 Activity

> The following are some examples of other medical investigations or treatments that frequently take place in a medical day unit. Look each of them up to see which body system they are concerned with and the types of conditions they diagnose or treat.

> Using the above case histories as a guide, consider what the role of the nurse might be in caring for patients attending the unit for these investigations or treatments:
> - Bronchoscopy.
> - Colonoscopy.
> - Venesection.
> - Suprapubic catheterisation.
> - Iron infusion.
> - Kidney biopsy.
> - Trial without catheter.

Examples of learning outcomes that are relevant will be any that concern communication, infection control, patient assessment, admission and discharge, medicines management and documentation. Some examples included in the NMC Standards for Pre-registration Education (2010b) are as follows:

- You must communicate safely and effectively to forge partnerships and build therapeutic relationships with people, family members and groups. You must take individual differences, capabilities and needs into account, and respond in a non-discriminatory way.

 Activity

> Look at your learning outcomes and competencies for your medical placement and identify which ones can be met while working in a medical day care or investigations unit.

- You must use verbal, non-verbal and written communication to listen, recognise, interpret and record people's knowledge and understanding of their needs. You must share information with others while respecting individual rights to confidentiality.

- You must maintain accurate, clear and complete written or electronic records using the right kind of language, avoiding jargon, and using plain English so that everyone involved in the care process understands the meaning.
- As an adult nurse, you must recognise the early signs of acute illness in young people, adults and older people, and accurately assess and start appropriate and timely management of those at risk of clinical deterioration, who are acutely ill or who need emergency care.
- As an adult nurse, you must safely use a range of diagnostic and clinical skills, complemented by existing and developing technology, to assess the nursing care of individuals undergoing therapeutic or clinical interventions.
- You must listen, recognise and respond to an individual's physical, social and psychological needs. You must then plan, deliver and evaluate technically safe, competent, person-centred care that addresses all their daily activities, in partnership with people and their carers, families and other professionals.

Summary

A placement on a medical day care or investigations unit can be a great opportunity to see a variety of medical diagnostic procedures, from gastroscopies to biopsies, and medical treatments, including blood transfusions, other drug infusions or insertion or removal of urinary catheters. It will give you the chance to revise your anatomy and physiology of several of the body systems and be able to relate these to how they are investigated and the potential problems and conditions patients are faced with.

There will be opportunities to understand the roles of the different health professionals working in the unit and those of nurses who have taken on extended roles,

such as clinical nurse specialists and nurse endoscopists. You will be able to care for a patient at each stage of their journey – admission, care and treatment, discharge – and it will require excellent communication skills because you will need to build rapport quickly with your patient as they will not be in the unit for very long.

References

Brooker, C., 2007. Promoting hydration and nutrition. In: Brooker, C., Waugh, A. (Eds.), Foundations of nursing practice. Mosby, Edinburgh.

Department of Health, 2009. Reference guide to consent for examination or treatment, 2nd ed. DH, London.

Holland, K., Hogg, C., 2010. Cultural awareness in nursing and healthcare. Hodder Arnold, London.

Howatson-Jones, L., Ellis, P., 2008. Outpatient, day surgery, and ambulatory care. Wiley–Blackwell, Oxford.

Nursing and Midwifery Council, 2010a. Essential skills clusters. NMC, London.

Nursing and Midwifery Council, 2010b. Standards for pre-registration nursing education. NMC, London.

Royal College of Nursing, 2004. Right blood, right patient, right time. RCN, London.

Skelly, M., Palmer, D., 2003. Conscious sedation in gastroenterology: a handbook for nurse practitioners. Whurr, Philadelphia.

Further reading

Department for Constitutional Affairs, 2007. Mental Capacity Act 2005: code of practice. The Stationery Office, London.

Dougherty, L., Lamb, J., 2008. Intravenous therapy in nursing practice, 2nd ed. Blackwell, Oxford.

Lynch, J., 2010. Consent to treatment. Medico-legal essentials. Radcliffe, Oxford.

Richards, S., Mughal, A.F., 2009. Working with the Mental Capacity Act 2005, 2nd ed. Matrix Training Associates, North Waltham.

Websites

NHS Choices Webpage with information aimed at patients about what a diagnostic gastroscopy is, why it is done and what it involves: http://www.nhs.uk/Conditions/Diagnosticendoscopyofthestomach/Pages/Introduction.aspx (accessed July 2011).

NHS Choices Webpage with information for patients about going into hospital. It includes a section about pre-admission and a short video of a nurse explaining what happens at a pre-admission assessment: http://www.nhs.uk/nhsengland/aboutnhsservices/nhshospitals/pages/going-into-hospital.aspx (accessed July 2011).

NHS Choices Webpage with information for patients about what a blood transfusion is and why it is given: http://www.nhs.uk/conditions/Blood-transfusion/Pages/Introduction.aspx (accessed July 2011).

Online *British National Formulary* – up-to-date reference on the selection, prescribing and administration of drugs used in the UK: http://www.bnf.org (accessed July 2011).

A US Website containing resources about culturally appropriate health care: http://ethnomed.org/ (accessed July 2011).

Link to the Royal College of Nursing's *Right Blood, Right Patient, Right Time* document: http://www.rcn.org.uk/__data/assets/pdf_file/0009/78615/002306.pdf (accessed July 2011).

12

The end of the journey: discharge from hospital and the experience of death

CHAPTER AIMS

- To enable the student to gain an understanding of the discharge process from hospital for the patient
- To enable the student to understand that the end of the journey for a patient might be death
- To understand what end of life care means for the patient and their family
- To explore sudden death and enable the student to reflect on their role when this happens
- To enable the student to identify their learning and development needs in relation to death and dying

Introduction

Wherever your medical placement is, your patients will ultimately be discharged home from the service they are currently using. So, if you are placed in a hospital ward or department, the patient will be discharged back to their home and, for some, this could mean a care home or similar environment. Sometimes patients are discharged home on the same day if you are in an investigations unit, or after a few days if you are on a medical ward. In an intermediate care setting or virtual setting (see Ch. 2), there may be a fixed length of time the patient will stay, for example 6 weeks, and then their care would be transferred elsewhere or they would be discharged home. Patients with long-term medical conditions may remain within the service, for example under the care of a medical consultant or clinical nurse specialist visiting out-patients, for the rest of their life.

Given the nature of medical placements, some of your patients will be acutely unwell and may die during their stay in hospital; others with long-term health conditions may be entering the end stages of their illness. Part of their care in a medical placement area will be to receive palliative or end of life care or be prepared for this in another setting such as their own home or a hospice.

This chapter will begin by looking at the normal process of the discharge home of a patient and the role of the nurse in discharge planning. It will then explore the end of life care that a patient may experience and, as a comparison, what can be a traumatic experience for nursing staff and patients' families – the sudden death of a patient in hospital.

Planning for discharge from hospital

As your patients will not expect or want to stay in hospital any longer than is necessary, it is essential that discharge planning begins on admission. Discharge planning should be an ongoing process throughout a patient's stay. It requires the multidisciplinary team to work together with the patient and their carer, if appropriate, to identify what will be required for the patient to be discharged home safely and in a timely manner – that is, as soon as they are medically well enough. The Nursing and Midwifery Council (NMC) Standards (2010) contain a number of competencies that are relevant to discharge planning, so should form part of your learning outcomes. They expect the following:

- You will understand the roles and responsibilities of other health and social care professionals and seek to work with them collaboratively for the benefit of all people in need of care.
- You will work with the person and others to make sure that they are actively involved in decision making in order to maintain their independence and take account of their ongoing intellectual, physical and emotional needs.
- You will use verbal, non-verbal and written communication to listen, recognise, interpret and record people's knowledge and understanding of their needs. You must share information with others while respecting individual rights to confidentiality.
- You will work closely with individuals, groups and carers, using a range of skills to carry out comprehensive, systematic and holistic assessments. These must take into account current and previous physical, social, cultural, psychological, spiritual, genetic and environmental factors that may be relevant to the individual and their families.
- You will recognise when the complexity of clinical decisions may need specialist knowledge and expertise and then consult or refer accordingly.
- You will work effectively across professional and agency boundaries, respecting and making the most of the contributions made by others to achieve integrated person-centred care.
- You will work as an independent practitioner as well as part of a team, taking a leadership role in coordinating, delegating and supervising care safely and appropriately while remaining accountable.

The more thorough your assessment on admission, the more you will understand what your patient will need in order to be discharged into a safe environment. An example may be their level of independence with certain activities of daily living. You will need to ensure your patients have reached independence by the time they are discharged or, if it seems likely that this will take a longer time than their stay in hospital, that sufficient provision is made for them to be able to maintain their activities of daily living at home and then rehabilitate further with support in the community.

The majority of discharges will be simple discharges – that is, those patients who are being discharged back to their own homes with simple ongoing needs that do not require any complex planning or delivery (Department of Health (DH) 2004).

 Activity

Discuss with your mentor which patients are likely to be simple discharges and which will be more complex discharges. Identify what role you could play in each type of discharge and the learning outcomes you could meet in doing this.

Some patients will be discharged to a care home setting. If this is their usual place of residence, it may be necessary for a nurse from the care home to assess the patient before they are discharged, to ensure that the staff in the care home are able to meet any ongoing needs the person has. Care homes are registered to provide different levels of care and it is essential that you are aware of the level of registration your patient's care home has to determine if their needs can be met there. A 'care home' will provide its residents with help with washing and dressing (personal care) and giving medication. A 'care home with nursing' has a registered nurse on duty 24 hours a day and will also provide personal care and give medications, but will be able to care for patients who are frailer, physically or mentally.

The following Website provides a useful glossary of terms and information on the various housing options available for older people:
http://www.housingcare.org/glossary.aspx (accessed July 2011).

The Department of Health (2010) has recommended 10 steps to help achieve a safe and timely discharge from hospital (see Box 12.1).

If your patient will require support at home, it will be part of your role as their nurse to ensure they have been adequately assessed by different members of the multidisciplinary team. This will involve identifying any needs they may have, during your ongoing assessment of their needs, and referring appropriately to the physiotherapist, occupational therapist,

---

Box 12.1 The 10 steps to achieve a safe and timely discharge from hospital (DH 2010)

1. Start planning for discharge or transfer before or on admission.
2. Identify whether the patient has simple or complex discharge and transfer planning needs, involving the patient and carer in your decision.
3. Develop a clinical management plan for every patient within 24 hours of admission.
4. Coordinate the discharge or transfer of care process through effective leadership and handover of responsibilities at ward level.
5. Set an expected date of discharge or transfer within 24–48 hours of admission, and discuss with the patient and carer.
6. Review the clinical management plan with the patient each day, take any necessary action and update progress towards the discharge or transfer date.
7. Involve patients and carers so that they can make informed decisions and choices that deliver a personalised care pathway and maximise their independence.
8. Plan discharges and transfers to take place over 7 days to deliver continuity of care for the patient.
9. Use a discharge checklist 24–48 hours prior to transfer.
10. Make decisions to discharge and transfer patients each day.

social worker and other members of the multidisciplinary team as necessary. An awareness of the services available in your local community to support people at home will help here. This should include statutory services provided in people's own homes and in residential accommodation, for example intermediate care services and services provided by local voluntary agencies. Communication between hospital and community services is essential for a 'seamless' approach to care delivery for the patient.

 Activity

Take some time to find out about the services available locally (that is, in your 'base trust' environment) to support patients once they have been discharged from hospital. Arrange to speak to the ward social worker and ask about the services available locally, which patients are eligible for them and how they are referred to each service. The physiotherapist will also be a good source of information about the rehabilitation services available in the community, for example community physiotherapy, home rehabilitation services and in-patient intermediate care services.

Expected (estimated) dates of discharge

You will find that an expected date of discharge is set early on during your patient's stay, sometimes even on admission. This is often quite easy to do once a diagnosis has been established. Expected dates of discharge are often based on the length of the therapy required to treat a particular condition and the amount of rehabilitation required to enable your patient to reach their pre-morbid functional level and leave hospital.

Of course, expected dates of discharge are initially based on the best case scenario, so if your patient does not recover as quickly as expected or suffers from any complications which cause a setback in their hospital stay, then their expected date of discharge will be reviewed accordingly.

 Activity

Find out from your mentor when expected dates of discharge are set for the patients in your area. Where are these documented and how often are they reviewed?

Over the course of your placement, can you see a pattern in the length of stay for patients with similar conditions?

Observe your mentor or another registered nurse talking to your patients and their families about their expected date of discharge and, if it is appropriate, see if you can get involved in the discussions.

The expected date of discharge will often be reviewed on the ward round or at a multidisciplinary meeting.

 Activity

Find out from your mentor which days the ward round and multidisciplinary meetings happen and arrange to attend to some of these rounds and meetings to see how the team decides on an expected date of discharge for each patient and arranges discharge plans.

As your patient approaches their expected date of discharge, there will be numerous things you will need to coordinate to ensure they are ready to be discharged as planned.

The checklist in Figure 12.1 includes many of the things that need to be

Discharge checklist	Date achieved	Signature
MDT agreed discharge date		
Patient aware of EDD		
Relatives/carers aware of EDD		
Residential/nursing home aware of EDD		
TTA medication prescribed		
TTA medication ordered		
OT specialist equipment ordered and delivered		
DN specialist equipment ordered and delivered		
Patient own transport confirmed		
Hospital transport booked		
Social services package confirmed		
Social services package start date/time		
Sickness certificate completed		
Property/valuables returned to patient		
District nurse referral faxed		
Anticoagulant advice/booklet given		
OPD appointment given		
OPD transport booked		
Mobility goals achieved		
Functional goals achieved		
Appropriate clothing available		
Keys available		
Heating working		
Food available at home		

Fig 12.1 Discharge checklist. MDT, multidisciplinary team; EDD, estimated/expected date of discharge; TTA, to take away

considered and confirmed before your patient is ready to go home. All of these will not necessarily apply to all patients.

 Activity

Your placement area is likely to have its own version of a discharge checklist, so ask your mentor where to find it so you can familiarise yourself with it. Try to identify a patient who is getting close to their estimated discharge date and, using your discharge checklist, assess whether all of their discharge needs have been met. If there is a service or item on the checklist that you are not familiar with, ask your mentor about it.

By the time your patient reaches their expected date of discharge, all of the items on the checklist should have been confirmed and any community services needed should be ready to start. On the day of discharge, your patient may need to be examined by their doctor to ensure they are well enough to leave hospital. Some wards may operate a nurse-led discharge system, where a senior nurse can assess the patient on the day of discharge to determine if they are ready to be discharged. Figure 12.2 shows some of the things a nurse will be required to check prior to discharging a patient under a nurse-led discharge system.

Preparing to leave hospital

An important aspect of the discharge process is to make sure that your patient is psychologically prepared to leave hospital. For most patients, once they have recovered from their acute illness they will be ready, but for others, especially those with long-term conditions or ongoing rehabilitation needs, they may have anxieties about leaving hospital. Remember that they have been used to having professionals around them 24 hours a day to call on for help, and the prospect of being at home, maybe alone, and having no one close by if they feel unwell can be a frightening prospect. It is for this reason that commencing discharge planning early is so crucial.

( ) Reflection point

Think of two patients you have looked after, one who was looking forward to getting home and another who may have been more reluctant or anxious about discharge.

1. What do you think influenced their feelings about being discharged home?
2. What support networks did they have at home?
3. How independent were they?
4. What ongoing needs did they have?

 Activity

Check with your mentor if nurse-led discharge operates in your department and familiarise yourself with any guidelines/checklists that are used. Which nursing staff are able to discharge patients? Did they have to undergo specific training or competency assessments in order to carry out nurse-led discharge? What might the benefits be for the patient being discharged by a nurse?

Discharge checklist	Achieved
Has the patient been informed?	Yes/No
Has the patient's relative/carer been informed?	Yes/No
Does the patient's status meet the identified criteria as stated in the notes?	Yes/No
Blood results within expected limits?	Yes/No/NA
Give details of blood results if required: (must also be documented in patient's case notes)	
TPR, B/P, and respirations are stable (within patient's normal limits)?	Yes/No
Early warning score 0 (if scoring seek advice and circle No)	Yes/No, Score:
Oxygen saturation within patient's normal limits?	Yes/ No
Urine output satisfactory (within patient's normal limits)?	Yes/No
Bowel care discussed on the date of discharge?	Yes/No
Pain controlled?	Yes/No
Analgesia prescribed?	Yes/No /NA
Eating and drinking?	Yes/No
Free from new or unexpected chest or calf pain?	Yes/No/ NA
Wound site checked?	Yes/No
Appears healthy and free from infection?	Yes/No
Sutures/clips removed or arrangements made for removal?	Yes/No/NA
Anti-embolic stockings supplied with advice?	Yes or NA
Verbal infromation given re: medical condition and aftercare advice?	Yes/No
Patient's standard of independence with mobility attained?	Yes/No or normally dependant
Multidisciplinary team aware of discharge and in agreement?	Yes/No/NA

Fig 12.2 Checklist for discharging a patient under a nurse-led discharge system

Continued

Fig 12.2—cont'd

Discharge checklist *(continued)*	Achieved *(continued)*
Discharge medication prescribed by doctor?	Yes/No date NA
Discharge medication discussed with patient?	Yes/No
Has the patient had cannula removed?	Yes/No/NA
Transport arranged?	Yes/No date NA
Patient has access to home?	Yes/No
Has the patient left the ward?	Yes – date/time
Patient's destination?	Home, discharge lounge, other

If your patients will need to manage ongoing medical problems themselves, then you need to ensure that they understand their condition and the treatment it requires. This may involve administering medication either orally or by injection (e.g. insulin) or monitoring their condition (e.g. peak flow or blood sugar monitoring) and then responding accordingly by adjusting medication or contacting their GP, practice nurse or clinical nurse specialist.

Assisting your patients to self-medicate and to start managing and monitoring their conditions while in hospital is a good way for you to be sure they understand what they need to do and are capable of doing it independently. If you or your patients have any concerns, these can then be addressed before they are discharged. Often, all your patients and their relatives or carers will need is reassurance that they are recovering and what to expect when they get home; also who to contact should they have any problems or feel unwell.

 Activity

With the help of your mentor, identify a patient who will need to manage an aspect of their ongoing health care themselves once they are discharged (e.g. taking their medication, administering their insulin, checking their blood sugar levels). Discuss with your mentor how you can be involved in educating your patient to do this. This may be something you could speak to a clinical nurse specialist about for advice (e.g. diabetes nurse specialist).

The following two articles will be useful to read as they discuss the importance of communication skills in giving information to patients and the many factors affecting a patient's ability to manage their own care:

Caress AL (2003). Giving information to patients. Nursing Standard 17(43):47–54.

Hughes SA (2004). Promoting self-management and patient independence. Nursing Standard 19(10):47–52.

End of life care

As mentioned previously, some patients may not be ending their time in hospital by going home, and will in fact be entering the end stages of their long-term condition and will require end of life care. For some patients, dying in hospital may be their preferred option, but for many, they may wish to die at home or in another organisation such as a hospice. Some of you may have a placement in a hospice, and more about this kind of care can be found in Howard and Chady (2012), another book in this series.

End of life care is an essential part of nursing and you can expect to encounter this experience in all areas you work in, both the hospital and the community.

There has been growing awareness of the need for good end of life care recently, and this has been supported by a number of initiatives and guidance from the Department of Health, most notably the *End of Life Care Strategy* (DH 2008).

The strategy and other resources aimed at helping health professionals to improve the quality of end of life care can be found at the National End of Life Care Programme Website:

http://www.endoflifecareforadults.nhs.uk/ (accessed July 2011).

The aim of these initiatives has been to ensure that all patients requiring end of life care receive the same standard of care and to ensure patients are involved as far as possible in planning for the end of their life, including where they would prefer to be when the time comes.

Take some time to look at the following Website on end of life care. This is aimed at people who may be nearing the end of their life and their carers and explains what they can expect from end of life care and the different places they can expect to receive it:

http://www.nhs.uk/planners/end-of-life-care/pages/end-of-life-care.aspx (accessed July 2011).

An important hospital and community team that you should make yourself familiar with is the palliative care team. This is a team of specialist nurses and doctors, often supported by therapists and social workers, who are experienced in managing end of life symptoms and helping patients and families come to terms with the fact that they or their loved one is near the end of their life.

☙ Activity

Ask your mentor about the palliative care team in your placement area and how to contact them. Try to arrange to spend some time with them while you are on placement, or ask to be involved when they are assessing a patient you are caring for.

What is palliative care?

The World Health Organization (WHO; 2011) defines palliative care as:

> an approach that improves the quality of life of patients and their families facing the problems associated with life threatening illness, through the prevention and relief of suffering by means of early identification and impeccable assessment and treatment of pain and other problems, physical, psychosocial and spiritual.

Palliative care aims to do the following (WHO 2011):

- Affirm life and regard dying as a normal process.
- Neither hasten nor postpone death.
- Provide relief from pain and other distressing symptoms.
- Integrate the psychological and spiritual aspects of patient care.
- Offer a support system to help patients live as actively as possible until death.

- Offer a support system to help the family cope during the patient's illness and their own bereavement.
- Use a team approach to address the needs of patients and their families, including bereavement counselling if indicated.
- Enhance quality of life, and may also positively influence the course of illness.
- Is applicable early in the course of illness, in conjunction with other therapies that are intended to prolong life, such as chemotherapy or radiation therapy, and includes those investigations needed to better understand and manage distressing clinical complications.

Palliative care is a process that may last for months or even years and supports anyone with a life-limiting illness, such as cancer, heart failure, dementia, neurological conditions and respiratory failure. Many of the patients you will care for who are in need of palliative care will be in the last few days, weeks or months of their lives. The management of their end of life requires a team approach and should involve the patient and their relatives as much as they are able to be involved. The following members of the multidisciplinary team are likely to be involved:

- Ward nurses.
- Specialist nurses.
- Consultants and doctors.
- Physiotherapists.
- Occupational therapists.
- Speech and language therapists.
- Chaplains or other religious leaders.
- Social workers.
- Psychologists.

A number of nationally recognised tools are used to ensure the standard of care provided at the end of life meets the needs of patients and relatives. Some of the ones used in your placement area may include the Liverpool Care Pathway, the Gold Standards Framework and the Preferred Place of Care (The Marie Curie Palliative Care Institute 2010). Ask your mentor if any of these are used in your area.

Liverpool Care Pathway

Care pathways are tools that are used to direct care for a particular group of patients or health problems, ensuring care is standardised, evidence-based and patient centred while also providing a method of monitoring the care given for clinical governance purposes (Vanhaecht et al 2011).

The Liverpool Care Pathway (LCP) is used to direct care in the last 2 to 3 days of someone's life. It provides guidance and prompts on the management of symptoms such as pain, agitation and nausea and also directs the nursing care the person may require. All care given in these last hours is documented in the pathway.

The following link will take you to more information about the LCP and a sample LCP. See also Chapter 2 in Ellershaw and Wilkinson (2011) for information on how the LCP should be used:

http://www.liv.ac.uk/mcpcil/liverpool-care-pathway/documentation-lcp.htm (accessed July 2011).

Activity

Try to find out the role each of these members plays in the end of life care for your patients. Speak to each of them about their role or talk to your mentor about it. Find out how you would refer a patient to one of these people if you needed to. Use this to enable you to achieve a learning goal of understanding how a multidisciplinary team works in an integrated way.

Gold Standards Framework

The Gold Standards Framework (GSF) aims to improve care for people who are admitted to hospital who are likely to be in the last year of their life. On a medical ward, this is most likely to be patients who have chronic conditions such as heart failure and respiratory failure. Identifying that a person is in the last year of their life helps the team to ensure that all the agencies necessary are involved in the person's care and plans can be made about how their condition can best be managed, helping to avoid unnecessary hospital admissions and the distress and increased risks this incurs.

Preferred Place of Care

The Preferred Place of Care (PPC) is a document that details the wishes of a person who is dying and their carers regarding where they would like to be cared for at the end of their life, for example in their own home or a hospice. This document would not usually be completed while a person is in hospital, but a patient may already have one of these when they are admitted so it is important that staff are aware of the document and the patient's wishes so that all efforts can be made to meet them.

 Activity

> Make yourself familiar with the LCP document. Look at the guidance provided about symptom control. Are you familiar with drugs that the guidance recommends? If not, look them up in the *British National Formulary*, find out how they are usually given and determine whether they are controlled drugs.

An excellent read is Chapter 3, *Symptom Control in Care of the Dying* by Glare et al (in Ellershaw &Wilkinson 2011). You may also find the following two articles useful as they discuss symptom control and common myths surrounding symptom control in end of life care that you may encounter:

Allmark P, Tod A (2009). End of life care pathways: ethical and legal principles. Nursing Standard 24(14):35–39.

Heming D, Colmer A (2003). Care of the dying patient. Nursing Standard 18 (10):47–54.

Whatever stage you are at in your training, you are likely to have learning outcomes that could be met caring for a patient at the end of their life. The NMC (2010) Standards for pre-registration education state that you must be able to do the following:

- Recognise and respond to the changing needs of adults, their families and carers during different phases of terminal illness. You must understand how you can help meet the needs of people receiving palliative care and how progressive illness, loss and bereavement may need different treatment goals at different stages. This should take account of the use of complementary and alternative approaches.
- Recognise and respond to the changing needs of individuals and their families and carers during different phases of life, including facing progressive illness and death, loss and bereavement.

 Activity

> Look at the nursing interventions in the LCP. Would you be able to carry out these interventions? If not, talk with your mentor about including some of them in your learning outcomes.

Many patients who are nearing the end of their life will be aware of what is happening to them. The extent to which they will want to be involved in making decisions about their care and receiving information about their condition and prognosis will vary between individuals and nurses must respect this. In some cases you may find that medical teams start to have conversations with patients about what they would like to happen at the end of their life, even if they are not currently in a terminal phase of illness. This is often called advance care planning and can be useful when patients have a long-term condition that is progressive that their wishes are respected if they are no longer able to make decisions for themselves.

The following link will take you to a guide, *Capacity, Care Planning and Advance Care Planning in Life Limiting Illness*, published by the National End of Life Care Programme (2011):
http://www.endoflifecareforadults.nhs.uk/publications/pubacpguide (accessed July 2011).

Resuscitation

One of the things that may be discussed with patients is if they would want to be resuscitated if they were to unexpectedly deteriorate and possibly have a cardiac arrest. Cardiac arrest means that the heart has stopped beating and there is no normal breathing. It is different from a myocardial infarction (MI or heart attack) or any other medical condition. It is a medical emergency and will result in death if untreated.

Resuscitation refers to the actions we may take in the event of cardiac arrest or if a patient is deteriorating, such as performing chest compressions, giving certain drugs or using a manual or automated defibrillator. The aim of these actions is to keep the brain and other important organs supplied with enough oxygen to prevent hypoxic damage and to restart the heart.

Some patients and relatives have strong views on what treatment they would or wouldn't want to receive, the quality of life they would find acceptable or whether they would want to be reliant on others. Some people may never have discussed this or find it too distressing. Although relatives and friends cannot make a decision about a patient's care, they may be able to give some insight into the patient's feelings and wishes so that a decision can be made in the patient's best interests. This will be particularly useful to the medical team caring for the patient if the patient is unable to discuss the decision themselves (e.g. because they are unconscious or too unwell). This shouldn't be a matter that you are asked to discuss with patients or relatives, although they may raise the subject with you, especially if you have built a particularly strong relationship with them.

The team caring for a patient might decide that if the patient's heart stopped it would not be best for the patient to attempt to restart their heart. This might be because the chances of successfully restarting the heart are very low or because the patient's quality of life would be too poor to be acceptable to them. In this case, a 'do not attempt resuscitation' (DNAR) decision will be made and recorded by the consultant in charge of the care of the patient, in order to prevent the patient having to undergo the indignity of resuscitation unnecessarily. However, 'do not attempt resuscitation' does not mean 'do not care'. Patients may still receive many other active treatments such as intravenous antibiotics or fluids or non-invasive ventilation. These should also be documented along with their resuscitation status.

Documentation will vary from one trust to another, but the DNAR form will usually be a short (one or two pages) document, often printed on coloured paper. In order to be valid, the DNAR form should include the patient's details, signature and name of the doctor completing the form, the patient's consultant and the time and date. DNAR forms are only valid for a limited amount of time – often 7 days – after which a new form must be completed.

It is really important that you know which, if any, of the patients you are

 Activity

Find out how resuscitation status is documented in your placement area and familiarise yourself with the form. Find out how resuscitation status is communicated – how will you know what your patient's resuscitation status is?

caring for have a valid DNAR document, so that in the event of a cardiac arrest you know whether to start basic life support or not.

Each patient's resuscitation status should be made clear at handover at the start of each shift, enabling the patient to have the most appropriate and dignified death possible. If you are unsure, ask! If you do find a patient in cardiac arrest but are unsure of their resuscitation status, you should start basic life support – you can always stop once you know otherwise.

Your exposure to cardiac arrests and resuscitation will be influenced by the areas you work in or go on placement to. Some student nurses will complete their training without attending a cardiac arrest; some may have been present at several.

Regardless of your experience, a cardiac arrest is an emotive event and affects everyone involved, and in very different ways. There is no right or wrong way to feel, and coping strategies that help your colleagues may not be helpful to you, and vice versa. Factors such as the age of the

The following article is the reflection of a third-year student nurse following a cardiac arrest situation during her placement on a cardiac ward where the decision to resuscitate the patient was not clear: Jones J (2007). Do not resuscitate: reflections on an ethical dilemma. Nursing Standard 21(46):35–39.

 Activity

Before you began your medical nursing placement you will have undergone resuscitation training or life support training. Take this opportunity to reread any notes you have about resuscitation algorithms.

Up-to-date resuscitation guidelines can be found on the Resuscitation Council (UK) Website:
http://www.resus.org.uk/SiteIndx.htm (accessed July 2011).

patient, whether you had cared for them, if cardiac arrest was unexpected, the reactions of the patient's family and friends and your own personal experience will all have an impact on how you react. You may feel differently during and after one cardiac arrest than another. It is important to remember that however you feel is normal and support is available to you from many sources.

You are likely to feel anxious about witnessing a cardiac arrest while on placement, even if you have been involved in one before. At this stage, it is useful to reflect on any past experiences involving a cardiac arrest, as some preparation before an event can increase your confidence and ability to deal with an emergency situation.

◑ Activity

Think about the following questions about cardiac arrest and discuss them with your mentor:

- If there was a cardiac arrest while you were on duty, how involved do you want to be? For example, would you like to perform chest compressions or would you rather observe from a distance?

- What other things are you able to do? How can you be useful in an emergency situation? Think about how the needs of other patients are met while a cardiac arrest is happening. It is very important that someone assures other patients and answers their questions in a confidential manner. Also a useful tip is always to make yourself aware of where everything is kept on the ward, such as IV fluids, special equipment and the resuscitation trolley. (See Hand & Banks (2004) for more understanding about the items commonly found on a resuscitation trolley.)

- What type of clinical area are you in? What is the likelihood of a patient having a cardiac arrest during your placement?

- Are there other people you could shadow for a day or other clinical areas you could arrange to visit where patients are at a higher risk of cardiac arrest, such as the critical care areas (accident and emergency department (A&E), coronary care unit or intensive care/high-dependency unit)? Find out how they manage a cardiac arrest and what is different from a ward situation.

- What are you competent to do? When did you last attend basic life support training? What will you say or do if you are asked to do something that you haven't been taught to do or don't understand?

- What do you want to achieve? Are you fulfilling any of the learning outcomes you need to achieve during your placement? What skills do you need to demonstrate to achieve these outcomes? What else can you learn from this experience?

- Who can support you and how? Is there someone who could stand with you in case you need help and to make sure you know what is happening? If you are asked to do something you are unsure about, who can you ask for help?

- Is this a situation that your mentor or other nursing staff encounter on a regular basis? Will they be able to offer you support or will they have other tasks to do?

- Who else is available to you with the appropriate knowledge to answer your questions or get you involved as part of the resuscitation team?

- Does it make a difference if it is during the day, night or weekend? Are there too many people to make it practical for you to be involved, such as other nursing or medical students, junior doctors?

Resuscitation officers

Each healthcare organisation will have a resuscitation officer (or equivalent) who is responsible for providing life support training, provision of resuscitation equipment and ensuring best practice in line with current guidelines (see Resuscitation Council at http://www.resus.org.uk). They are specialists in resuscitation medicine and an invaluable resource to you.

Activity

Find out who the resuscitation team/officer is for your placement area and how to contact them. Arrange to spend some time with them during your placement if possible. They may be holding training sessions that you could attend or may even organise specific training for you and a group of your colleagues. Many students obtain a certificate of attendance at these kinds of training days and include them in their learning portfolios along with a reflection summary. Ask if they can suggest any other learning opportunities that might be appropriate for you. Your resuscitation officer may be the ideal person to get you involved during a cardiac arrest. Discuss with them what you would like to do if the opportunity arises.

What to do in the event of a cardiac arrest

It is possible that you may be the one to find a patient in cardiac arrest or be one of the first responders on the scene. Your university will have provided basic, or possibly more advanced, life support training, however a real life clinical emergency can be very different to the calm environment of the classroom. It is normal to feel anxious or scared – this is because your body releases adrenaline and is part of the way we respond to an emergency. However, a normal response along with your basic or advanced knowledge and skills will give you the confidence to make decisions. It is surprising how many qualified nurses will tell you that, even though they carried out highly competent and expert practice, once the situation has been resolved they often cannot recall completely how they made their decisions and actions.

If you are outside of a hospital setting, you may need to call the emergency services for an ambulance (999 or 112 are the emergency services numbers throughout Europe, including the UK; make sure you know the emergency number for the country you are in!). If you are in a hospital, you may be asked to call the resuscitation team and your call will be answered as a priority (to do this, dial 2222 from any internal phone; this is a standardised number so will be the same in all acute NHS trusts in England and Wales; make sure you know the number for the resuscitation team if you are in a different country). Speak clearly stating the team you require and your location:

"Adult cardiac arrest, Oak Ward!"
The telephone operator will then repeat back your request and the call can be terminated. Don't try to give any more information or details about the patient or be specific about what you need; giving irrelevant information will only cause a delay in getting help to you and your patient.

 Activity

Think about your placement area. How would you summon help if you found someone in cardiac arrest? Imagine a situation where your patient has a cardiac arrest in the bathroom, or the day room where there are other patients in the vicinity.

Discuss with your mentor whether this is the right way to summon help in your area. Discuss the role of the nurse and what would be expected of you as a student nurse while waiting for help to arrive. Agree various decision-making scenarios with your mentor to give you confidence.

Once you have called for help, if the cardiac arrest is in a hospital setting, you can expect a team of people to arrive. Cardiac arrests may look disorganised to someone who has not seen one before but it is often thought of as organised chaos! There are several key roles that people will undertake in a cardiac arrest situation within the resuscitation team (see Box 12.2). These roles may be performed by different people, or one person may do more than one role. Ideally the team leader will allocate these roles as team members arrive. This will, of course, depend on the area in which the cardiac arrest has occurred and the policy of the hospital.

If at any point during or after a resuscitation you become too distressed or upset to stay, it is acceptable to leave the area to compose yourself. If you have been asked to do something, make sure you hand it over to someone else who will be able to complete it before you leave the area. Speak to someone you feel comfortable with to discuss what upset you so much and how you could cope with a similar situation were you faced with it in the future. This might be something you discuss during debriefing or you may prefer to talk it over in private with your mentor. It is important to note that it is not only students who this happens to, and it may be that the situation can be a 'trigger' for other members of the team as well. Learning the skills for reflection on significant events is an important part of your programme of study, and this type of situation is an excellent example of where the practical value can be seen. It is not simply for writing your reflection of situations but the actual value of learning in practice with your mentor.

Witnessed resuscitation

In some circumstances, relatives and friends may wish to be present during a resuscitation attempt. There are many benefits for relatives who witness their loved one being resuscitated; they can see that all efforts are made to revive their loved one and, if the resuscitation is unsuccessful, they have the opportunity to say goodbye before compressions are stopped. This is often seen in the resuscitation room in A&E when a patient has been admitted having had a cardiac arrest on the street and the relatives arrive at the department. This is an unexpected situation where relatives feel they need to be present in case they have to say goodbye to the patient. In this kind of situation, however, it is essential that relatives remaining in the resuscitation room are supported by a senior member of staff who can explain what is happening and answer questions. In a ward situation, this becomes more difficult because of the position of the beds, the equipment needed, the space involved and the needs of other patients. The team leader or other senior person available will make a decision about this on an individual basis. Often this is a time when relatives may need a great deal of support and, if they are present, being aware of their changing needs is an important part of the ongoing events. Read the RCN (2002) *Witnessed Resuscitation: Guidance for Nursing Staff* for more information.

Outcomes

At some stage, the resuscitation will come to an end, either when the patient's heart starts beating independently or because a decision is made by the team that further resuscitation would not be in the patient's best interest. This decision is made on a combination of clinical evidence at the time and the patient's health problems and needs.

Return of spontaneous circulation (ROSC) means the patient's heart begins to beat independently and is the start of the post-resuscitation care phase. Sadly, many patients will not regain a ROSC despite the best efforts of all involved; many of those whose heart does restart may also go on to die in the next few days due to irreparable damage to important organs like the brain.

Box 12.2 Roles in a cardiac arrest

Team leader

This could be a resuscitation officer, doctor, nurse or other healthcare professional with the relevant training. They will usually stand at the foot end in order to get an 'overview' of everything that is happening. The team leader should give instructions and lead the resuscitation, collating the information he/she receives from the team.

Anaesthetist

The anaesthetist generally stands at the patient's head and will be a doctor trained in advanced airway skills who will manage the patient's airway to prevent aspiration of stomach contents into the lungs.

Chest compressions

Anyone who has attended life support training can perform chest compressions and it is good practice to swap with other people regularly to avoid becoming fatigued and therefore less effective. When changing over, there should be minimal interruption. Compressions are performed at a different ratio once the patient has a secure airway (e.g. intubated with an endotracheal tube). For recommendations on basic and advanced in-hospital life support, see http://www.resus.org.uk (accessed July 2011).

Monitoring

If the patient is not already attached to a monitor then they will need to be attached to the defibrillator and other cardiac and respiratory monitoring equipment. Most of the monitoring equipment needed will be available on the resuscitation trolley; patients in cardiac arrest will not have a blood pressure so do not go in search of an electronic blood pressure monitor or sphygmomanometer unless specifically asked to.

Defibrillator

An appropriately trained person will be allocated to use the defibrillator. They will deliver a shock, if required, and be responsible for the safety of everyone around. A defibrillator delivers a large dose of electricity into the chest via sticky pads in an attempt to 'shock' the heart back into a working rhythm. However, it is sufficient to shock a healthy, beating heart into cardiac arrest if inadvertently delivered to the wrong person (e.g. a member of the cardiac arrest team), so it is essential that you listen to the safety commands given. If you are told to 'stand clear' or similar, ensure you are not in contact with the patient or with anything they are in contact with (bed or trolley, bag of fluids, etc.) as this could result in the shock being passed to you. Do not touch the patient until the shock has been delivered and chest compressions have restarted. The defibrillation pads will remain on the patient's chest throughout the cardiac arrest. This is to enable a series of shocks to be delivered quickly and easily throughout the resuscitation.

Continued

Box 12.2 Roles in a cardiac arrest—cont'd

Vascular access and bloods

Someone will be needed to gain vascular access and take blood samples. Often an intravenous (IV) cannula will be used, however, if it is very difficult to get IV access, you may see an intraosseous (IO) device being used. This is a type of access device which, instead of sitting in the vein like an IV cannula, is sited to sit in the bone, usually just below the knee or upper arm/shoulder (see Fenwick 2010). There are various different types of IO device available, but they all work in a similar way; a large needle is sited so it goes through the bone and into the bone marrow inside. Some are applied manually; others have a driver or 'gun' to site it. Drugs and fluids can be given through IO access and bloods taken from it can be sent to the lab for testing.

Drugs

Certain medications may need to be prepared and will need to be administered to the patient. Many of the first-line drugs used are pre-prepared, however additional drugs may be requested, some of which require careful calculations and complicated preparation. Often more than one person is required to deal with drugs – this may be any member of staff who is usually able to give medications. Check local policy (before it happens, not during!) on whether you are able to check drugs with a registered nurse or doctor. The team leader will ensure that a record is managed of medication given during a cardiac arrest.

Scribe

As with all patient care, accurate documentation is essential. It is easy to lose track of everything that happens during a cardiac arrest. One member of the resuscitation team will keep a written account of details such as how many shocks are given and the number of cycles of cardiopulmonary resuscitation as well as the medication given and any other related treatment or activity. This then becomes part of the patient's documentation and gives a time-specific record of cardiac arrest management. In some circumstances, this record is vital if any inquiry is conducted around the cardiac arrest situation and, as a student, you need to become familiar with the NMC (2009) *Record Keeping: Guidance for Nurses and Midwives.*

It may be that the team makes a decision to stop the resuscitation attempt as it is so unlikely that the patient's heart will restart. Many factors are taken into account while making this decision: the length of time in cardiac arrest, whether the arrest was witnessed at its onset (linked to the time when the heart first stopped) and whether basic life support was given immediately in order to restore cardiac and respiratory function are all important considerations, as is the patient's health and quality of life prior to the cardiac arrest. Although the team leader is ultimately responsible for the patient's care, this should be a team decision.

After a cardiac arrest

What happens once a resuscitation attempt is finished depends on whether the patient has survived and, if so, what the planned management and treatment is. If the patient has regained a pulse, the first priorities are to stabilise the patient and prevent further damage to the important organs such as the brain. If the cardiac arrest has happened in A&E or a ward, the patient may need to be transferred to another area or even to another hospital, usually to a high-dependency area where they can be provided with specialist one-to-one nursing care. They may need further blood tests, body scans or images like a chest X-ray or an electrocardiogram tracing recorded, and treatments such as therapeutic hypothermia (where the patient's temperature is deliberately lowered using cooled fluids, ice or 'cooling blankets') may be started.

The following article describes the role of the nurse before, during and after a cardiac arrest in hospital along with the care of a patient following a successful resuscitation: Spearpoint K (2008). Resuscitating patients who have a cardiac arrest in hospital. Nursing Standard 23(14):48–57.

If the resuscitation has been stopped as it was no longer in the patient's best interest, cardiopulmonary resuscitation will be stopped and the time of death will be noted; at this point, many of the team members might leave.

After a patient dies there are many things that need to be done, and you will find that, as many of the cardiac arrest team are not in attendance, you may well be asked to help with some of these.

If you have any immediate questions or problems, don't be afraid to speak up – have a quiet word with your mentor, the nurse caring for the patient or the nurse in charge and explain your concerns. If you want to discuss the details of the event, or have clinical questions about what happened, try to speak to one of the nursing or medical staff involved. Bear in mind, though, that immediately following resuscitation may not be the best time. It is important, however, not only for your personal experience but also your developing professional practice, that you reflect on the event first, discuss it with someone if that is something that you would like to do and also identify all the things you learnt from the situation. You could use the NMC (2010) Domains, professional values and nursing practice and decision making, as a framework to identify how your involvement helped you to achieve some important learning outcomes and competencies in your placement.

Administration and documentation

If you are working alongside your mentor or other qualified nurse who is responsible for documenting the care given to the patient, ask to learn and contribute to the record keeping. You need to ensure that your documentation is completed and thorough. Wherever possible, record any actions, treatments or interventions by staff of any discipline as they occur. Don't leave yourself in a position where the patient is ready to be transferred to the mortuary or other department and you haven't written anything down. As with all your documentation, the record of cardiac arrest management is entered into the patient's notes and forms part of the patient's documentation. Any of your documentation could potentially one day be used in a court of law in the event of an untoward incident or complaint – get into the habit of thinking whether this would stand up as evidence (see Ch. 8 for more information on documentation and NMC 2009).

Debriefing

Debriefing is a way of enabling those involved in an event or incident to deal with their feelings and discuss any concerns they have. It is often used following an emotive event such as a cardiac arrest, especially if it was particularly distressing or stressful. It can be a useful tool to identify positive aspects and areas to learn from. If you were involved in the cardiac arrest, even just as an observer, it will be useful for you to attend the debrief.

A debrief is usually led by the resuscitation officer and will be attended by everyone who played a part in the cardiac arrest. Other staff who may be able to provide support to the team (e.g. chaplain, occupational health nurse) may also attend. This may happen not long after the event, if particularly needed, or 1 or 2 days later. If you have reflected on the situation in which you were involved, this will help during a debrief, as most debriefing has both a structured 'let's go through the event' approach and a more reflective exploration of 'how we feel' approach. Whoever leads this meeting /discussion will be experienced at doing so, enabling positive resolution for the majority of the team.

The death of a patient

At some point during your medical placement you may experience the death of a patient. This could be following a cardiac arrest but it could be a patient who has been receiving end of life care in your placement area. Roper et al (2000) view dying as the final activity of life and, as such, caring for the dying patient or the patient who has died is a very important aspect of nursing to learn as a student nurse. Many students worry about this and the issues raised in this chapter. Therefore, the most important thing you can do is to prepare your knowledge base prior to going to any placement. Then, in the eventuality of needing to know how to manage the dying experience with the patient and/or relatives and also after death, you will be confident that there are some things you know and are able to do as a student nurse.

The chapter on dying by Roberts in Holland et al (2008) explains more about the process of dying and this would be a good place to start in preparing your knowledge base.

⟨⟩ Reflection point

Have you ever been present at the death of a patient? Have you assisted in providing care for a patient after they have died, for example washing the body (usually called last offices), or dealt with bereaved relatives?

Your needs and the support you require following the death of a patient will depend partly on your experience in the situation. It will also depend on your personal circumstances. Have you experienced a bereavement yourself recently? Reflect on your current situation and then discuss with your mentor the support you may require should one of your patients die. Think about who is available to support you in this while you are on placement – your mentor, your link lecturer and personal tutor from university, your practice experience facilitator or occupational health services at the university/hospital.

Breaking bad news

Following the death of a patient, a member of staff will need to inform the patient's next of kin, family and/or friends that they have died. They may have been present at the patient's death but they will still require the support of a senior member of staff to confirm that the patient has died and to explain what happens next. This is usually the role of a senior nurse in the ward/ department. In the case of a sudden death or cardiac arrest situation, this responsibility may be with the doctor who was present or who is the patient's named consultant or team member.

 Activity

> Your placement area may have its own guidelines on breaking bad news; see if you can find them.

There are many sets of guidelines that can be accessed via a search on the Internet. For example:

http://www.cen.scot.nhs.uk/files/4c-breaking-bad-news-nhs-yorkshire.pdf (accessed July 2011).

Breaking bad news is not just about the death of a patient but also relates to giving someone an unwelcome diagnosis or talking about approaching the end of life. Read up on some of the literature around breaking bad news and consider what your learning needs may be in relation to this. Speak to your mentor and see if you can identify an opportunity for you to observe a senior member of staff breaking bad news.

The following articles may help you to reflect on strategies used to break bad news and also help to prepare you if you are in a situation where bad news has just been given to a patient or family/carers:

McGuigan D (2009). Communicating bad news to patients: a reflective approach. Nursing Standard 23(31):51–56.

Read S (2002). Loss and bereavement: a nursing response. Nursing Standard 16 (37):47–53.

There is no one right or wrong thing to say or do when caring for bereaved relatives, whatever the age of the patient. Each family and each situation will be different; it will require all your nursing skills to decide on the best approach. Where possible, relatives and friends should be offered somewhere private

to sit, facilities for contacting others and tissues, and it may be worth offering to make tea – there are very few situations you will encounter as a nurse where the offer of tea is not appreciated!

Last offices

Last offices is the name attributed to the care given to a patient after they have died. There will be a specific set of tasks that need to be completed to comply with local policy and procedure and also the law.

 Activity

> Find out what the policy and procedure for last offices are within your placement area and any documentation that accompanies them. What role could you play in assisting with last offices? Discuss this with your mentor.

You may be asked to assist with washing and changing the patient, and listing valuables or clothing. Lots of people are anxious or scared about encountering a dead body, especially if it is the first time; if you are worried, talk to the nurses you are working with – they have probably felt the same way at some point. While with the patient, some people will talk to them as though they are alive, some people are quiet and others might chat about last night's football and take-away. Don't feel that you have to behave in a certain way just because someone else does, but try to remember that all of these reactions are coping mechanisms. What might seem strange to you might be someone else's way of dealing with an emotive event.

The following articles by Pattison describe both the practical aspects of caring for a patient after they have died and the support and psychological needs of those around the patient:

Pattison N (2008). Care of patients who have died. Nursing Standard 22(28):42–48.

Pattison N (2008). Caring for patients after death. Nursing Standard 22(51):48–56.

You will also find details about what to do during last offices in many clinical skills books, for example Nicol (2008) and in the guide produced by The National End of Life Care Programme which can be found at:

http://www.endoflifecareforadults.nhs.uk/
assets/downloads/
Care_After_Death___guidance.pdf
(accessed July 2011).

Cultural and religious considerations

Different cultures and religions may have specific actions to be taken or rites to be followed in the event of death. This may be prayers to be are said or arrangements for the funeral to be held within 24 hours. You need to be aware of the cultural and religious needs of your patients (see Holland (2010) for more about the meaning of death and bereavement in different cultures).

The best thing you can do is ask your patient (if appropriate) or their family if there is anyone, such as a religious or spiritual leader, they would like you to contact or if they have any special requirements or needs that you need to be aware of. Patients and their families will appreciate you asking, and if they have any specific requirements they will be happy to tell you. There are a number of texts, such as Neuberger (2004), that may help you to understand the different practices and beliefs of people of different faiths at the time of death (see also Further reading list), but it is important to not make the assumption that all people of the same faith would want the same things in the event of their death.

The hospital chaplaincy service can be an invaluable source of support, for both family and staff members, in the event of a death or when caring for a dying patient. Representatives from most religions, be that a vicar, priest or imam, are available throughout the day or night, and will come into the hospital to support relatives. They may be able to advise you on the requirements of different religions but they may not want to meet a family unless you have already spoken to them about contacting a religious leader. Imagine someone who isn't particularly religious being approached by a priest to talk about dying; this may provoke anxiety, fear and distress for your patient and their family. The members of the chaplaincy service are also there for you to talk to if you feel that would be helpful. Alternatively, you may want to talk to the religious leader at your own church or place of worship.

 Activity

Find out how to contact the chaplaincy service in your organisation, as this is something you may be asked to do if a patient or relative requests support. Find out what resources are available in your placement area to meet the cultural or religious needs of a patient and their family when someone dies or is dying.

Summary

Successfully discharging a patient or caring for a patient and their loved ones at the end of life will require considerable skill and knowledge, particularly in your communication skills. A good knowledge and understanding of the members of the multidisciplinary team will also be essential. As part of your learning outcomes or competencies, communication and team working or multidisciplinary care will feature prominently whatever level of training you are in, so there will be plenty of opportunities for you to meet these outcomes during your medical placement.

End of life care and the death of a patient can be a difficult time for a first-year student but you can use this opportunity to think about your learning needs for subsequent placements where you are likely to encounter similar situations.

All of the skills you gain here in discharge and end of life care will be transferable to other placement areas.

References

Department of Health, 2004. Achieving timely 'simple' discharge from hospital. DH, London.

Department of Health, 2008. End of life care strategy. DH, London.

Department of Health, 2010. Ready to go? Planning the discharge and the transfer of patients from hospital and intermediate care. DH, London: Online. Available at: http://www.dh.gov.uk/prod_consum_dh/groups/dh_digitalassets/@dh/@en/@ps/documents/digitalasset/dh_113951.pdf (accessed July 2011).

Ellershaw, J., Wilkinson, S., 2011. Care of the dying: a pathway to excellence, 2nd ed. Oxford University Press, Oxford.

Fenwick, R., 2010. Intraosseous approach to vascular access in adult resuscitation. Emergency Nurse 18 (4), 22–25.

Glare, P., Dickman, A., Goodman, M., 2011. Symptom control in care of the dying. In: Ellershaw, J., Wilkinson, S. (Eds.), Care of the dying: a pathway to excellence, second ed. Oxford University Press, Oxford.

Hand, H., Banks, A., 2004. The contents of the resuscitation trolley. Nursing Standard 18 (44), 43–52.

Holland, K., 2010. Death and bereavement: a cross cultural perspective. In:

Holland, K., Hogg, C. (Eds.), Cultural awareness in nursing and healthcare: an introductory text, 2nd ed. Hodder Arnold, London.

Howard, P., Chady, B., 2012. Placement learning in cancer and palliative care nursing. Baillière Tindall, Edinburgh.

Neuberger, J., 2004. Caring for dying people of different faiths, 3rd ed. Radcliffe Medical Press, Oxford.

Nicol, M., 2008. Essential nursing skills, third ed. Mosby, London.

Nursing and Midwifery Council, 2009. Record keeping: guidance for nurses and midwives. NMC, London.

Nursing and Midwifery Council, 2010. Standards for pre-registration nursing education. NMC, London.

Roberts, D., 2008. Dying. In: Holland, K., Jenkins, J., Solomon, J., Whittam, S. (Eds.), Applying the Roper, Logan, Tierney model in practice, 2nd ed. Churchill Livingstone, Edinburgh.

Roper, N., Logan, W., Tierney, A., 2000. The Roper–Logan–Tierney model of nursing. Churchill Livingstone, Edinburgh.

Royal College of Nursing, 2002. Witnessed resuscitation: guidance for nursing staff. RCN, London.

The Marie Curie Palliative Care Institute, 2010. What is the Liverpool Care Pathway for the dying patient (LCP)? TMCPCI, Liverpool. Online. Available at: www.liv.ac.uk/mcpcil/liverpool-care-pathway/Updated%20LCP%20pdfs/What_is_the_LCP_-_Healthcare_Professionals_-_April_2010.pdf (accessed July 2011).

The National End of Life Care Programme, 2011. Guidance for staff responsible for care after death (last offices). TNELCP, London. Online. Available at: http://www.endoflifecareforadults.nhs.uk/assets/downloads/Care_After_Death___guidance.pdf (accessed July 2011).

Vanhaecht, K., Panella, M., van Zelm, R., et al., 2011. What about care pathways?

In: Ellershaw, J., Wilkinson, S. (Eds.), Care of the dying: a pathway to excellence, 2nd ed. Oxford University Press, Oxford.

World Health Organization, 2011. WHO definition of palliative care. WHO, Geneva. Online. Available at: http://www.who.int/cancer/palliative/definition/en/ (accessed July 2011).

Further reading

Booth, S., Edmonds, P., Kendall, M., 2010. Palliative care in the acute hospital setting: a practical guide. Oxford University Press, Oxford.

Foster, J., Turner, M., 2007. Implications of the Mental Capacity Act on advance care planning at the end of life. Nursing Standard 22 (2), 35–39.

General Medical Council, 2010. Treatment and care towards the end of life: good practice in decision making. Guidance for doctors (GMC/EOL/0510)GMC, London. Online. Available at: http://www.gmc-uk.org/End_of_life.pdf_32486688.pdf (accessed July 2011).

Holloway, M., Adamson, S., McSherry, W., et al., 2011. Spiritual care at the end of life: a systematic review of the literature. Department of Health, London.

Jevon, P., 2009. Care of the dying and deceased patient. Essential clinical skills for nurses. Wiley–Blackwell, Oxford.

Kennedy, C., Lockhart, K., 2007. Loss and bereavement. In: Brooker, C., Waugh, A. (Eds.), Foundations of nursing practice. Mosby Elsevier, Edinburgh.

Komaromy, C., 2004. Cultural diversity in death and dying. Nursing Management 11 (8), 32–36.

Lees, L., 2007. Nurse facilitated hospital discharge. M&K Update, Cumbria.

Mootoo, J., 2005. A guide to cultural and spiritual awareness. RCN Publishing Company, London.

Royal College of Nursing, 2010. Standards for infusion therapy. RCN, London.

Sheikh, A., Gatrad, A.R., 2008. Caring for Muslim patients, 2nd ed. Radcliffe, Oxford.

Spitzer, J., 2003. Caring for Jewish patients. Radcliffe, Oxford.

Thakrar, D., Das, R., Sheikh, A., 2008. Caring for Hindu patients. Radcliffe, Oxford.

Wood, J., Wainwright, P., 2007. Cardiopulmonary resuscitation: nurses and the law. Nursing Standard 22 (4), 35–40.

Websites

Housing Care, an organisation providing advice on housing options to older people. It contains a useful glossary with different types of accommodation available to older people: http://www.housingcare.org/glossary.aspx (accessed July 2011).

The National End of Life Care Programme has access to numerous guides and factsheets for healthcare professionals and patients about end of life care issues: http://www.endoflifecareforadults.nhs.uk/ (accessed July 2011).

The Resuscitation Council (UK): http://www.resus.org.uk (accessed July 2011).

Section 3. Case studies

13 Case study of a patient with heart failure

Introduction

This chapter provides you with an example of the nursing care that a patient with heart failure may require. The heart failure care plan (Fig. 13.1) has been written by a senior charge nurse for coronary care, Rafael Ripoll, and outlines care for the four stages of heart failure. The case history for

Martha will then guide you through the assessment, nursing action and evaluation of a patient with heart failure.

Patient profile

Martha is a 60-year-old lady who is admitted to accident and emergency (A&E) with breathlessness – her respiratory rate is 40 per minute and her oxygen saturation is 89%. On admission, her pulse is 175 beats per minute (bpm) and irregular. Her blood pressure is 90/50 mmHg. Martha is put on high-flow oxygen, a continuous cardiac monitor, hourly observation of vital signs and an intravenous cannula is inserted. Martha is administered intravenous digoxin and furosemide in A&E and is catheterised to

 Activity

A definition of heart failure was given in Chapter 1 and asked you to revise your anatomy and physiology (see Montague et al 2005). Before reading the case study, find out the following:

1. What are some of the symptoms of heart failure?
2. What health education could you provide for a patient with heart failure?

You can find out the answers to these questions by following the link below. The British Heart Foundation provides free booklets to download:

http://www.bhf.org.uk/heart-health/conditions/heart-failure.aspx (accessed July 2011).

Fig 13.1 Heart
failure care plan
(Reproduced with
permission of Rafael
Ripoll)

Heart Failure Care Plan	Name: ....
Stage 1	**Stage 2**
On inotropes	On frusemide infusion +/– GTN infusion
High flow oxygen	Oxygen therapy
Continuous cardiac monitor	Continuous cardiac monitor
Continuous SpO$_2$ monitor	Continuous SpO$_2$ monitor
Central line ± CVP monitoring	Peripheral canula
Remove all peripheral IV cannulas	Date/time inserted: ....
Observations documented hourly and PRN, weight if possible	Observation documented 2nd hourly and PRN, daily weight
Fluid balance chart	Fluid balance chart
1 litre fluid restriction	1 Litre fluid restriction
Urinary catheter, hourly measures	± Urinary catheter, hourly measures
Assist with all personal care	Assist with personal care as required
Assess and evaluate all potential sites of pressure areas	Sit out of bed, mobilise around bed space
Sit out of bed as able	Advise low salt diet
Low salt diet	
Bloods:	**Bloods:**
Ensure daily U&Es ordered,	Ensure daily U&Es ordered,
Monitor results	Monitor results
Assess suitability for heart failure clinic referral	Assess suitability for heart failure clinic referral
Date/sign	**Date/sign**

Continued

Fig 13.1—cont'd

Heart Failure Care Plan *(continued)*

Stage 3	Stage 4
On intermittent IV diuretics	Oral diuretics
± Oxygen therapy	PRN oxygen therapy
Cardiac monitor as condition dictates	Discontinue monitor
QDS and PRN observations. Include SpO$_2$ Daily weight	TDS and PRN observations, Include SpO$_2$ Daily weight
Fluid balance chart	Discontinue fluid balance chart
1 Litre fluid restriction	Assess for fluid restriction and advise accordingly
Assist with personal care as required	
Full mobilisation	
Advise low salt diet	
Bloods: Monitor U&Es	Bloods: Monitor U&Es
Assess suitability for heart failure clinic referral	Assess suitability for heart failure clinic referral
Date/sign	Date/sign

R.Ripoll CCU 2005

enable accurate fluid balance. Martha is married with three grown-up children and smokes 20 cigarettes a day. Martha is then transferred to a medical ward with a cardiac specialty.

Assessment on admission

Martha is breathless and on oxygen therapy 35% via the mask. She has peripheral oedema and is fluid overloaded. Furosemide is being administered intravenously. She is on stage 2 (see Fig. 13.1) of the heart failure care plan but is not receiving glyceryl trinitrate (GTN) due to hypotension.

Martha is tachycardic and attached to a cardiac monitor which is showing atrial fibrillation between 110 and 115 bpm. Urinary output is greater than 70 mL/hour.

Martha is very distressed but knows where she is and why. She is unable to eat or drink at the moment due to her breathlessness. She is a life-long smoker. She lives with her husband in a third-floor flat with a lift. She still works part time as a cleaner for a local company.

Activity

See Appendix 4 in Holland et al (2008) for possible questions to consider during the assessment stage of care planning.

Many organisations will have a care plan pathway, and Figure 13.1 is an example of one by R. Ripoll (2005 unpublished). This is to ensure that the care of the patient is explicit and standardised. This does not mean that the care becomes less individualised.

Martha's problems

Based on your assessment of Martha, the following problems should form the basis of your care plan:
- Martha is breathless.
- Martha is cardiovascularly unstable due to her condition.
- Martha is frightened and distressed.
- Martha has a urinary catheter.
- Martha is unable to eat or drink adequately due to her condition.
- Martha is a life-long smoker and cannot smoke in hospital.

Martha's nursing care plans

1. Problem: Martha is breathless.

   Goal: To restore normal breathing pattern.

Nursing action	Rationale
Assess Martha's breathing, respiratory rate and keep oxygen saturation >95% Observe for signs of cyanosis Administer prescribed oxygen Inform the nurse in charge of any changes to Martha's condition	To observe for any signs of deterioration To ensure that Martha does not become hypoxic Oxygen is a drug and must be prescribed

Continued

Nursing action	Rationale
Encourage Martha to sit upright supported by pillows	To maximise lung expansion and gaseous exchange To increase comfort
Administer any medication as prescribed and ensure that Martha is fully informed about the medication and any side effects For example, explain to Martha why she needs to keep her oxygen mask on	Martha is much more likely to comply with her medication if she understands why she needs to have it
Refer Martha to the physiotherapist and liaise	To maximise gaseous exchange To prevent complications from immobility To ensure consistent treatment from nurses and physiotherapists

2. Problem: Martha is cardiovascularly unstable due to her condition.

   Goal : To stabilise Martha.

Nursing action	Rationale
Martha needs continuous cardiac monitoring of her condition until it has stabilised Ensure that alarm limits are set within appropriate limits Hourly observations of pulse and blood pressure Inform the nurse in charge and doctor regarding any changes in observations and discuss the frequency of observations required	To detect any change in Martha's condition as soon as possible To be able to respond to these changes and for the team to be informed
To check blood urea and electolytes	Abnormal potassium levels will increase the risk cardiovascular instability

3. Problem: Martha is frightened and distressed.

   Goal : To try to relieve Martha's distress.

Nursing action	Rationale
Spend time with Martha using verbal and non-verbal communication to reassure her	Being alone will increase Martha's distress
Always introduce Martha to the nurse who is relieving you or taking over your shift	Knowing who is looking after her will help Martha to relax

Continued

Nursing action	Rationale
If you need to go to another area, explain to Martha who will be looking after her Explain to Martha how the call bell system works and make sure that it is in easy reach	Knowing where her nurse is is important as Martha will know that there is someone identified who is looking after her needs If Martha cannot see her nurse she will understand how to summon help
Communicate with Martha's family and significant others with her permisssion	Family and friends may find the environment and equipment daunting Information will help them to understand about Martha's condition Nurses should never presume that a patient wants her family to know about their condition and it is important to respect Martha's wishes

4. Problem: Martha has a urinary catheter.

   Goal: To monitor fluid balance accurately and to prevent infection.

Nursing action	Rationale
Explain to Martha why she requires urinary catheter. Hourly measurements of urine: if below 30 mL/h or above 200 mL/h, report to the nurse in charge and liaise with the doctors when reducing the frequency of the urine output measurements Document urine output on a fluid balance chart	To accurately monitor Martha's fluid balance. Martha is at risk of fluid overload due to her cardiac condition
Provide catheter care and hygiene Check the colour of the urine each shift Report any changes to the nurse in charge Provide privacy when providing catheter care	To prevent infection To detect any signs of infection or trauma To ensure that Martha's privacy and dignity needs are met
Monitor temperature, pulse and blood pressure and respirations four times a day while Martha has an indwelling urinary catheter Take a catheter specimen of urine for microscopy, culture and sensitivity testing if Martha's temperature is >37.5°C and inform the nurse/doctor	To detect any infection and treat as soon as possible

5. Problem: Martha is unable to eat or drink adequately due to her condition.

   Goal: For Martha to have adequate fluid and dietary intake.

Nursing action	Rationale
Ensure a malnutrition risk assessment is undertaken in the first 24 hours (see Ch. 9)	To determine Martha's nutritional status
Maintain strict food and fluid balance monitoring Martha may be on fluid restriction Inform Martha about this and provide her with rationale Inform the nurse in charge or doctor if Martha's diet or fluid intake are below the normal limits	Due to her cardiac failure, Martha is at risk of fluid overload To ensure that Martha receives adequate fluids and nutrition To prevent complications of dehydration To ensure that there is effective communication within the multidisciplinary team
Ensure that nutritional supplements are explained to Martha and encourage her to drink them	To keep Martha fully informed
Monitor and document observations of her vital signs (see Ch. 7)	To detect any deterioration/improvement
Administer intravenous therapy as prescribed and ensure that a cannula care plan is in place for this (see Ch. 9)	To reduce the risk of cannula-associated infection/complications
Keep Martha informed of her condition	To promote and enhance communication

6. Problem: Martha is a life-long smoker and cannot smoke in hospital.

   Goal: To help Martha deal with any cravings or withdrawal symptoms.

Nursing action	Rationale
To discuss with Martha how she is feeling and discuss prescribing nicotine supplements with the medical team	To prevent Martha from suffering from nicotine withdrawal symptoms
Once Martha is feeling better, discuss how she feels about smoking after discharge and whether she would accept a referral to the cardiac rehabilitation/heart failure team or smoking cessation team Provide verbal and written information for Martha and her husband	To provide health education and promotion to Martha and her family

How Martha progressed

Once Martha had been given digoxin loading doses, the atrial fibrillation subsided and, in turn, this relieved her heart failure as her heart was now able to pump effectively. With this, her breathing eased and gradually her oxygen was reduced and then removed. Her cardiac monitor was discontinued and gradually her observations were reduced to four times per day. During the acute phase, Martha required a lot of psychological support as she was very frightened and said that she thought she was going to die. She was very shocked that she had become so ill and the multidisciplinary team took time to explain what had happened and how to prevent reoccurrence.

Martha began to improve and, prior to her discharge date, was informed about her need to stay on oral digoxin and furosemide. She was referred to the heart failure nurse, given an out-patient appointment and referred to the smoking cessation clinic. Her husband was also a smoker and the nurses spent time with them both explaining the risks of smoking and reinforced this with leaflets.

Unfortunately, Martha's condition became unstable the night before her discharge and, despite being actively treated, she died 2 days later.

References

Holland, K., Jenkins, J., Solomon, J., et al., 2008. Applying the Roper, Logan, Tierney model in practice, 2nd ed. Churchill Livingstone, Edinburgh.

Montague, S., Watson, R., Herbert, R., 2005. Physiology for nursing practice, 3rd ed. Elsevier, Edinburgh.

Further reading

British Heart Foundation, 2007. Risking it: how to reduce your risk of coronary heart disease. British Heart Foundation, London.

Department of Health, Coronary Heart Disease Policy Team, 2009. The coronary heart disease national service framework: building on excellence, maintaining progress. Progress report for 2008. DH, London.

Hatchett, R., Thompson, D.R., 2007. Cardiac nursing: a comprehensive guide, 2nd ed. Churchill Livingstone, Edinburgh.

Jowett, N.I., Thompson, D.R., 2007. Comprehensive coronary care, 4th ed. Elsevier, Edinburgh.

Lindsay, G., Gaw, A., 2004. Coronary heart disease prevention: a handbook for the healthcare team. Churchill Livingstone, Edinburgh.

Rawlings-Anderson, K., Johnson, K., 2007. Oxford handbook of cardiac nursing. Oxford handbooks in nursing. Oxford University Press, Oxford.

Thompson, D.R., Webster, R.A., 2004. Caring for the coronary patient, 2nd ed. Elsevier, Edinburgh.

Woods, S.L., Froelicher, E.S., Motzer, A., et al., 2010. Cardiac nursing, 6th ed. Wolters Kluwer Health/Lippincott Williams & Wilkins, Philadelphia.

14 Case study of a patient who has been diagnosed HIV positive

Brian Thornton

CHAPTER AIMS

- To provide you with a case study of a patient who is living with a diagnosis of HIV together with the rationale for care
- To encourage you to research and deepen your knowledge of HIV/AIDS

Introduction

This chapter provides you with an example of the nursing care that a patient with HIV might require. The case study has been written by an HIV nurse specialist and provides you with a patient profile to enable you to understand the context of the patient. The case study aims to guide you through the assessment, nursing action and evaluation of a patient with HIV together with the rationale for care.

Patient profile

Ms Jessie Chitalwa is a 27-year-old Nigerian lady who has lived in the UK since the age of 22. She is doing a business studies degree at a local university. She attended accident and emergency (A&E) with a 2-week history of increasing shortness of breath and lethargy. She tested HIV positive on a point of care test in A&E. Her working diagnosis is pneumocystis pneumonia and she has been prescribed intravenous co-trimoxazole to treat this. She arrived on the ward overnight, at 11 p.m., and you are her nurse for the morning shift, starting at 7.15 a.m.

 Activity

A definition of HIV was given in Chapter 1 and asked you to revise your anatomy and physiology (see Montague et al 2005). Before reading the case study, try to find out how HIV affects the immune system. What key issues did you discover for how HIV affects the immune system?

This comprehensive article may help you to research this:

Flannigan J (2008). HIV and AIDS: transmission, testing and treatment. Nursing Standard 22(34):48–56. Online. Available at: http://nursingstandard.rcnpublishing.co.uk/archive/article-hiv-and-aids-transmission-testing-and-treatment (accessed July 2011).

Assessment on admission

When greeting and introducing yourself to Ms Chitalwa, you notice she is very anxious and visibly upset. Her vital signs are: pulse 118 regular, respiratory rate 28, temperature 37.3°C tympanic, oxygen saturation 94% (receiving 2-L oxygen via nasal specs). She is in a bay with five other patients on your medical ward.

During your assessment discussion with Ms Chitalwa, using the Roper, Logan and Tierney (Roper et al 2000) model of activities of daily living, you note that she is normally totally independent in all activities of daily living (see Table 14.1).

Ms Chitalwa's problems

Based on your assessment of Ms Chitalwa, the following problems should form the basis of your care plan:

- Jessie is unable to independently maintain a safe environment.

 Activity

See Appendix 4 in Holland et al (2008) for possible questions to consider during the assessment stage of care planning.

- Jessie has reduced communication ability, partly due to shortness of breath and partly due to her current psychological state and fear of her HIV diagnosis being discovered.
- Jessie has pneumonia.
- Jessie has reduced blood oxygen saturation levels and is short of breath.
- Jessie has reduced appetite and is at risk of inadequate nutritional intake.
- Jessie has reduced mobility and is at risk of deep vein thrombosis and other hazards of prolonged immobility.
- Jessie is unable to walk to the bathroom.
- Jessie is tired but unable to sleep.
- Jessie is worried that she is going to die.
- Jessie has an intravenous cannula in situ, and is receiving intravenous therapy.

Jessie's nursing care plans

1. Problem: Jessie is unable to independently maintain a safe environment.

   Goal: To ensure a safe environment.

Nursing action	Rationale
Ensure the call buzzer is within reach at all times	So Jessie is able to summon assistance as required and not attempt to do things beyond her current level of capability, potentially causing her condition to deteriorate or for her to fall
Ensure Jessie is aware that she should summon assistance and not try to push herself to do things which she is not currently capable of	To re-enforce to Jessie that she is unwell and that it is OK for her to ask for assistance

Table 14.1 Assessment of Ms Chitalwa using the Roper, Logan and Tierney model

Maintaining a safe environment	She requires assistance due to reduced mobility and lethargy. Local hazards include the oxygen tubing for her nasal specs and the drip stand and tubes for her intravenous co-trimoxazole
Communicating	She is fluent in English, which is her second language. Shortness of breath is reducing her sentence length. Recent HIV diagnosis has been a shock to her and she appears to be upset and withdrawn. She is very worried that her HIV status will be discovered by the other patients in her bay, as well as by her flatmates when they come to visit her. She seems reluctant to communicate about her HIV diagnosis. She has spent a lot of her time reading her bible. She is happy to be called Jessie
Breathing	Jessie becomes short of breath easily. She is receiving oxygen therapy via a humidification system and nasal specs. She finds it difficult to have a deep breath, and starts coughing
Eating and drinking	Her appetite has been reduced for the last week. She is a vegetarian. She feels nauseous when she tries to eat
Eliminating	She is too weak to walk to the bathroom, even with assistance
Personal cleansing and dressing	She is able to wash herself with a bowl at the bedside. She has been unable to bathe or shower for the last 3 days due to her lethargy and shortness of breath
Controlling body temperature	Currently no problems
Mobility	Severely reduced. Can barely manage five steps without becoming distressed. Oxygen and IV therapy are continuous so her range is already restricted due to the length of the tubes and IV lines
Working and playing	Does not want to discuss this right now
Expressing sexuality	Does not want to discuss this right now
Sleeping	Feels tired but has had a very unsettled night. Has not slept properly for several days, cannot remember how long
Dying	She is convinced that she is dying. The recent HIV diagnosis has made her resign herself to this fact. She has seen people die of HIV in Nigeria when she was younger and remembers the pain and suffering they went through, as well as the stigma for them and their families

Evaluation:

Jessie's environment remained safe throughout her hospital stay and recovery.

2. Problem: Jessie has reduced communication ability, partly due to shortness of breath and partly due to her current psychological state and fear of her HIV diagnosis being discovered.

   Goal: To ensure optimum communication with Jessie.

   Goal: To support Jessie psychologically with her recent HIV diagnosis.

Nursing action	Rationale
Try to ask closed questions, if possible	To reduce the need for Jessie to feel she has to respond with long answers
Ensure privacy for discussions, taking Jessie to a private room as soon as this is feasible	Jessie will hopefully be more able to have conversations about HIV infection in a private setting, when she is aware that the rest of the patients will not be able to overhear
Make Jessie aware of the good prognosis and longevity for people with HIV infection	To reduce her fears of death or pain because of her HIV infection To enable Jessie to realise that she should recover and lead a normal life, but will have to take medicines every day
Refer to psychology service	To ensure an appropriately trained health professional is able to assess and support Jessie with her concerns and worries
Ensure all healthcare professionals are aware of Jessie's concerns over confidentiality of her HIV infection	To reduce the risk of her HIV status being mentioned or discussed either in front of her, therefore disclosing to the other patients in her bay, or in public areas where the discussions could be overheard by other patients or visitors

Evaluation:

The first two nursing actions may seem to contradict one another, but the nurse needs to be able to ensure information is passed on to Jessie in a way that her psychological state is improved, and information about the expected good recovery prognosis is shared with her, but at the same time giving her the ability to ask questions and express her concerns. As Jessie's condition improves with treatment and good nursing care, the conversations can be more in depth. A psychology referral should be made, if a psychologist is available, to assist with this. The HIV clinical nurse specialist will have a key role in this.

During her hospital stay, Jessie learned more about HIV infection and accepted that she should lead a normal, healthy life, supported by HIV medicines and routine follow up at the HIV clinic.

3. Problem: Jessie has pneumonia.

    Goal: The pneumonia will resolve and she will return to a normal state of health.

Nursing action	Rationale
Ensure all medicines are given as prescribed and on time	To ensure the maximum efficacy of medication
Routine 4-hourly observations of vital signs, reporting abnormalities to the registered nurse	To quickly detect deterioration, and to record improvement in condition
Ensure Jessie is aware of what pneumonia is, what the treatment is and what the expected course of her recovery is	To ensure Jessie has appropriate expectations of her recovery and treatment process
Refer to physiotherapist or teach appropriate breathing exercises	To ensure that Jessie is supported and starts to recover from the pneumonia

Evaluation:
Jessie's recovery was as expected. Within 7 days she was feeling much better. Deep breathing became easier and she did not develop any further infection in her lungs.

4. Problem: Jessie has reduced blood oxygen saturation levels and is short of breath.

    Goal: To maintain saturation and tissue perfusion.

    Goal: To reduce episodes of shortness of breath.

Nursing action	Rationale
Administer oxygen as prescribed, using appropriate humidification and warming system	To ensure adequate oxygen saturation in blood and adequate tissue perfusion To prevent drying and damage of nasal and respiratory passages from unhumidified oxygen administration
Daily check of Jessie's nose	To reduce risk of damage to nose from nasal oxygen prongs
Reduce physical exertion which requires greater oxygen use	To reduce the risk of shortness of breath occurring
Try to ensure Jessie remains calm	To reduce anxiety and associated increase in respiratory rate and oxygen use

Evaluation:
Oxygen therapy remained for 3 days. There were episodes of increased anxiety and times when Jessie tried to do things beyond her capability, resulting in acute shortness of breath, but nursing support and care ensured these episodes were minimised.

5. Problem: Jessie has reduced appetite and is at risk of inadequate nutritional intake.

    Goal: To ensure adequate nutritional intake.

Nursing action	Rationale
Undertake appropriate dietary/nutritional assessment	To ensure a baseline is recorded and adequate planning can be made for any necessary dietary support
Refer to dietician	To ensure appropriate supplements are ordered and obtained To provide nursing staff with expert advice and support on the best way to care for Jessie's nutritional needs
Ensure assistance, as appropriate, with completing menu request forms	To ensure that Jessie is able to request the most appetising and edible meals for herself, in order to try to get her to eat as much food as she needs

Evaluation:
Jessie's appetite was reduced for 7 days, during which time she was prescribed food supplements via the dietician. She was reluctant to order food at first, but nursing staff encouraged and supported her. Appropriate nutritional food and fluid intake was ensured.

This article may be of interest to you:
Ward D (2002). The role of nutrition in the prevention of infection. Nursing Standard 16 (18):47–52. Online. Available at: http://nursingstandard.rcnpublishing.co.uk/archive/article-the-role-of-nutrition-in-the-prevention-of-infection-3141 (accessed July 2011).

6. Problem: Jessie has reduced mobility and is at risk of deep vein thrombosis and other hazards of prolonged immobility.
   Goal: To prevent hazards of prolonged immobility.

   Goal: To encourage controlled recovery to normal mobility.

Nursing action	Rationale
Refer Jessie to a physiotherapist	To ensure expert assessment of current reduced mobility To ensure structured plan for assistance to improve and return to normal levels of mobility To ensure appropriate exercises/limb movements/deep breathing are taught and observed
Ensure Jessie is updated on goals of improving and increasing mobility	To ensure maximum engagement in her care management

Continued

Nursing action	Rationale
Complete appropriate risk assessments, e.g. falls, pressure ulcer risk, making appropriate referrals as necessary	To ensure potential hazards are identified and rectified To reduce risk of adverse events To ensure that the falls nurse and tissue viability nurse are involved if necessary to provide expert input and advice
Encourage regular position movement and standing	To reduce the risk of tissue breakdown
Administer any prescribed antiembolus medicines or stockings as prescribed	To reduce the risk of deep vein thromboses

Evaluation:

Jessie's skin remained intact. She did not develop any associated hazards of prolonged immobility. For the first 2 days her mobility was greatly reduced, and she was frustrated, but as time went on she recovered as expected.

7. Problem: Jessie is unable to walk to the bathroom.

   Goal: To maintain Jessie's privacy and dignity when eliminating.

Nursing action	Rationale
Ensure the call buzzer is within reach	To ensure Jessie can summon assistance if she needs help getting to the bathroom
Use a wheelchair to transport Jessie to the bathroom	Jessie is unable to walk to the bathroom and she is reluctant to use a commode at the bedside Her privacy and dignity are maximised by ensuring she is taken into the bathroom when she needs to eliminate

Evaluation:

Jessie was happy that her privacy was maintained as she was able to use the bathroom every time she needed to eliminate.

8. Problem: Jessie is tired but unable to sleep.

   Goal: To ensure adequate rest and sleep.

Nursing action	Rationale
Make Jessie as comfortable as possible in bed	She is more likely to sleep if she is comfortable

Continued

Nursing action	Rationale
Facilitate afternoon quiet times on the ward	Reducing noise, visitors and visits by clinical staff can cause an environment conducive to rest and relaxation
Administer any prescribed sedative or sleeping medication	To support Jessie in having rest and sleep

Evaluation:

Jessie found it difficult to sleep, but the afternoon 'quiet times' were helpful to her. As she started to recover from the pneumonia and her psychological state improved, she found it was easier, but never had a good, full night's sleep in hospital.

9.   Problem: Jessie is worried that she is going to die.

   Goal: To support Jessie psychologically.

   Goal: To try to alleviate Jessie's fears and concerns.

Nursing action	Rationale
Ensure a private place is available for conversations with Jessie	Discussing personal or sensitive information should always be undertaken in the right environment Jessie is more likely to engage if she is not worried about other people overhearing and discovering her private, personal information
Ensure Jessie is aware of her condition and the potential recovery from her current infection as well as HIV and HIV therapy	To ensure Jessie has realistic expectations for recovery and prognosis To ensure Jessie is able to appreciate what HIV infection is, what it does to the body, how it is controlled and to stress that she is expected to recover and live to be an old woman, as long as she takes the prescribed therapy
Refer to a psychologist	To offer expert assessment of Jessie's psychological state To ensure expert planning for managing and supporting Jessie
Refer to HIV specialist team members as appropriate	The HIV nurse specialist and other team members can provide expert input and support, and can work alongside ward staff to assist in patient care

Evaluation:

Jessie was upset and convinced she was going to die for several days, but with appropriate input she realised that HIV is a treatable condition and she had an excellent prognosis for recovery.

10.   Problem: Jessie has an intravenous cannula in situ, and is receiving intravenous therapy.

Goal: To prevent infection at the cannula site and other associated problems of an IV cannula.

Nursing action	Rationale
Complete and maintain a cannula care plan	To ensure that appropriate recording of insertion and inspection of cannula/cannula site is maintained (see page 171 for an example of a phlebitis score)

Evaluation:
Jessie received IV therapy for 7 days, during which time she was cannulated four times. All sites were regularly inspected and she did not develop thrombophlebitis or any other associated risks.

Summary

Jessie's previous experience of people with HIV, who were untreated and who died horrible deaths, had affected her psychological acceptance of her own HIV infection and this required a lot of input from all healthcare professionals. Associated with worries of stigma and being rejected from her community, Jessie could initially see no positive outcome. However, excellent team work and providing the right information at the right time ensured that Jessie could realise the truth about HIV and current HIV therapy and realise and accept that she is expected to be fit and healthy, with minimal interference from her HIV infection.

When patients are admitted with pneumocystis pneumonia, they are very weak and need a lot of physical and emotional support (see Ch. 14 in Holland et al 2008). Assisted respiration, such as continuous positive airway pressure, is often needed if the presentation to the hospital is late in the infection, and sometimes ventilation and intensive care admission are needed. Appropriate nursing care and management, including quickly identifying any deterioration, are vital.

It is easy for healthcare workers to forget the sensitivity of personal information, such as HIV infection, and discuss things at the nurses' station where other patients and visitors can overhear. The nurse must remain vigilant at all times and challenge colleagues in such situations.

Cases such as this one can provide ideal learning opportunities for student nurses around communication skills, giving 'bad news', interviewing and counselling skills, as well as learning about current developments in treatments, such as treatments for HIV infection.

References

Holland, K., Jenkins, J., Solomon, J., et al., 2008. Applying the Roper, Logan, Tierney model in practice, 2nd ed. Churchill Livingstone, Edinburgh.

Montague, S., Watson, R., Herbert, R., 2005. Physiology for nursing practice, 3rd ed. Elsevier, Edinburgh.

Roper, N., Logan, W., Tierney, A., 2000. The Roper–Logan–Tierney model of nursing. Churchill Livingstone, Edinburgh.

Websites

HIV insight e-tutorials for nurses. Free online learning modules from basic to more advanced HIV information, including patient management learning: http://www.hivinsight.co.uk/ (accessed July 2011).

National HIV Nurses Association. Includes national competencies for HIV nurses, study and training days, news and updates in HIV nursing and management: http://www.nhivna.org/ (accessed July 2011).

British HIV Association. Includes UK guidelines for diagnosis, care and management of individuals with HIV infection, as well as national conference information, news and updates: http://www.bhiva.org/ (accessed July 2011).

HIV Treatment Information Base. Patient-centred Website to provide support and information for those affected by HIV infection. Includes easy-to-read educational leaflets, news, personal views and new developments in HIV care: http://i-base.info/home/ (accessed July 2011).

As well as the above resources, putting HIV and your area of interest into an online journal database will produce a number of articles for you to review. There is a wealth of information about HIV infection and I suggest that you consider your specific requirement when you do online searches (e.g. HIV infection AND faith, or HIV infection AND depression, or HIV infection AND cure, etc.).

15 Case study of a patient with tuberculosis

Maria Mercer

CHAPTER AIMS

- To provide you with a case study of a patient who has been diagnosed with pulmonary tuberculosis (TB) together with the rationale for care
- To encourage you to research and deepen your knowledge of TB

The following article may help you:
William VG (2006). Tuberculosis: clinical features, diagnosis and management. Nursing Standard 20(22):49–53. Online. Available at:http://nursingstandard. rcnpublishing.co.uk/archive/article-tuberculosis-clinical-features-diagnosis-and-management (accessed July 2011).

Introduction

This chapter provides you with an example of the nursing care that a patient with pulmonary TB might require. The case study has been written by a TB nurse specialist and provides you with a patient profile to enable you to understand the context of the patient. The case study aims to guide you through the assessment, nursing action and evaluation of a patient with pulmonary TB together with the rationale for care.

Patient profile

Mr Patel is a 21-year-old gentleman who lives in a shared flat with friends and studies English at a local college. He is a new arrival to the UK having arrived from Bangladesh in October 2009. There are six adults, including Mr Patel, who share a two-bedroom flat. They share three adults to a room. He was referred to accident and emergency (A&E) via his GP with a 2-month history of a productive cough (no episodes of haemoptysis), associated fevers, drenching night sweats, loss of

 Activity

In Chapter 1 you were asked to revise the normal anatomy and physiology of the respiratory system (see Montague et al 2005) and a brief definition of TB was given. Before reading the case study below, find out how pulmonary TB would affect the respiratory system and what symptoms a patient with TB might present with.

appetite and a 5-kg weight loss. In the last 7 days his symptoms have worsened and warranted the admission via A&E.

been reported as abnormal: 'Patchy shadowing seen in left upper lobe? Pulmonary TB.'

Assessment on admission

Mr Patel has a pyrexia of 38.5°C, he is cachectic and has pleuritic chest pain. His respiratory rate is slightly raised at 18 per minute and he has a tachycardia of 114 beats per minute. Blood pressure is normal. Inflammatory markers – erythrocyte sedimentation rate (ESR) and C-reactive protein (CRP) – are raised at 72 mm/h and 65.4 mg/L. A chest X-ray has

 Activity

See Appendix 4 in Holland et al (2008) for possible questions to consider during the assessment stage of care planning.

Mr Patel's problems

Based on your assessment of Mr Patel, the following problems should form the basis of your care plan:
- Mr Patel has a potential diagnosis of pulmonary TB which can be an infectious disease and public health risk.
- Mr Patel feels stigmatised because of respiratory isolation measures and the potential diagnosis of TB.
- Mr Patel has a temperature, raised inflammatory markers, a slightly elevated respiratory rate and a tachycardia.
- Mr Patel is nutritionally compromised because of a 5-kg weight loss due to anorexia.
- Mr Patel has pleuritic chest pain associated with coughing and expectoration of sputum.

Mr Patel's nursing care plans

1. Problem: Mr Patel has an infection. Pulmonary TB is felt to be the primary diagnosis.

   Goal: To limit transmission of TB to other patients and staff and ensure prompt treatment is commenced.

Nursing action	Rationale
Mr Patel to be isolated in a side room with bathroom facilities with respiratory isolation measures in place immediately	To reduce the risk of TB transmission to other patients and staff
The door to the side room must be shut at all times Appropriate face masks (FFP2 or FFP3, depending on risk assessment – refer to infection control/TB policy) should be worn when entering Mr Patel's room and he should wear the appropriate face mask if he needs to leave the side room for investigations Gloves and aprons do not need to be worn unless handling bodily secretions	

Continued

Nursing action	Rationale
Liaise with bed managers and infection control team to expedite bed availability as necessary	
Collect three consecutive sputum specimens for acid-fast bacilli (AFB) Send one sputum specimen urgently on day of admission	To ascertain diagnosis and ensure the appropriate treatment is commenced promptly
Ensure Mr Patel is aware that sputum specimens need to be collected consecutively. Label 3 sputum pots clearly and leave in side room. Instruct Mr Patel to inform the nurse caring for him when the sputum for each day is ready so it can be collected and sent to the Laboratory as soon as possible.	To ascertain diagnosis and ensure the appropriate treatment is commenced promptly.
Contact the TB nurses to perform a Mantoux test if prescribed by the medical staff.	To facilitate prompt diagnosis and obtain specialist nursing advice and support
Ensure effective communication with Mr Patel explaining why the above measures are necessary and providing reassurance and support	To alleviate fear and anxiety

Evaluation:

Mr Patel was diagnosed with pulmonary TB when his first sputum specimen returned from microbiology 12 hours after admission as AFB smear positive. Tuberculosis treatment was prescribed. A referral was made to the TB nurses in the community.

2. Problem: Mr Patel was diagnosed by microbiology as having AFB smear positive sputum.

Goal: To ensure Mr Patel understands the rationale for the commencement of TB treatment.

Nursing action	Rationale
Mr Patel will be seen by a TB nurse and have the rationale for commencing TB treatment explained and reiterated The TB nurses have time to spend talking to Mr Patel and will prove support and reassurance	To ensure Mr Patel understands fully the rationale for his TB diagnosis and agrees to adhere to TB treatment to ensure cure
Mr Patel will have the side effects of the TB medications explained fully	To ensure he informs nursing staff of any side effects promptly and appropriate interventions will be instigated

Continued

Nursing action	Rationale
Mr Patel will have the importance of adherence to TB medications explained Barriers to adherence will be assessed by the TB nurse This assessment will be used to consider if Mr Patel requires directly observed therapy instigated on discharge from hospital	To facilitate cure of TB and prevent any risks of drug resistance occurring due to non-adherence
Mr Patel will have the TB nurse discuss TB contact tracing of household, close social and college contacts and instigate the appropriate screening appointments	To identify any individuals with active or latent TB infection and implement the appropriate interventions Prevent and control TB in the population
The TB nurse will explain to Mr Patel that TB is a notifiable disease A consultant in communicable disease control will be informed of Mr Patel's diagnosis via a referral to the health protection unit Reassure Mr Patel that this information is confidential	To monitor control and management of TB in the place where Mr Patel lives, and in the wider UK

Evaluation:

Mr Patel was linked into the community TB service for follow up on discharge from hospital (after 2 weeks of TB treatment). The allocated TB nurse will case manage all subsequent appointments, repeat prescriptions, support and supervision. There were no barriers to adherence identified on discharge and directly observed therapy did not need to be implemented.

3. Problem: Mr Patel feels isolated and neglected in the side room. He also feels stigmatised because staff have to wear a mask when they enter his room.

    Goal: To reduce Mr Patel's feelings of isolation, neglect and stigma.

Nursing action	Rationale
Ensure Mr Patel has regular nursing interventions performed and that nursing staff communicate fully with him so he does not feel neglected in the side room	To ensure Mr Patel feels safe and cared for
Ensure that the side room Mr Patel is placed in has bathroom facilities so that he is not forced to leave his room with a face mask unnecessarily	To maintain and promote dignity
Ensure Mr Patel has access (as appropriate) to stimuli, e.g. television, radio, CD/iPod, books, etc.	

Continued

Nursing action	Rationale
Ensure staff offer to go to the hospital shop for Mr Patel if he requires newspapers, magazines and snacks	To limit boredom, promote wellbeing and reduce feelings of social isolation
Ensure Mr Patel is fully aware of why it is necessary to isolate him Reassure him that he will be assessed after 2 weeks of TB medications (with no adherence issues identified) to ensure that he is rendered non-infectious	To keep Mr Patel fully informed that he will not be in respiratory isolation for an unlimited period of time
Inform Mr Patel that TB is non-discriminating and can affect anyone at any time	To provide reassurance and reduce feelings of fear/stigma/isolation

Evaluation:
Mr Patel was rendered non-infectious after 2 weeks of TB medications. He was discharged home with no requirement to have any isolation measures continued in the community.

4. Problem: Mr Patel has a temperature, raised inflammatory markers, a slightly elevated respiratory rate and a tachycardia. These symptoms could be related to pulmonary TB but other sources of infection need to be excluded.

   Goal: To establish no other cause for signs of infection other than pulmonary TB.

Nursing action	Rationale
4-hourly vital signs, report any abnormal recordings to the nurse in charge	To monitor condition and note signs of deterioration and/or improvement
Administer prescribed antipyretic medications and monitor effect with the above recordings of vital signs	To promote Mr Patel's comfort and monitor condition
Ensure a routine urinalysis is performed If any traces of protein or blood, collect a mid-stream specimen of urine	To establish any other cause of infection
Ensure a routine sputum specimen is collected for culture and sensitivity	To establish any other cause of infection
Obtain a fan for Mr Patel's use and/or tepid sponging	To promote comfort

Evaluation:
Mr Patel's temperature and heart rate returned to within normal parameters and inflammatory markers began to reduce on TB medications. No other source of infection was found.

5. Problem: Mr Patel has lost 5 kg in 2 months and has a depleted appetite. He is leaving meals untouched because he does not feel hungry at meal times.

   Goal: To increase appetite, maintain nutritional requirements and facilitate weight gain.

Nursing action	Rationale
Ensure Mr Patel is weighed and height measured on admission to establish baseline weight and body mass index (BMI) Ensure a malnutrition risk assessment performed	To establish baseline weight and BMI and calculate what Mr Patel's healthy weight gain and BMI should be
Refer to dietician re nutritional supplements and (high-protein) healthy eating advice Encourage friends to bring in foods that Mr Patel would prefer to encourage appetite	To obtain specialist advice to encourage healthy weight gain and ensure further weight loss does not occur during hospital stay
Weigh Mr Patel at least weekly during admission and more frequently if necessary	To monitor weight gain and/or weight loss
Ensure Mr Patel is not suffering with any symptoms of nausea either as a result of his TB or side effects of medications If yes, ensure medical staff prescribe an antiemetic and monitor effectiveness	To establish if there is another cause of anorexia and treat accordingly
Maintain a fluid balance chart and food chart ensuring they are filled in correctly and regularly	To ensure adequate hydration and nutrition

Evaluation:
Mr Patel gradually gained his appetite during his hospital stay and began to gain weight with supplements and encouragement to eat small, frequent meals throughout the day. He did not require an antiemetic.

6. Problem: Mr Patel has pleuritic chest pain associated with coughing and expectoration of sputum.

   Goal: To reduce pain and promote comfort.

Nursing action	Rationale
Assess severity of pain by using a pain assessment tool	To establish the type and severity of the pain so that the appropriate analgesics can be prescribed to alleviate pain

Continued

Nursing action	Rationale
Ensure medical staff prescribe analgesia and that it is administered regularly (and as prescribed) by the nursing staff Use a pain assessment tool to assess effectiveness	To alleviate pain and promote comfort
Ensure Mr Patel has enough pillows to be able to sit upright in bed to maintain respiratory expansion	To ensure that no further respiratory complications develop
Ensure that Mr Patel does not sit out of bed for more than an hour at a time	To reduce the risk of further pressure damage

Evaluation:
Mr Patel was given regular ibuprofen with effect. The physiotherapist provided advice for effective positioning that facilitated comfort and reduced pain.

References

Holland, K., Jenkins, J., Solomon, J., et al., 2008. Applying the Roper, Logan, Tierney model in practice, 2nd ed. Churchill Livingstone, Edinburgh.

Montague, S., Watson, R., Herbert, R., 2005. Physiology for nursing practice, 3rd ed. Elsevier, Edinburgh.

Further reading

British Thoracic Society, 2000. Control and prevention of tuberculosis in the UK: code of practice. BTS, London. Online. Available at: http://www. brit-thoracic.org.uk/guidelines/ tuberculosis-guidelines.aspx (accessed July 2011).

Department of Health, 2004. Stopping tuberculosis in England: an action plan from the Chief Medical Officer. DH, London. Online. Available at: http://www.dh.gov.uk/en/ Publicationsandstatistics/Publications/ PublicationsPolicyAndGuidance/DH_ 4090417 (accessed July 2011).

Health Protection Agency, 2009. Tuberculosis in the UK: annual report on tuberculosis surveillance in the UK 2009. HPA, London.

Marais, F., 2002. Tuberculosis control: a nurse-led model with case management. The Foundation of Nursing Studies, London.

Mayho, P., 2006. The tuberculosis survival handbook. Merit Publishing International, Weybridge, Surrey.

National Institute for Health and Clinical Excellence, 2006. TB guidelines: clinical diagnosis and management of tuberculosis, and measures for its prevention and control. NICE, London. Online. Available at: http://guidance.nice. org.uk/CG33 (accessed July 2011).

Pratt, R., Grange, J., Williams, V., 2005. Tuberculosis. A foundation for nursing and healthcare practice. Holder Arnold, London.

Rom, W.R., Garay, S.M., 2004. Tuberculosis, 2nd ed. Lippincott Williams and Wilkins, Philadelphia.

World Health Organization, 2008. Tuberculosis. WHO, Geneva. Online. Available at: http://www.who. int/gho/tb/en/ (accessed July 2011).

16

Case study of a patient living with diabetes mellitus

Anne Claydon

CHAPTER AIMS

- To provide you with a case study of a patient who is living with diabetes together with the rationale for care
- To encourage you to research and deepen your knowledge of diabetes

Being in this community of practice has also enlightened me about diabetes as we come across many patients with diabetes. I have since learnt different ways of diabetes management. I can also give advice to patients suffering from diabetes bearing in mind that this is evidence based.
(Patricia Moyo, third-year student nurse)

Introduction

This chapter provides you with an example of the nursing care that a patient with type 1 diabetes might require. The case study has been written by a diabetes nurse specialist and provides you with a patient profile to enable you to understand the context of the patient. The case study aims to guide you through the assessment, nursing action and evaluation of a patient with type 1 diabetes together with the rationale for care.

The following paper outlines the latest guidelines for the care of patients with diabetic ketoacidosis (DKA). It would be useful to read these guidelines before you read the case study:

Joint British Diabetes Societies Inpatient Care Group (2010). The management of diabetic ketoacidosis in adults. NHS Diabetes, London. Online. Available at: http://www.bsped.org.uk/professional/guidelines/docs/DKAManagementOfDKAinAdultsMarch20101.pdf (accessed July 2011)

 Activity

Chapter 1 gives a brief definition of diabetes and asks you to revise the normal anatomy and physiology of the endocrine system (see Montague et al 2005). How can diabetes affect the body and what happens within the body when a person's blood sugars become unstable?

Patient profile

Lucy is an 18-year-old university student in her first year and is living in student accommodation. Lucy has had type 1 diabetes since the age of 13. Her parents are very supportive but naturally worried about her leaving home.

Lucy had a take-away chicken meal 2 days ago and since then she has been vomiting and has diarrhoea. She stopped taking her insulin as she is not eating. She has been admitted with DKA.

Assessment on admission

Lucy is apyrexial and has not vomited for 6 hours. Her vital signs are: pulse 96 beats per minute, blood pressure 130/80 mmHg, respiratory rate slightly raised at 18 per minute. Due to her diarrhoea and vomiting, she is dehydrated. Ketones are +2 on a standard urine stick, her blood glucose is 16 mmol/L and her venous pH is 7.2.

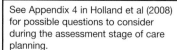 **Activity**

See Appendix 4 in Holland et al (2008) for possible questions to consider during the assessment stage of care planning.

Lucy's problems

Based on your assessment of Lucy, the following problems should form the basis of your care plan:
- Due to DKA, Lucy is dehydrated and has electrolyte imbalance.
- Lucy lacks knowledge about the precipitating factors of DKA and how to prevent it.

Lucy's nursing care plan – acute stage (first hour)

The most important therapeutic intervention for DKA in the acute stage is appropriate fluid replacement followed by insulin administration.

Problem: Due to DKA, Lucy is dehydrated and has electrolyte imbalance.

Goal: Lucy will maintain urine output >30 mL hour. Lucy will have elastic skin turgor and moist, pink mucous membranes.

Nursing action	Rationale
Measure and record urine output hourly Report urine output <30 mL for 2 consecutive hours Catheterise Lucy Provide catheter care	Lucy may undergo osmotic diuresis and have excessive urine output Measure fluid output accurately Maintain catheter hygiene at all time to prevent infection
Administer intravenous therapy as prescribed and ensure that a cannula care plan is in place for this	To prevent infection/complications around the cannula site

Continued

Nursing action	Rationale
Assess Lucy for signs of dehydration Assess Lucy's skin turgor, mucous membranes and complaints of thirst	Testing the skin; dry membranes and thirst are all signs of dehydration
Continuous measurement of Lucy's vital signs during this acute stage of DKA	As Lucy has DKA and is dehydrated, compensatory mechanisms take place that may result in peripheral vasoconstriction which is characterised b a weak thready pulse, hypotension and Lucy may look pale
Monitor Lucy's neurological state Observe and document how awake Lucy is Assess how alert and orientated Lucy is to time and place	Mental status in DKA can be altered due to severe volume depletion and electrolyte imbalance
Monitor Lucy's blood glucose levels every 15 minutes, then hourly as long as the insulin infusion continues Remember to wash Lucy's hands to remove any contaminants that might alter the results	Glucose levels need to be reduced gradually to prevent the risk of cerebral oedema Intravenous insulin therapy needs to continue until ketoacidosis is resolved
Assess Lucy for signs of hypokalaemia, for example muscle weakness, shallow respirations, cramping and confusion	DKA can cause excretion of potassium Insulin therapy results in intracellular movement of potassium resulting in low potassium levels
Lucy may have signs of hyperkalaemia Assess Lucy for any weakness or irritability, ECG changes such as tall, peaked T waves, QRS and prolonged PR intervals may suggest this Potassium levels should be kept between 4 and 5 mmol/L	As ketoacidosis resolves, potassium levels can rise quickly causing hyperkalaemia Ensure that the ECG leads are connected correctly and that the pads are not causing discomfort to Lucy's skin
Assess Lucy for signs of metabolic acidosis Lucy may show signs of being drowsy, she may have Kausmaul respirations, confusion and her breath may smell of pear drops	Lucy may have metabolic acidosis due to a build up of ketones in her blood
Measure Lucy's serum ketone levels using a hand-held ketones meter Check ketones 4 hourly	Blood glucose should be checked by a hand-held ketones meter This provides direct results for DKA to be resolved Ketonaemia has to be suppressed
Lucy will need intravenous insulin during the acute stage Lucy will require fixed-rate intravenous infusion of insulin calculated on 0.1 units/kg	Aim for a reduction of blood ketone concentration by 0.5 mmol/L/hour Insulin has the following effects: ● Reduction of blood glucose

Continued

Nursing action	Rationale
The fixed rate of insulin may have to be adjusted in insulin resistance if the ketone concentration does not fall fast enough	• Correction of electrolyte imbalance • Suppression of ketogenesis
Keep Lucy informed of her condition With Lucy's permission, communicate with her parents	To promote good communication and to provide Lucy with information
Refer Lucy to the diabetes team	The team are experts in treating DKA and the diabetes nurse specialist needs to educate Lucy

Evaluation:

Lucy had no serum ketone and her dehydration and electrolyte imbalance were corrected. Once this occurred, Lucy was changed from intravenous insulin to subcutaneous insulin.

Lucy's nursing care plan – long term

Problem: DKA is preventable. Currently Lucy lacks knowledge about the precipitating factors of DKA and how to prevent it.

Goal: Lucy will understand and be able to discuss with the nurse why she should never have stopped her insulin therapy. Lucy will understand and discuss the need for sick day management. Follow up will be arranged with the community diabetes nurse specialist and a diabetologist to help support Lucy in the future.

Nursing action	Rationale
Determine Lucy's learning needs and her self-management skills If Lucy agrees, this discussion would be better if it takes place with her parents so that they can be educated too	An initial assessment should be done to ascertain what Lucy already knows and about her educational needs
Lucy should be counselled about the precipitating factors and warning signs of DKA Lucy must seek medical advice if she experiences the following: • Excessive thirst and urine • Stomach pain • Sickness and vomiting • Drowsiness • Visual disturbances	Precipitating factors of DKA are to be discussed such as infection or omission of insulin injections Advise Lucy to seek medical advice if she experiences any of the symptoms as she may be developing DKA

Continued

Nursing action	Rationale
• Difficulty in breathing • Cracked lips or dry mouth (signs of dehydration) Lucy must be taught the 'sick day rules' and must devise a sick day plan Continue to take all diabetes medicine The golden rule is – always take insulin Lucy must monitor her glucose levels 2–4 hourly Lucy must know how to test her urine for ketones if blood glucose levels rise above 16 mmol or she vomits persistently	Lucy's insulin requirements will increase with any infection or illness as this increases blood glucose If Lucy monitors more frequently, she will be guided on the treatment she requires The lack of insulin causes fat to be broken down in the body and this leads to increased acid production (ketones)
Lucy needs to drink plenty of water – about a glass an hour or frequent sips If Lucy cannot eat, advise her to drink sweet fluids such as fruit juice, lucozade or soup	Lucy will need to supplement her intake of fluids to prevent dehydration Lucy must still take her insulin as these fluids will stop her blood glucose from falling and causing hypoglycaemia
Before discharge, establish goals with Lucy for glucose levels and haemoglobin A1c (HbA_{1C}) targets	Glucose control should be between 4–6 mmol/L fasting and 5–7 mmol/L post-prandial HbA_{1C} ideally should be between 6–6.5% (both these targets are difficult to attain in teenagers)
Refer to the community diabetes team	Lucy will need support during these difficult years

Evaluation:

Lucy knew that she must always take her insulin and she now knows when to ask for medical advice. Lucy was able to verbalise the 'sick day rules' and what to do if she ever became ill again. Lucy had learnt the signs and symptoms for DKA and was able to explain them. Lucy had support in the community from the diabetic nurse specialist and saw a diabetologist every 6 months.

References

Holland, K., Jenkins, J., Solomon, J., et al., 2008. Applying the Roper, Logan, Tierney model in practice, 2nd ed. Churchill Livingstone, Edinburgh.

Montague, S., Watson, R., Herbert, R., 2005. Physiology for nursing practice, 3rd ed. Elsevier, Edinburgh.

Further reading

Dunning, T., 2009. Care of people with diabetes: a manual of nursing practice, 3rd ed. Blackwell, Chichester.

Featherstone, H., Whitham, L., Chambers, M., 2010. Incentivising wellness: improving the treatment of long-term conditions. Policy Exchange, London.

Hillson, R., 2008. Diabetes care: a practical manual. Oxford care manuals, Oxford University Press, Oxford.

Holt, T.A., Kumar, S., Watkins, P.J., 2010. ABC of diabetes, ABC series 6th ed. Wiley–Blackwell/BMJ, Chichester.

Joint British Diabetes Societies Inpatient Care Group, 2010. The management of diabetic ketoacidosis in adults. NHS Diabetes, London. Online. Available at: http://www.bsped.org.uk/professional/ guidelines/docs/DKAManagement OfDKAinAdultsMarch20101.pdf (accessed July 2011).

Liburd, L.C., 2009. Diabetes and health disparities: community-based approaches for racial and ethnic populations. Springer, New York.

Pickup, J., Williams, G., 2003. Textbook of diabetes, 3rd ed., vol. 1. Blackwell Science, Oxford.

Pickup, J., Williams, G., 2003. Textbook of diabetes, 3rd ed., vol. 2. Blackwell Science, Oxford.

Section 4. Consolidating your learning

17 Revision and future learning

CHAPTER AIMS

- To establish current knowledge base about a range of health problems
- To identify future learning needs
- To provide you with some revision questions to test your knowledge
- To encourage you to reflect on your medical placement and to consider how this will impact on your future learning experiences

Introduction

Having completed your medical placement, it is important that you consolidate your learning which helps you to develop a lifelong learning approach to nursing experience. You need to spend some time making sense of what you have experienced and learnt, and every placement furnishes you with new knowledge. It is important that you transfer this new knowledge to other placements and contexts.

Developing good practice in learning

So how can you ensure that you capture what you have learnt? There is a variety of techniques that help you to capture your learning, and identifying some aspects of your learning may be easy. For example, if you have been placed on a respiratory medical ward, it is anticipated that your knowledge of respiratory conditions, the medical treatments and nursing care of patients with respiratory problems will have increased. Some learning will have developed more slowly, however, and you may struggle to articulate exactly what you have learnt.

It is important that you look back at your first meeting with your mentor and think about what you identified as your learning outcomes. Were your learning objectives specific, measurable, achievable, realistic and timely (SMART)? Did you meet your learning objectives? If not, why not? Did anything get in the way of your learning, for example ill health or lack of ongoing contact with your mentor? Students and their mentors are expected to work and learn together in various ways for 40% of their placement learning (Nursing and Midwifery Council (NMC) 2010). Recent guidance from the NMC (2011) states that an appropriate registered professional can also assess you as long as they have been suitably prepared. For example, your mentor could ask a physiotherapist to assess you in positioning a patient or assisting them to mobilise. If you did not work with your mentor enough, it is important to explore why that happened. Did you have other commitments or did your mentor work mainly nights or have to take sudden leave? Did you prefer to work with your associate mentor? How did you deal with this? If this was to happen to you again on another placement, what could you do differently?

◖◗ Reflection point

If you did experience any of the difficulties above, think about how you dealt with the situation at the time and how you might deal with it if it arose on another placement experience.

It may be helpful to consider the following points:
- If your mentor was unavailable for more than a week, did you inform anyone, e.g. placement manager, key mentor, practice experience facilitator, link lecturer, personal tutor?
- If you worked with your associate mentor more than your main mentor, you need to think about why this happened.
- Did you feel uncomfortable working with your mentor or associate mentor? If so, did you report this to anyone, e.g. placement manager, key mentor, practice experience facilitator, link lecturer, personal tutor?
- How will your assessment and documentation meet the required standards of your university and professional body (NMC 2008, 2011)?

Often the answer is to ensure effective communication. If you have other commitments, it is important that your next hospital or community placement understands what these are and to find out whether they are able to accommodate your requests for particular shift times or to work on specific days. If they can accommodate your requests, they will then allocate you a mentor who is most likely to work the same shifts as you. It is essential that the university (i.e. your personal tutor) is aware of any special circumstances that may affect your ability to work in your placement area or adjustments that you require when in placement.

If you missed placement time due to ill health or personal reasons, you now need to think about how you are going to negotiate making up this time. The NMC (2010) requires each student nurse to undertake 4600 hours of learning during their pre-registration nurse training programmes. Fifty per cent of these hours must be undertaken within clinical practice. Clinical skills simulation can contribute towards this but cannot exceed 300 hours over the entire pre-registration programme.

You also need to think about how you are feeling now and whether you need to think about making an appointment with your personal tutor or occupational health service.

In Chapter 3 we discussed how you would prepare for your placement and what you could expect from your mentor. Now look back at your initial meeting with your mentor; you will have identified some learning needs and agreed them together. It is important that your identified learning needs were closely linked to your curriculum documentation learning outcomes. At your mid-point meeting with your mentor, a review of your learning objectives identified in your initial meeting should have taken place to ensure you were on track. At this meeting, you may have realised that you had met those initial learning outcomes and identified some more learning objectives with your mentor. In the final meeting with your mentor, you should be able to see what you learnt, areas of strength and some areas for future development. It is important that you take this forward to your next placement as a continual record of your learning.

Evaluating your learning post-placement

Another helpful tool is the 'strengths, weaknesses, opportunities and threats' (SWOT) analysis which helps you to identify your strengths and weaknesses, the opportunities and threats that may present themselves. Some students undertake this before and after each placement as they find it useful to understand some of the areas which they need to focus on and the barriers that might prevent them from getting there.

It can be helpful to think about your first day on your medical placement and what you actually knew then and what you know now. If it is your first ward, you may have felt completely lost and worried about approaching a patient, undertaking essential skills and fitting in with the team. By the end of your first placement, you should feel much more confident in all of those areas. As a senior student, you may have worried about undertaking the shift handover for a group of patients and prioritising your workload. It is important that you check your learning in this area and think about what you still need to do and how you can achieve it.

See Table 17.1 for examples of some SWOT analysis comments made by students.

When you return to university, you will be asked to complete an evaluation form about your placement. Different methods may be used to evaluate your placement – some universities will use a combination of group discussion and formal written feedback and in other universities your evaluation may be completed electronically.

This evaluation is fed back to your placement anonymously to allow placement staff to understand what is going well and to take action where areas for development have been highlighted.

It is important that learning is quality assured and enhanced for future students. The evaluations are usually linked to national educational standards that are incorporated into clinical learning environment audits for the placement area. This audit is usually reviewed annually for each placement area. It is important that you identify what was good about the placement so that the area is aware of its strengths regarding student learning. It is equally important for the ward placement area to understand how learning could be enhanced for future students.

This feedback is shared with the placement areas, educational leads in the hospitals, senior nurses, lecturers and the programme directors. There is usually a trust and university committee where the feedback is discussed and action agreed and disseminated. If a ward has received outstanding feedback, there may be an award ceremony which incorporates a reward for the best placement.

Some universities also encourage students to nominate exceptional placements and mentors for various awards and tributes. If your placement has been outstanding, it is important they receive that recognition because they often go above and beyond what is expected of them despite having heavy workloads. Your feedback is vital to ensure that the practice learning experience continues to be enhanced.

Developing your role as a nurse

The role of the nurse within the medical placement was discussed in Chapter 1, and the fact that this placement should

Table 17.1 Examples of some SWOT analysis comments made by students

Strengths	Teamwork
	Linking abbreviations
	Confidence increased
	Coping with activities of daily living
	Coping with stress
	Bed making
	Applying theory to practice
	Time management
	Communication
	Eating and drinking
	Universal precautions
	Helpful mentor
	Able to maintain confidentiality and dignity
	Good link lecturer
	Lots of learning opportunities
	Working under pressure
	Time keeping
	Building relationships with patients and staff
	Being independent
	Being assertive
	Good library
	Being accepted as a student
	Giving good care to patients
	Always asking consent and explaining treatment to patients
Weaknesses	Spelling
	Vital signs
	Language
	Doctors' notes illegible
	Not enough computers
	Mentor not familiar with curriculum documentation
	Not enough time
	Balancing placement with academic demands
	Not enough available time with mentor
	Time management
	Not feeling part of the team
	Not enough staff on ward
	Working under pressure
	Not enough time to provide quality care to patients
Opportunities	Given opportunity to meet learning outcomes
	Doing dressings under supervision
	Observing drug rounds
	Writing nursing notes
	Involvement in admission and discharge

Table 17.1 Examples of some SWOT analysis comments made by students—cont'd

	Meeting and working with different members of the multidisciplinary team
	Seeing a cardiac arrest
	Taking part in last offices
	Working with experienced staff
	Caring for my own patient and handing over verbally and in writing
	Escorting patients to X-ray
	Attending multidisciplinary team meetings
	Being challenged
	Giving injections under supervision
	Reading patients' notes
	Meeting people from different backgrounds
Threats	Doctors not understanding how junior we are and our level or knowledge
	Keeping up with academic work
	Not able to complete learning outcomes
	Losing manual skills by relying on electronic equipment
	Mentors not having time for us
	Feeling tired, not having enough sleep
	Not realising own limitations
	Being asked difficult questions by patients

furnish you with transferable skills that you can take forward to your next placement or into your preceptorship period was discussed in Chapter 3. Now that you have come to the end of your placement, it is important to reflect upon how you have developed your role as a student nurse during your time on the medical ward. If this was your final placement, you will need to consider what your learning needs might be as a newly qualified nurse commencing your preceptorship period. The Department of Health (DH; 2010a) and the NMC (2006) recommend preceptorship for all newly qualified nurses.

The NMC (2006) states that:

Preceptorship is about providing support and guidance enabling 'new registrants' to make the transition from student to accountable practitioner to:

- *practise in accordance with the NMC code of professional conduct: standards for conduct, performance and ethics;*
- *develop confidence in their competence as a nurse, midwife or specialist community public health nurse.*

  To facilitate this, the 'new registrant' should have:
- *learning time protected in their first year of qualified practice; and*
- *have access to a preceptor with whom regular meetings are held.*

(Preceptorship guidelines, NMC 2006)

Whether you are at the end of your first, second or third year, you will have had learning objectives to ensure that you gradually develop your nursing role in line with the NMC requirements. Your curriculum documentation will have incorporated the NMC domains for professional values, communication and interpersonal skills, nursing practice and decision making, and leadership, management and team working (NMC 2010). Those of you on the NMC 2004 regulations and competencies will consider the domains of professional and ethical practice, care delivery, care management, and personal and professional development (NMC 2004).

Wherever you are in your training, you should have sat and discussed the care that you were giving and the rationale behind it with your mentor. You will have spent time following the nursing process of assessment, planning, implementation and evaluation (Habermann & Uys 2005). You will have used all of these phases of the nursing process during your time on the ward and now is the time to look back and think about what you have learnt about care giving and what you can transfer to your next placement.

Activity

How have you been involved in following the nursing process during your placement? Write a reflective account using a reflective framework of your choice about an episode of care where you used the nursing process (see Ch. 3 for an example of a reflective framework). Think about what you learnt from this and how this affected/ enhanced your ability to plan care for your patients.

This should highlight your knowledge and identify areas for development for you to take forward in your role as a caregiver.

As a final-year student, your mentor will have expected you to be familiar with the nursing process and care planning and will have allocated you a group of patients under supervision. Initially this can seem

challenging, but as a more senior student, your skills of assessment, planning, implementation and evaluation will have steadily improved during your placements. You may have struggled sometimes with goal setting as patients in a medical placement are rarely straightforward and can often present with a multitude of complex health problems. As your placement progressed, you should have started to feel more confident and felt your dependence on your mentor reducing. Combining your knowledge of anatomy and physiology within the context of your patients' conditions will have allowed you to be more proactive in suggesting nursing actions, reviewing and evaluating care for your patients.

The nursing team will have had a good working knowledge of their patients, and as a first- or second-year student you will have been allocated one or two patients to care for to enable you to develop person-centred holistic care. You will have needed to know your patients well, their care and treatment and progress made and been able to communicate this among the team.

Activity

If you are a final-year student, think about a group of patients that you looked after and how you planned their care for a shift. Did you feel confident when writing their documentation and were you able to set realistic goals? What can you take forward to your next placement?

If you are a first- or second-year student, think about an individual patient that you looked after and how you planned their care for a shift. Did you feel confident when writing their documentation and were you able to set realistic goals? What can you take forward to your next placement?

Nurses need to have good interpersonal skills, not just with a patient but with everyone involved in the care of that patient, and many would argue that good communication is the cornerstone of good care (Sully & Dallas 2010). Within your curriculum documentation for practice, communication will have been identified as a learning outcome whether you are a junior or senior student. In fact, in the NMC (2010) competencies, communication and interpersonal skills are now a major domain for becoming 'fit for practice' as a qualified nurse. This major shift is due to the substantive evidence base linking effective communication and quality of patient care delivery (Lynch et al 2008, McGilton et al 2009, DH 2010b).

A unique factor of the nurses' role is their 24-hour presence in the care environment, as a member of the nursing team is always present in the ward environment. Within day care, intermediate care or the virtual ward, the nurse is probably going to be the professional most involved in the care of patients.

As a third-year student, you will have contributed to discussions with the multidisciplinary team and made referrals under supervision. The importance of relaying information clearly, logically and appropriately may have seemed challenging at times, but as you look back on the experience it is important to reflect on what went well and to identify areas for development that you can take forward to your next placement. There may have been more junior student nurses who required support during your practice experience and, at this point, you could consider how it felt to advise and support more junior colleagues (Gilmour et al 2007).

As you near your final placement, you will have been given the opportunity to shadow the shift coordinator and may have been able to act as a shift coordinator under supervision. You will have needed to share information with the team, been adaptable and flexible. This opportunity will have greatly enhanced your team working and coordinating skills.

 Activity

> Think back to the shifts that you worked during your placement and your observations of how continuity of care was maintained. In what ways did you improve the way in which you provided continuity of care for your patients?

 Reflection point

> Reflect on a situation that required your coordinating skills. If you came across this situation again, would you do anything differently?

Everyone on the ward coordinates care to some degree. All students will be helping patients to navigate their way through their healthcare journey. As a more junior student, you may have observed third-year students and registered nurses liaising with the multidisciplinary team, learnt about their roles and communicated with them about any patients within your care.

 Reflection point

> Overall, how do you think you have developed in your role as a student nurse? What aspects of your role would you like to develop on your next placement? Consider what the following student who just qualified said about her experience.

Overall I believe working on an acute and busy medical ward as a newly qualified nurse is a great and valued experience. It allows me to care for a wide range of acutely ill patients with a whole variety of conditions, enables me to develop myself as a nurse who is able to work under pressure and in demanding situations, and also gives me the opportunity to work alongside various other healthcare professionals, for example physiotherapists, social workers, clinical nurse specialists.

All of this I believe will be excellent experience for my nursing career.

(Nicola Cooper, newly registered staff nurse)

If this was your final placement and you are now preparing to complete your registration as a staff nurse, the following text may be interesting for you to read:

Siviter B (2008). The newly qualified nurses' handbook. Baillière Tindall, Edinburgh.

Also the Flying Start Website is dedicated to helping your transition from student to newly qualified health professional through resources and learning activities: http://www.flyingstartengland.nhs.uk/ (accessed July 2011).

Testing learning and knowledge

This section will help you to identify how your knowledge has developed during your placement and where you may still have further areas to develop. There are some multiple choice questions, exercises and exam scenarios to help you to bridge theory and practice.

? Quiz: test your knowledge

(Answers on p. 283.)

17.1. What are the key areas you need to consider when communicating?
   a. The relationship with the patient and significant others
   b. Professional relationships
   c. Record keeping
   d. All of the above.

17.2. Name four health professionals that you have liaised with while on your medical placement.

17.3. Medical ward handovers will often incorporate an office handover and a bedside handover: true or false?

17.4. COPD means:
   a. Chronic obstructive pancreatic disease
   b. Constant obstructive pulmonary disorder
   c. Care of the patient's discharge
   d. Chronic obstructive pulmonary disease.

17.5. SBARR is:
   a. A chronic disease
   b. A communication tool
   c. A piece of equipment
   d. A part of the duodenum.

17.6. A low blood pressure and raised pulse could signify:
   a. Fluid overload
   b. Pain
   c. Normal vital signs
   d. Dehydration.

17.7. Which of the following could cause a raised respiratory rate?
   a. Heart failure
   b. Chest infection
   c. Opiate overdose
   d. Sepsis.

17.8. Normal oxygen saturations are?
   a. 85–90%
   b. 90–93%
   c. 95–100%
   d. 88–96%.

17.9. Normal peak flow readings depend on which of the following?
   a. Age
   b. Height
   c. Sex
   d. All of the above.

17.10. Which of the following observations is normally incorporated in an early warning score?
   a. Weight
   b. Temperature

    c. Pulse

    d. Blood pressure

    e. Oxygen saturations

    f. AVPU

    g. Urine output

    h. Skin colour.

17.11. What do you need to consider before discharging a patient home?

17.12. What waterlow score would prompt you to take action?

    a. 17

    b. 3

    c. 7

    d. 11.

17.13. What is CAM?

    a. Confusion assessment method

    b. Chronic/acute medical problems

    c. Coordinate and manage

    d. Chronic/acute mastitis.

17.14. Does a patient who is on diuretic therapy require a fluid balance chart?

17.15. Does a patient who is having enteral feeding require a fluid balance chart?

17.16. Does a patient who has just been admitted with a fall and confusion require a fluid balance chart?

17.17. What would you look for when inspecting a cannula site?

17.18. How often would you inspect a cannula site?

    a. Once day

    b. Never

    c. On removal

    d. Every shift.

17.19. Why is it important to have vitamins in our diets?

17.20. What are the main causes of slips and trips accidents?

    a. Inappropriate or lack of footwear

    b. Obstructions

    c. Wet and slippery floors

    d. All of the above.

17.21. What actions should be taken first when a patient falls?

    a. Inform the doctor

    b. Assess the patient and record the observations of vital signs

    c. Ensure that the patient is safe

    d. Complete and incident form and falls risk assessment.

17.22. Bed rails are used to restrict a patient from climbing out of bed. Yes or no?

17.23. If another student asked you what the following conditions were, what would your answers be?

    a. Epilepsy

    b. Left ventricular failure

    c. Cerebral vascular accident

d. Ulcerative colitis
e. Sickle cell anaemia.

17.24. Who are registered nurses accountable to?

17.25. When should a MUST tool be used?
a. On patients who are obese
b. On patients who are obviously underweight
c. For all patients within the first 3 days of admission
d. For all patients within 24 hours of admission.

17.26. Can you list the seven broad categories of abuse?

17.27. Does every patient need to be weighed?

17.28. What are the normal temperature ranges?

17.29. What is a normal respiratory rate?

17.30. What factors could affect the saturation reading?

17.31. What could cause a patient to have an abnormal respiratory rate?

? Quiz – medications

(Answers on p. 284.)

17.32. Convert 1100 mg to g.

17.33. Convert 20 mg to µg.

17.34. Convert 55 µg to mg.

17.35. Convert 68 mg to g.

17.36. Convert 250 mL to L.

17.37. Convert 6.5 L to mL.

17.38. Convert 80 µg to mg.

17.39. Convert 72 µg to mg.

17.40. Convert 3.5 g to mg.

17.41. A patient is prescribed 20 mg of morphine. The stock ampoule contains 50 mg in 2 mL. What volume would you draw up?

17.42. A patient is prescribed 12.5 mg of haloperidol. The stock ampoule contains 50 mg in 1 mL. What volume would you draw up?

17.43. A patient is prescribed 200 mg of amiodarone. The stock ampoule contains 150 mg in 3 mL. What volume would you draw up?

17.44. A patient is prescribed 250 mg of digoxin. The stock ampoule contains 500 mg in 2 mL. What volume would you draw up?

17.45. A patient is prescribed 120 mg of furosemide. The stock ampoule contains 50 mg in 5 mL. What volume would you draw up?

17.46. A patient is prescribed temazepam 20 mg. The tablets in stock are 10 mg. How many tablets would you need?

17.47. Calculate the following in drops per minute:
   a. 250 mL normal saline over 4 hours via a standard giving set
   b. 360 mL blood over 4 hours via a blood giving set
   c. 1000 mL 5% dextrose over 12 hours via a standard giving set
   d. 240 mL plasma over 3 hours via a blood giving set.

17.48. Which of the following *must* be checked prior to administering medications?
   a. Patient's hospital ID number
   b. Patient's allergies
   c. Prescription chart
   d. All of the above.

17.49. What clinical observations should you check prior to giving beta blockers?

17.50. What would be the indications for prescribing warfarin?

17.51. What are the potential side effects of warfarin?

17.52. What is the normal dose of cyclizine?

17.53. What would be the indications for administering diclofenac?

Exam scenarios

All nursing programmes will incorporate varied assessment methods, with at least one written exam. The following exam scenarios are based on the type of question you could expect to receive in an exam. When reading an exam question it is important to pay attention to the marking criteria, for example critical analysis of an appropriate framework may account for 20% of the total mark, 10% for accurate and appropriate referencing.

You may find the following study skills text useful:
Ely C, Scott I (2007). Essential study skills for nursing, Mosby, Edinburgh

Exam scenario 17.1

Mr Henry is a 62-year-old man who presents with a hemiplegia. He has a past medical history of hypertension and raised cholesterol levels. He is married with three grown-up sons and is currently employed as a delivery driver for a homeware store. He smokes 20 cigarettes a day and drinks 20 units of beer a week. He has no known allergies.

On admission, his temperature is 37.4°C, pulse 64 beats per minute irregular, blood pressure 170/110 mmHg, respiratory rate 13 per minute and oxygen saturation 95% on air. He is slightly drowsy but responding to voice and his speech is slightly slurred, his pupils are equal and reacting to light and his Glasgow Coma Score (GCS) is 12. He has a severe weakness on his left side affecting his arm and leg. He is currently nil by mouth awaiting a swallow assessment.

Exam scenario 17.2

Mr Imrad is a 29-year-old man who has been admitted to the medical admissions unit with a 2-week history of epigastric pain followed by 24 hours of haematemesis. He is married with two young children, has a stressful job working long hours and has a high alcohol intake. He is currently nil by mouth and is awaiting an urgent gastroscopy. His haemoglobin is 9 mmol and his vital signs are: blood pressure 105/60 mmHg, pulse 95 per minute regular, respiratory rate 19 per minute, oxygen saturation 92% on air, temperature 36.7°C.

Mr Imrad is anxious about having an endoscopy, being away from work and worried about his family. He has been cross-matched for 4 units of blood and the first unit of blood is on the ward ready to commence.

 Activity

Critically discuss the care that Mr Imrad will require pre- and post-gastroscopy using an appropriate framework and evidence base.

A care plan aimed at meeting Mr Imrad's needs can be found on page 291. Your university may also expect you to include the following in your answer:

- Show understanding of the anatomy and physiology of the upper gastrointestinal system.
- Show understanding of haematemesis and a gastroscopy.
- Show understanding of the risks associated with a gastroscopy and how you would maintain patient safety throughout the pre- and post-procedure period through evidence-based nursing care.
- Rationale for the framework you have used.
- Up-to-date and appropriate references.

 Activity

Using an appropriate framework, critically discuss the initial assessment you would make for the first 24 hours of admission. You should include the role of the nurse and other healthcare professionals who might be involved in Mr Henry's care using evidence to support your decisions.

A care plan aimed at meeting Mr Henry's needs can be found on page 285.

Your university may also expect you to include the following in your answer:

- Show understanding of the anatomy and physiology of a stroke.
- Show understanding of the roles of the multidisciplinary team within stroke care and the importance of this.
- Rationale for the framework you have used.
- Critical discussion of the initial assessment including its impact on Mr Henry and his family.
- Evidence-based clinical decision making in relation to your assessment of his needs.
- Up-to-date and appropriate references.

Summary

We hope that this chapter has helped you to establish your current knowledge base and identify any areas for future development. Reflecting on your medical placement and consolidating your knowledge is an essential process to fully equip you for your next placement learning experience, wherever that may be, or for your first destination post as a newly registered nurse. Nursing is a process of lifelong learning and this is only the start of your journey. You will continue to develop and learn, both as a student nurse and as a qualified practitioner, and hopefully your medical nursing placement will have provided you with a solid base of skills and knowledge for your career as a nurse.

References

Department of Health, 2010a. Preceptorship framework for newly registered nurses, midwives and allied health professionals. DH, London.

Department of Health, 2010b. Essence of care benchmarks. DH, London. Online. Available at: http://www.dh.gov.uk/prod_consum_dh/groups/dh_digitalassets/@dh/@en/@ps/documents/digitalasset/dh_119970.pdf (accessed July 2011).

Gilmour, J., Kopeikin, A., Douche, J., 2007. Student nurses as peer-mentors: collegiality in practice. Nurse Education Today 7 (1), 36–43.

Habermann, M., Uys, L.R., 2005. The nursing process: a global concept. Churchill Livingstone, Edinburgh.

Lynch, L., Hancox, K., Happell, B., et al., 2008. Clinical supervision for nurses. Wiley–Blackwell, Oxford.

McGilton, K.S., Boscart, V., Fox, M., et al., 2009. A systematic review of the effectiveness of communication interventions for health care providers caring for patients in residential care settings. Worldviews Evidence Based Nursing 6 (3), 149–159.

Nursing and Midwifery Council, 2004. Standards of proficiency for pre-registration nursing education. NMC, London.

Nursing and Midwifery Council, 2006. Preceptorship guidelines. NMC, London. Online. Available at: http://www.nmc-uk.org/Documents/Circulars/2006circulars/NMC%20circular%2021_2006.pdf (accessed July 2011).

Nursing and Midwifery Council, 2008. Supporting assessment and learning in practice. NMC, London.

Nursing and Midwifery Council, 2010. Standards for pre-registration nursing education. NMC, London.

Nursing and Midwifery Council, 2011. Advice and supporting information for implementing NMC standards for pre-registration nursing education. NMC, London.

Sully, P., Dallas, J., 2010. Essential communication skills for nursing and midwifery, Essential skills for nurses' series, 2nd ed. Mosby, Edinburgh.

Further reading

Aston, L., Wakefield, J., McGowan, R., 2010. The student nurse guide to decision making in practice. Open University Press, Maidenhead.

Burton, R., Ormrod, G., 2011. Nursing: transition to professional practice. Oxford University Press, Oxford.

Intercollegiate Stroke Working Party, 2008. National clinical guideline for stroke. Royal College of Physicians, London.

Richards, A., Edwards, S., 2008. A nurse's survival guide to the ward. Churchill Livingstone, Edinburgh.

Smith, G., Wilson, R., 2005. Gastrointestinal nursing. Blackwell, Oxford.

Williams, J., Perry, L., Watkins, C., 2010. Acute stroke nursing. Wiley–Blackwell, Oxford.

Answers to quizzes

Test your knowledge

17.1 d

17.2 You should have been able to list four of the professionals mentioned in the Who's who in Chapter 1.

17.3 True.

17.4 d

17.5 b

17.6 d

17.7 a, b and d

17.8 c

17.9 d

17.10 b, c, d, f and g

17.11 You could consider: patient education about their condition and medications, help to maintain their activities of daily living at home, referrals to health professionals in the community, how they will get home and access to their property, the conditions at home, carers' needs, information for their GP, out-patient follow up appointments.

17.12 a and d

17.13 a

17.14 Yes.

17.15 Yes.

17.16 Yes.

17.17 Redness, inflammation, pain, swelling, tracking, whether the dressing is clean and dry and date of insertion.

17.18 d

17.19 They are essential to maintain a healthy immune system, formation of antibodies, maintain a healthy nervous system, formation of collagen, aid the absorption of iron, maintain capillaries, promote absorption of calcium and maintain healthy teeth and bones, formation of red blood cells, good sight.

17.20 d

17.21 c

17.22 No.

17.23
   a. Epilepsy is a tendency to have recurrent seizures (fits) caused by a sudden burst of electrical activity within the brain disrupting the normal communication between brain cells.
   b. Heart failure is a result of the heart no longer pumping effectively, usually as a result of damage to the heart muscle (e.g. a heart attack). This results in an accumulation of blood and fluid within organs and tissues. Some patients may

       have either left-sided heart failure (left ventricular failure) or right-sided heart
       failure, depending on where the damage to the heart muscle is.

  c. A cerebral vascular accident or stroke happens when the blood supply to a part of
     the brain is interrupted by either a clot (ischaemic stroke) or a bleed (haemorrhagic
     stroke) resulting in the brain cells in that part of the brain dying.

  d. Ulcerative colitis is a chronic inflammatory condition affecting the lining of the
     large intestine causing diarrhoea and rectal bleeding.

  e. Sickle cell anaemia is a genetic disorder where red blood cells can become hard, sticky
     and sickle (crescent) shaped causing premature death of the blood cells and anaemia.

17.24 Patients, employers, profession (NMC), public.

17.25 d

17.26 Physical, psychological, financial, sexual, neglect and acts of omission,
       discriminatory, institutional.

17.27 Yes.

17.28 36–37.5°C.

17.29 12–16 breaths per minute.

17.30 Machine faulty, peripherally cold, nail varnish, carbon monoxide poisoning.

17.31 Chest infection, fluid overload, sepsis, anxiety, pain, sedation, opiate medication,
       head injury.

Medications

17.32 1.1 g

17.33 20000 μg

17.34 0.055 mg

17.35 0.068 g

17.36 0.25 L

17.37 6500 mL

17.38 0.08 mg

17.39 0.072 mg

17.40 3500 mg

17.41 0.8 mL

17.42 0.25 mL

17.43 4 mL

17.44 1 mL

17.45 12 mL

17.46 2 tablets.

17.47

    a. 29 drops per minute
    b. 22/23 drops per minute
    c. 28 drops per minute
    d. 20 drops per minute.

17.48 d

17.49 Pulse and blood pressure.

17.50 Pulmonary embolus (PE), deep vein thrombosis (DVT), atrial fibrillation (AF).

17.51 Bruising, bleeding.

17.52 50 mg three times a day (tds).

17.53 Moderate pain and inflammation.

Answers to exam scenarios

Exam scenario 17.1

The following are the problems we would expect you to indentify through an assessment of Mr Henry, an example of the nursing care he would require in the first 24 hours and his ongoing care and rehabilitation.

Mr Henry's problems

- He is neurologically unstable and drowsy and his airway will need to be maintained.
- He is unable to take food or fluids orally due to drowsiness.
- He is unable to communicate fully due to a reduced level of consciousness and dysphasia.
- He is unable to meet his hygiene needs due to left-sided weakness.
- He is at risk of complications associated with immobility and developing spasticity in his affected limbs.
- He is catheterised and incontinent of faeces.

Mr Henry's immediate nursing care plans

Problem: He is neurologically unstable and drowsy and his airway will need to be maintained.

Goal: To promptly detect, report and treat any signs of deterioration.

Nursing action	Rationale
Nurse Mr Henry in the recovery position if he is unable to maintain his airway, use airway adjuncts as appropriate and maintain saturations above 95% Administer oxygen if prescribed	To keep Mr Henry's airway clear and ensure adequate oxygenation
Hourly GCS recording until instructed otherwise Report any changes in GCS to medical team	To detect deterioration in condition

Problem: He is unable to take food or fluids orally due to drowsiness.

Goal: To maintain adequate nutrition and hydration.

Nursing action	Rationale
Keep nil by mouth until GCS improves and then refer to speech and language for swallow assessment	To prevent aspiration and ensure prompt assessment as condition improves
Give intravenous fluids as prescribed and maintain cannula care	To ensure adequate fluid intake and prevent complications from cannula site
Ensure accurate fluid balance monitoring of intake and output	To prevent dehydration and fluid overload
Pass nasogastric tube for administration of medication and/or enteral feed. Ensure position of tube is checked by aspirating fluid before administration of medication or feed	To allow medication to be administered and enteral feed if appropriate and prevent aspiration
Provide regular mouth care	To prevent Mr Henry from developing complications of dry mouth and enhance comfort
Ensure MUST assessment is completed and dietician referral made as needed	To assess risk of malnutrition

Problem: He is unable to communicate fully due to a reduced level of consciousness and dysphasia.

Goal: To employ alternative strategies to ensure we are able to communicate fully with Mr Henry.

Nursing action	Rationale
Always explain what you are going to do to Mr Henry. Use verbal and non-verbal communication	To ensure Mr Henry understands what is happening to him and is able to communicate his needs. To reduce isolation
Avoid jargon and speak slowly and clearly to Mr Henry. Recognise that tiredness and poor concentration may affect his ability to communicate	So Mr Henry understands what is being said
Refer to speech and language therapist	To ensure prompt assessment when condition improves and assessment of swallowing function when alert

Problem: He is unable to meet his hygiene needs due to left-sided weakness.

Goal: To keep Mr Henry clean, dry and comfortable while maintaining his dignity.

Nursing action	Rationale
Always explain what you going to do to Mr Henry	To prevent isolation and ensure that Mr Henry always knows what is happening
Ensure the environment is private and use signage to prevent unwanted interruptions	To maintain dignity
Ensure hygiene needs are met as required and skin condition is checked regularly and documented	To keep Mr Henry comfortable and promptly identify any deterioration in skin integrity

Problem: He is at risk of complications associated with immobility and developing spasticity in his affected limbs.

Goal: To prevent complications associated with immobility.

Nursing action	Rationale
Ensure risk assessments for nutrition, venous thromboembolism, pressure ulcers, falls and bed rails are completed and appropriate action taken and documented Review as required	To identify risk and ensure prompt action to prevent complications
Liaise with physiotherapist re correct positioning for affected limbs and passive limb exercises	To prevent spasticity and dependent oedema
Handle Mr Henry's affected shoulder carefully, avoiding pulling the joint	To prevent subluxation of the shoulder joint

Problem: He is catheterised and incontinent of faeces.

Goal: To prevent complications of catheterisation and constipation.

Nursing action	Rationale
Hourly measurements of urine: if below 30 mL/h or above 200 mL/hr report to the nurse in charge and liaise with the doctors when reducing the frequency of the urine output measurements Document urine output on a fluid balance chart	To accurately monitor Mr Henry's fluid balance

Continued

Nursing action	Rationale
Provide catheter care and hygiene Check the colour of the urine each shift Report any changes to nurse in charge Provide privacy when providing catheter care	To prevent infection To detect any signs of infection or trauma To ensure that Mr Henry's privacy and dignity needs are met
Monitor temperature, pulse and blood pressure and respirations four times a day while Mr Henry has an indwelling urinary catheter Take a catheter specimen of urine for microscopy, culture and sensitivity if Mr Henry's temperature is >37.5°C and inform the nurse/doctor	To detect any infection and treat as soon as possible
Review need for catheter as Mr Henry's condition improves	To ensure catheter is removed as soon as no longer necessary to help regain urinary continence
Monitor bowel movements and document on each shift Give laxatives as prescribed	To identify and prevent constipation
Use continence aids, e.g. pad and pants, appropriately Check skin condition regularly and provide regular personal hygiene while maintaining privacy and dignity at all times	To prevent complications and keep Mr Henry clean and comfortable

Rehabilitation of the stroke patient starts on the day of admission, however, once Mr Henry's condition stabilises and he is fully conscious, he can be fully assessed by the multidisciplinary team and intensive rehabilitation can commence.

Two weeks later, Mr Henry is transferred to the rehabilitation stroke unit. He is now fully awake and alert. After a full assessment and a discussion with Mr Henry, you determine that his nursing needs now are:
- To be able to engage with therapists and his rehabilitation programme.
- To be able to communicate effectively with the team and his family and friends.
- To maintain his food and fluid intake.
- To manage his urinary incontinence.

Mr Henry's ongoing nursing care plans

Problem: Mr Henry has a left-sided weakness affecting his arm and leg.

Goal: To be able to engage with therapists and his rehabilitation programme.

Nursing action	Rationale
Involve Mr Henry in planning his therapy sessions with the physiotherapist and occupational therapist and in goal setting	Mr Henry knows what is planned and can feel in control of his rehabilitation
Assist Mr Henry to be ready for his therapy sessions, e.g. assisting with washing and dressing, transferring into wheelchair	To ensure therapy sessions are not delayed and to reduce anxiety
Liaise with the physiotherapist and occupational therapist to find out how best to facilitate and encourage Mr Henry to continue his therapy during his activities of daily living	Rehabilitation continues 24/7
Ensure Mr Henry gets adequate rest during the day and sleep at night so that he can maximise his energy during therapy sessions	To ensure Mr Henry gets the most out of his therapy sessions
Encourage Mr Henry to acknowledge his affected side, including taking care of affected limbs, e.g. ensuring arm isn't hanging down at his side, foot not properly placed on footplate of wheelchair/floor	To increase awareness of affected limbs and prevent injury to affected limbs

Problem: Mr Henry has expressive dysphasia.

Goal: To be able to communicate effectively with the team and his family and friends.

Nursing action	Rationale
Liaise with the speech and language therapist to discuss the best way to communicate with Mr Henry, using communication aids, e.g. picture boards, as appropriate	To optimise communication with Mr Henry
Allow plenty of time when communicating with Mr Henry and use prompts and aids as required	To ensure Mr Henry has the opportunity to communicate his needs and reduce frustration and maintain dignity
Provide education and support to the family and friends of Mr Henry	To enable them to communicate with Mr Henry and feel supported in this

Problem: Mr Henry has dysphagia and requires thickened fluids and a soft diet.

Goal: To maintain his food and fluid intake.

Nursing action	Rationale
Liaise with dietician and speech and language therapist to ensure Mr Henry is receiving the correct diet and his swallowing function is regularly assessed	To prevent aspiration and ensure optimum nutritional intake
Ensure Mr Henry understands the type of diet he needs and why	To enhance compliance with special diet and increase his feeling of control over his situation
Ensure all the nursing and support staff on the ward are aware of Mr Henry's dietary needs and that thickener is readily available at his bed side	To prevent aspiration and ensure optimum nutritional intake
Monitor Mr Henry's food and fluid intake on a daily basis, discuss any issues with Mr Henry to ensure he enjoys the food he is receiving	To detect inadequate dietary intake and allow prompt action to be taken
Explain Mr Henry's needs to his family and encourage them to bring in soft foods he may like to eat	To allow a variety of foods and choice for Mr Henry and increase his enjoyment of eating
Encourage Mr Henry to sit at a table when eating and use any communal areas available on the ward and encourage family to join him if possible	To promote socialisation and an environment that is closer to that which he would experience at home

Problem: Mr Henry has urge incontinence.

Goal: To manage his urinary incontinence.

Nursing action	Rationale
Maintain dignity and privacy at all times when attending to Mr Henry and use continence aids, e.g. pads, as appropriate	To maintain dignity and ensure Mr Henry has confidence that his problem will be handled sensitively
Keep a bladder diary for a minimum of 3 days, documenting when Mr Henry is incontinent, and use this and his fluid chart to establish a toileting regime Ensure all of the multidisciplinary team are aware of this	To determine a toileting regime to manage continence
Prompt and assist Mr Henry to use the toilet at regular intervals (determined by bladder diary) and review regime regularly	To promote continence

Continued

Nursing action	Rationale
Ensure call bell is close at hand at all times and encourage Mr Henry to call for assistance as soon as he feels the need to urinate	To ensure prompt attention and maintain dignity
Educate Mr Henry about why he has urge incontinence and what can be done to help him regain his continence	For Mr Henry to understand that his incontinence can be managed and may improve with bladder retraining
Liaise with continence specialist to discuss bladder retraining	To ensure continence management is effective and continues after discharge

Evaluation:

Mr Henry was ready to be discharged home after 6 weeks in the rehabilitation unit. Regular goal setting meetings were held with Mr Henry and his family during his stay and this enabled both him and his family to prepare for life at home. His care was managed at home by the stroke community team which included nurses, physiotherapists, occupational therapists, speech and language therapists and social workers. He was also followed up by the psychologist to help him come to terms with the fact that he could not return to his previous job and to help him adapt to his new lifestyle. He and his family also joined the local stroke support group and he attended an aphasia group every month. His GP and practice nurse continued to monitor his vascular risk factors on a regular basis to optimise stroke prevention.

Exam scenario 17.2

Based on your assessment, Mr Imrad has the following problems which should form the basis of your care plan.:

- He has the potential to become cardiovascularly unstable.
- He requires a blood transfusion.
- He is nil by mouth.
- He has epigastric pain and vomiting.
- He is anxious about being in hospital.
- He is awaiting an endoscopy.

Mr Imrad's nursing care plans

Problem: Mr Imrad has the potential to become cardiovascularly unstable.

Goal: Early prevention and detection of deterioration.

Nursing action	Rationale
Hourly recording of vital signs Recording of early warning score Immediate notification of any abnormal results to senior nurse	Prompt detection of deterioration
Strict fluid balance monitoring, input and output	To detect deterioration
Observe for any vomiting – volume, colour, consistency, frequency	To detect bleeding and to prevent hypovolaemia
Inform medical team of any haematemesis (coffee ground vomiting)	
Ensure that patient has large-gauge venous access	In case of sudden deterioration

Problem: Mr Imrad is to receive a blood transfusion.

Goal: For blood transfusion to take place without complication.

Nursing action	Rationale
Check that the blood has been prescribed correctly	To avoid error in identification and administration of blood
Explain rationale for transfusion to Mr Imrad and gain his consent to receive the transfusion	To reassure the patient, give an opportunity to answer any questions Verbal consent must be gained before any blood transfusion
Ask the patient to state their name and date of birth, check this against the blood and the prescription	Pre-transfusion checks should take place at the patient's bedside Use of open-ended questions to check identity prevents the patient saying 'yes' to a question they may not have heard or understood
Check the blood group, unit number and expiry date on the blood unit Check the quality of the unit	To ensure that the blood is the correct type, has not expired and has not been damaged
Check the name, date of birth and hospital number on Mr Imrad's ID band against the demographics on the blood unit	To ensure the right unit of blood is being given to the right patient
Second staff member checks the name, date of birth and hospital number on the ID band against the demographics on the blood unit, independently of the first checker	Two members of staff must check to avoid error Checks must be made independently to avoid staff relying on each other to check the details

Continued

Nursing action	Rationale
Carry out a baseline set of vital signs	To allow changes in vital signs to be quickly identified
Wash hands using six-stage technique and dry thoroughly Wearing gloves, prime the giving set and start the transfusion according to the prescription	To reduce the incidence of infection when manipulating the cannula
Explain to Mr Imrad the importance of alerting staff if he begins to feel unwell	To aid the early identification of a transfusion reaction
Observe Mr Imrad throughout the transfusion for signs of a reaction – fever, chills, tachycardia, hyper- or hypotension, collapse, rigors, flushing, urticaria, bone, muscle, chest and/or abdominal pain, shortness of breath, nausea, generally feeling unwell, respiratory distress Stop transfusion immediately if Mr Imran has a transfusion reaction and contact medical team	To aid the early identification of a transfusion reaction
Monitor and record vital signs as per hospital policy	Blood pressure, temperature, pulse and respirations should be measured pre-transfusion, 15 minutes into the transfusion and at the end of each unit as a minimum The observations should be done more frequently in certain situations (e.g. if the patient cannot communicate/has significant cardiovascular disease/is in a side room/transfusion is happening at night)
Ensure the transfusion is completed in the correct time frame	Maximum time for a red cell transfusion is 4 hours
Ensure traceability documentation is completed as per hospital policy	It is the law that hospitals are able to trace all blood components administered A record of all transfusions must be kept in the hospital lab for 30 years

Problem: Mr Imrad is nil by mouth.

Goal: To ensure adequate hydration and comfort while nil by mouth.

Nursing action	Rationale
Explain the reason for being nil by mouth to Mr Imrad and give an indication as to how long he will need to remain nil by mouth	To increase his concordance with nil by mouth and reduce anxiety
Ensure Mr Imrad has access to mouth care, e.g. toothbrush, toothpaste, and encourage him to carry out regular mouth care, providing assistance where necessary	To prevent drying and damage to oral mucosa
Ensure nil by mouth status is reversed as soon as is clinically indicated	Prolonged periods of fasting may result in dehydration, hypoglycaemia, hypotension or other adverse metabolic consequences
Ensure any medication prescribed can be given via an alternative route, e.g. IV, or check if OK to be given orally	To ensure all medication is received as prescribed despite nil by mouth status
Administer intravenous fluids as prescribed	To prevent dehydration
Maintain strict fluid balance	To allow prompt identification of hypovolaemia

Problem: Mr Imrad has epigastric pain and vomiting.

Goal: To relieve pain and vomiting.

Nursing action	Rationale
Ensure regular analgesia is prescribed with an appropriate route (e.g. IV/IM if nil by mouth)	To relieve pain
Assess pain levels before and after administration of analgesics	To assess effectiveness of analgesia
Ensure regular antiemetics are prescribed with an appropriate route (e.g. IV/IM if nil by mouth)	To relieve nausea and vomiting
Encourage Mr Imrad to use any non-pharmacological pain relief methods that may work for him (e.g. positioning in bed)	To maximise pain relief
Administer proton pump inhibitor drugs as prescribed	To inhibit gastric acid secretion
Provide Mr Imrad with information about food/drink that are likely to exacerbate dyspepsia	To educate the patient to improve health and wellbeing once discharged from hospital

Problem: Mr Imrad is anxious about being in hospital.

Goal: To relieve anxiety as far as possible by keeping Mr Imrad informed and involved in his care.

Nursing action	Rationale
Ensure all procedures, medications and tests or investigations are fully explained to Mr Imrad and he is given an opportunity to ask questions, and informed consent is given	To relieve anxiety associated with not understanding what is happening or why and allow opportunities for questions to be answered
Ensure Mr Imrad is kept up to date with progress on test results, discharge plans, etc.	To allow him to make plans with his work and family
Ensure Mr Imrad is able see his family and have contact with family or employer as often as he needs to	Increased anxiety will exacerbate pain and delay recovery
Encourage Mr Imrad to use any relaxation techniques that work for him, e.g. walking, listening to music, reading, etc.	For Mr Imrad to be proactive in managing his anxiety and increase his control over the situation
Allow Mr Imrad time to talk about his anxieties and ask any questions he has about his condition or treatment	To increase understanding of his condition and treatment

Problem: Mr Imrad is awaiting an endoscopy.

Goal: For Mr Imrad to have his endoscopy without complications.

Nursing action	Rationale
Ensure Mr Imrad is fully informed about the endoscopy and informed consent has been gained	Written informed consent is a legal requirement before such a procedure
As per hospital protocol, keep Mr Imrad nil by mouth as necessary prior to the procedure	To avoid complications during the endoscopy
Liaise with endoscopy unit re date and time of procedure and keep My Imrad informed	To relieve anxiety and ensure that he is prepared
Ensure any pre-procedure checklist (as per hospital protocol) is completed	To identify any possible complications and ensure the patient is fully prepared for the procedure
Give a full handover to the receiving nurse in endoscopy	To ensure good communication between professionals

Continued

Nursing action	Rationale
On return from endoscopy, ensure a full handover is given, regarding any problems or complications during and after procedure, sedation or other medication given, special instructions re eating/drinking/medication, vital signs, results of tests	To ensure good communication and identification of any problems
Monitor vital signs as often as necessary on return from procedure, with attention to conscious levels if sedation was given	To promptly identify any signs of deterioration

Evaluation:
Following his endoscopy, Mr Imrad was told that he had a gastric ulcer which had been bleeding. He was commenced on appropriate medication and given advice about managing his stress levels, alcohol intake and diet to avoid a recurrence of the ulcer.

Glossary

Acute

Of a short-lived condition, in contrast to a chronic condition; this sense also does not imply severity.

Anaemia

A reduction in the quantity of haemoglobin carrying oxygen in the blood.

Anaesthetic

Administration of a regimen of drugs and/or gases and/or volatile agents to abolish the sensation of feeling.

Analgesics (also known as painkillers)

Group of drugs used to relieve pain.

Anorexia

Lack or complete loss of appetite, which may result in malnutrition and/or starvation.

Antacid

A substance which buffers, neutralises or absorbs the effects of hydrochloric acid in the stomach.

Antiemetic

A drug that is effective against vomiting and nausea.

Antiseptics

Solutions which are intended to inhibit the proliferation of pathogens.

Aperient

Mild laxative medication that stimulates a bowel action.

Arrhythmia

An abnormal heart rhythm that may be regular or irregular.

Asepsis

Prevention of wound contamination by using only sterile instruments and solutions.

Bacteraemia

Presence of bacteria in the blood.

Biopsy

Tissue removed for laboratory examination.

Bronchoscopy

Endoscopic examination of the main bronchi.

Cannula

A tube that can be inserted into the body, often for the delivery or removal of fluid.

Capillary refill

The time taken for capillaries to refill – usually tested by pressing on an area with a finger (to occlude the capillaries) and then releasing the pressure.

Care plan

A documented (paper or electronic) record of the care planned to address an actual or potential problem of an individual patient which is reviewed and updated at set times.

Care planning meeting

A meeting held to discuss a plan of ongoing care for a patient, either in hospital or after discharge, with all members of the multidisciplinary team, the patient and their carers/significant others.

Catheterisation

Insertion of a hollow tube into the bladder for the purpose of draining urine or installation of medication into the bladder; can be urethral (via urethra) or suprapubic (via the abdomen).

Chemotherapy

A systemic cytotoxic drug treatment.

Chronic

Prolonged or slow to heal. The opposite of acute.

Colonoscopy

The examination of the colon using a colonoscope.

Cyanosis

Bluish discoloration of the skin caused by a relative decrease in oxygen saturation levels within the capillaries.

Dyscalculia

Difficulty with calculating.

Dyslexia

Difficulty with reading and abstract thinking.

Dysphagia

Difficulty with swallowing.

Dyspnoea

Difficulty with breathing.

Dysuria

Painful urination.

Electrocardiogram

Electrical tracing of the heart using an electrocardiograph.

Embolism

Obstruction of blood vessels by impaction of a solid body (e.g. thrombi, fat or tumour cells).

Endoscopy

Visualisation of hollow structures and organs using an endoscope.

Enteral nutrition

May refer to food or fluids taken orally or via a tube placed within the gastrointestinal tract.

Exacerbation

Increased severity of symptoms.

Gastroscopy

An examination of oesophagus, stomach and duodenum using an endoscope.

Gastrostomy

Incision into the stomach. A tube is placed within the incision; often used for feeding.

Haematemesis

Vomiting blood.

Handover

A set time when clinical information about patients is communicated from nurse to nurse.

Hyperpyrexia

A fever with an extreme elevation of body temperature greater than or equal to 41.5°C.

Hypovolaemia

Diminished quantity of total blood.

Hypoxia

Lack of oxygen to the tissues and body organs.

Infection

The presence of microorganisms in sufficient numbers to cause a host reaction.

Intravenous

A dose of medicine administered from a drip, down through a hollow needle inserted into a vein.

Ischaemia

Lack of blood supply to a part of the body.

Isolation

The separation of a patient suffering from a contagious disease from contact with others.

Jejunostomy

A surgically-made fistula between the jejunum and abdominal wall. A fine tube is placed within the fistula, usually for feeding.

Ketoacidosis

Acidosis due to the accumulation of ketone bodies.

Ketosis

An abnormal amount of ketones in the blood and urine as a result of inefficient metabolism of carbohydrates.

Malignant

Term used to describe a severe and progressively worsening disease.

Malnutrition

A condition that arises when the body's nutrition becomes depleted.

Melaena

Faeces are coloured black with altered blood, as a result of bleeding into the lower part of the digestive system.

Multidisciplinary team

A team of different professionals involved in the care of a patient, e.g. nurse, doctor, physiotherapist, occupational therapist.

Nurses' station

Usually a central desk in a clinical area used by nurses to complete documentation, answer the telephone, use the computer and keep nursing-related documentation.

Observations (vital signs)

A collection of clinical measurements used to assess a patient's health status, e.g. blood pressure, pulse, temperature, respirations.

Off duty (rota)

Usually a paper or electronic record of the shifts allocated to each member of staff in a clinical area.

Glossary

Oxygen saturation (SaO₂)

Measurement of the percentage of oxygen bound to haemoglobin; normal range is 95–99%.

Percutaneous

An invasive approach through the skin.

Percutaneous endoscopic gastrostomy (PEG)

An endoscopic medical procedure in which a tube (PEG tube) is passed into a patient's stomach through the abdominal wall.

Pernicious anaemia

Anaemia caused by the lack of absorption of vitamin B_{12}.

Phlebitis

Inflammation of a vein, which is often associated with clot formation (thrombophlebitis).

Pulse oximeter

An instrument that uses arterial pulsation to detect the level of oxygen saturated on haemoglobin.

Pyrexia

A fever characterised by an elevation of temperature above the normal range of 36.5–37.5°C.

Radiologically-inserted gastrostomy

A feeding tube inserted into the stomach using radiology.

Renal dialysis

The use of dialysis to remove waste products from the blood in the case of kidney failure.

Self-esteem

The outcome of the process of self-evaluation and self-worth, i.e. thinking favourably of oneself; evaluation of one's self-worth.

Septicaemia

Presence of bacteria in the bloodstream, accompanied by symptoms of infection and illness.

Shift

A set time period when you are expected to be at work. In nursing – early shifts, late shifts, night shifts, long day shifts.

Sluice

A designated area for all types of waste, dirty linen, bed pans and commodes.

Spirometry

The measurement of the volume of air that a person can move into and out of the lungs, using a spirometer.

Stress incontinence

Incontinence caused by increased abdominal pressure, e.g. in coughing.

Tachypnoea

Abnormally rapid breathing.

Total parenteral nutrition

The provision of full nutritional support via routes (intravenous or subcutaneous) other than the mouth or rectum.

Transfusion

The transfer of blood or blood products from one individual to another.

Treatment room (clinical room)

A designated area for aseptic procedures such as intravenous drug preparation, wound dressings.

Treponemal syphilis serology

Blood test for syphilis.

Urgency

Overwhelming desire to pass urine immediately.

Urinary frequency

Voiding frequency, e.g. up to 10–12 times per day.

Urinary incontinence

Absence of voluntary control over the passing of urine.

Venesection

The opening of a vein, either to withdraw blood or for letting blood.

Ward round

A set time when the doctors of the team caring for patients, usually led by the consultant and accompanied by a nurse, review all of the patients on a ward.

Wound

An injury that causes tissue damage and may result in the loss of continuity of the skin or tissue.

Index

Note: Page numbers followed by *b* indicate boxes, *f* indicate figures, and *t* indicate tables, and *ge* indicate glossary terms.

Index

Index

Index